FORM AND FUNCTION IN THE HUMAN LUNG

SBN 443 00565 6

PRINTED IN GREAT BRITAIN

Form and Function in the Human Lung

Proceedings of a Symposium
held in the University of Birmingham
April 5th 6th and 7th, 1967

Edited by

GORDON CUMMING
B.Sc., Ph.D., M.B., Ch.B., M.R.C.P., F.R.I.C.
Senior Lecturer in Medicine in the University of Birmingham
Consultant Physician to the United Birmingham Hospitals

and

L. B. HUNT
M.A., M.B., B.Chir., D.P.H.
Medical Director, Lederle Laboratories Division
Cyanamid of Great Britain Ltd

E. & S. LIVINGSTONE LTD
EDINBURGH AND LONDON
1968

LEDERLE INTERNATIONAL
SCIENTIFIC SYMPOSIUM

Lederle

CYANAMID

PREFACE

OVER the past few years it has become apparent to those interested in the study of the lung that a great need exists for freer communication and greater understanding between workers in different disciplines. Clinicians interested in chest disease find themselves faced on the one hand with physiologists whose concepts of function seem to have little relevance to their own experience with patients, and on the other with morbid anatomists whose views on structure often fail to relate to the processes of disease during life.

This volume records the proceedings of a symposium held in April 1967 in an attempt to bring together a number of those most closely concerned with these problems from different specialised angles in the hope that from their meeting would spring a useful cross-fertilisation of ideas and a greater degree of mutual comprehension.

That this conference was held in the University of Birmingham arises quite naturally from the fact that there have developed in the Departments of Medicine and Pathology there, a number of working groups actively studying various aspects of these problems. We were fortunate moreover, in obtaining the sponsorship of Lederle Laboratories whose support covered not only the accommodation and catering but also contributed handsomely to the travel expenses of those visiting from abroad. We were also fortunate in the number of distinguished visitors from universities in continental Europe and America, as well as from other parts of the United Kingdom, who were able to participate.

The proceedings were planned in five self contained sessions, each one covering an aspect of pulmonary function or disease of special interest at this time or around which some controversy centres. The attempt to find some correlation between the structural changes induced in the lung by disease and the disturbances we observe clinically in the patient became our principal preoccupation throughout the meeting and constituted the guiding thread along which successive discussions took place. We were concerned with circulatory problems as well as those of ventilation and gas-exchange. The papers in each session provided an opportunity for the presentation of original work at the 'growing points' of each speciality and also an informal forum for the development of new and sometimes speculative theories. Reference to the contents list will indicate the full range of subjects covered. Papers attributed to multiple authorship were presented at the meeting by the first-named. Reference lists will be found at the end of each session.

Unanimous agreement on subjects of dispute is rarely reached at meetings of this kind and our symposium was no exception. All agreed however, that a most valuable interchange of views took place. The discussion was open-ended and often quite prolonged, offering the opportunity for the confrontation, if not the resolution, of divergent views.

G.C.
L.B.H.

ACKNOWLEDGMENTS

THE organisers wish particularly to record their gratitude to Dr F. C. Ottati, the Director of Lederle Laboratories' International Medical Research Department for his support of this project. Special thanks are also due to the Halls Administrator of Birmingham University, the competence and courtesy of whose staff made the visitors' stay in Lake Hall a pleasurable one.

Miss P. J. Buckland, M.P.S. assisted with the preparation of the index and Miss S. Wall rendered secretarial assistance.

LIST OF PARTICIPANTS

W. MELVILLE ARNOTT, T.D., M.D., F.R.C.P., Professor of Medicine, University of Birmingham, Physician, United Birmingham Hospitals.

DAVID V. BATES, M.D., F.R.C.P.(C)., M.R.C.P., Director of Joint Cardiorespiratory Service, Royal Victoria Hospital, Professor of Experimental Medicine, McGill University, Montreal, Canada.

E. BERGLUND, M.D., Karolinska Institutet, Thoracic Surgery Research Laboratory, Stockholm, Sweden.

J. M. BISHOP, M.D., D.Sc., F.R.C.P., Professor of Medicine, University of Birmingham, Physician, Queen Elizabeth Hospital, Birmingham.

D. B. BREWER, M.D., Professor of Pathology, University of Birmingham.

R. A. L. BREWIS, M.D., M.R.C.P., Lecturer in Medicine, University of Manchester.

E. J. M. CAMPBELL, M.D., F.R.C.P., Senior Lecturer in Medicine, Royal Postgraduate Medical School, Physician, Hammersmith Hospital, London.

J. E. COTES, M.A., D.M., M.R.C.P., Medical Research Council Pneumoconiosis Research Unit, Llandough Hospital, Penarth, Glamorgan.

G. CUMMING, B.Sc., Ph.D., M.B., Ch.B., M.R.C.P., F.R.I.C., Senior Lecturer in Medicine, University of Birmingham, Consultant Physician, Queen Elizabeth Hospital, Birmingham.

M. S. DUNNILL, M.A., M.D., M.R.C.P., Department of Pathology, The Radcliffe Infirmary, Oxford.

G. F. FILLEY, M.D., Associate Professor of Medicine, University of Colorado Medical Centre, Clinical Physiologist, The Webb-Waring Institute for Medical Research, Denver, Colorado, United States of America.

A. P. FISHMAN, M.D., Director, The Cardiorespiratory Laboratory, College of Physicians and Surgeons of Columbia University, New York, United States of America.

C. M. FLETCHER, *C.B.E.*, M.A., M.D., F.R.C.P., Reader in Clinical Epidemiology, Royal Postgraduate Medical School, Physician, Hammersmith Hospital, London.

J. GEORG, M.D., Rigshospitalet, Copenhagen, Denmark.

A. GUZ, M.D., M.R.C.P., Reader in Medicine, Charing Cross Hospital Medical School, Physician, Fulham Hospital, London.

PETER HARRIS, M.D., Ph.D., F.R.C.P., Simon Marks Professor of Cardiology, University of London, Director, Institute of Cardiology, Physician, National Heart Hospital, London.

P. S. HASLETON, M.D., Research Fellow in Pathology, University of Birmingham.

DONALD HEATH,[1] Ph.D., M.D., M.R.C.P., M.C.Path., Reader in Pathology, University of Birmingham.

A. G. HEPPLESTON, D.Sc., M.D., F.R.C.P., F.C.Path., Professor of Pathology, University of Newcastle-upon-Tyne.

[1] Subsequently appointed to the George Holt Chair of Pathology in the University of Liverpool.

K. HORSFIELD, M.D., M.R.C.P., Lecturer in Medicine, University of Birmingham.

NORMAN L. JONES, M.D., M.R.C.P., Department of Medicine, Royal Postgraduate Medical School, Hammersmith, London.

J. G. LEOPOLD, M.B., B.Ch., M.C.Path., Senior Lecturer in Pathology, The Welsh National School of Medicine.

P. T. MACKLEM, M.D., Research Associate, McGill University Clinic, Royal Victoria Hospital, Montreal, Canada.

C. B. MCKERROW, M.D., M.R.C.P., Medical Research Council Pneumoconiosis Research Unit, Llandough Hospital, Penarth, Glamorgan.

JERE MEAD, M.D., Professor of Physiology, Harvard University School of Public Health, Boston, United States of America.

J. MILIC-EMILI, M.D., Assistant Professor of Physiology and Assistant Professor of Experimental Medicine, Department of Physiology and Cardiorespiratory Service, Royal Victoria Hospital, McGill University, Montreal, Canada.

D. C. MUIR, M.D., M.R.C.P., Research Fellow, Clinical Respiratory Physiology Research Group, Royal Post Graduate Medical School, Hammersmith Hospital, London.

SOLBERT PERMUTT, M.D., Professor of Environmental Medicine, The Johns Hopkins University, Baltimore, United States of America.

F. J. PRIME, M.D., Reader in Applied Physiology, Institute of Diseases of the Chest, The Brompton Hospital, London.

LYNNE REID, F.R.A.C.P., M.R.C.P., F.C.Path., Professor in Experimental Pathology, Institute of Diseases of the Chest, The Brompton Hospital, London.

JOSEPH C. ROSS, M.D., Professor of Medicine, Department of Medicine, Director, Pulmonary Disease Division, Indiana University Medical Centre, Indianapolis, Indiana, United States of America.

S. J. G. SEMPLE, M.D., M.R.C.P., Reader in Medicine, St. Thomas's Hospital Medical School, London.

C. H. STUART-HARRIS, *C.B.E.*, M.D., F.R.C.P., Professor of Medicine, University of Sheffield.

L. B. STRANG, M.D., F.R.C.P., Professor of Paediatrics, University College Hospital, Medical School. Consultant Paediatrician, University College Hospital.

W. M. THURLBECK, B.Sc., M.B., Professor of Pathology, McGill University, Montreal, Canada.

O. L. WADE, M.A., M.D., F.R.C.P., Professor of Therapeutics and Pharmacology, Queen's University, Belfast.

J. B. WEST, M.D., Ph.D., Director, Clinical Respiratory Physiology Research Group, Lecturer, Department of Medicine, Royal Postgraduate Medical School, Consultant Clinical Physiologist, Hammersmith Hospital, London.

W. WHITAKER, M.D., B.Sc., F.R.C.P., Senior Lecturer in Clinical Medicine, University of Leeds, Consultant Cardiologist, United Leeds Hospitals.

J. WIDIMSKY, M.D., C.Sc., Institute for Cardiovascular Diseases, Prague, Czechoslovakia.

J. P. WYATT, M.D., Department of Pathology, University of Manitoba, Winnipeg, Canada.

CONTENTS

SESSION ONE

THE STRUCTURE OF THE LUNG AND THE CHANGES INDUCED BY DISEASE

Chairman : W. MELVILLE ARNOTT

CHAIRMAN'S OPENING REMARKS

LADIES AND GENTLEMEN : It is my first duty to welcome you all here to this Symposium. The whole question of Form and Function is one of absorbing interest to all of us. Both have been studied for a long time and a great deal of data has been accumulated. The problem, a very real problem, is to define the significant associations between dynamic and static characteristics.

I am sure none of us need any reminding of the importance of measurement in understanding pulmonary function. I think if we had to approach the problem of the lung not from the standpoint of studying a product of selective evolution but from the standpoint of a brief for the construction of a functional device according to certain laid-down specifications, to exchange so much oxygen and so much CO_2 over such and such a range, at such and such a temperature in varying circumstances—if all that were written down it would at once be obvious that to fulfill that specification would require all the resources of physicists, engineers, chemical engineers, and mathematicians. There would be no question of any inspired deduction or anything of that sort. So I think from that angle it should be very plain that applied physiology and applied medicine in this respect is a technology made up of those various disciplines. I hope that this Symposium—if it doesn't solve many of the problems—will at least delineate the areas of difference and areas of agreement and act as a stimulus for further work.

I must also say how indebted we all are to Messrs Lederle for having provided the sinews for this Symposium and to Dr Hunt, for having made so many material provisions and arrangements, and to Dr Cumming along with him, for arranging what one might call the academic side.

THE FORM AND NOMENCLATURE OF THE AIR SPACES OF THE HUMAN LUNG

D. B. Brewer

Studies on the quantitative anatomy of the respiratory system seem to have been first undertaken by that brilliant eighteenth century eccentric Stephen Hales (1731). The fruits of his genius were many and varied. They ranged from the first measurements of blood pressure in animals, to the devising of the technique for preventing pie crusts from sinking in by supporting them with an inverted teacup. Using a method very similar in principle to the linear dimensions method of Weibel (1963) he estimated the internal surface area of a calf's lung to be 289 sq. ft. (27 m^2).

Since that time there have been many other estimates of the total internal surface area of the lung and also of the total number of alveoli. A variety of methods have been used and the published results vary widely. The results for human lungs have been collected together by Weibel (1963). The figures for internal surface area vary between 5 and 200 m^2. For the total number of alveoli the figures lie for the most part between 725×10^6 and 66×10^6 with two markedly discrepant figures of $1{,}800 \times 10^6$ and $5{,}000 \times 10^6$.

Using the method of the mean linear intercept described in Weibel's book, but first applied to the study of lungs by Duguid *et al.* (1964) it is possible to get consistent and reliable results on both normal and abnormal lungs. Thus for 5 normal cases Weibel obtained a range for internal surface area of from 68·1–83·4 m^2 (results corrected to a standard lung volume of 6,000 ml. by the method of Duguid *et al.*, 1964). Our results (Hicken *et al.*, 1966), again for five normals, give a range of 59·9–83·4 m^2 and the results of Duguid *et al.* (1964), obtained by a semi-automatic scanning method of determining the mean linear intercept, give a range of 76–88 m^2.

Weibel (1963) has described two further methods of obtaining estimates of the internal surface area. These are independent of the mean linear intercept method and of each other so that it is possible to obtain three different estimates of the internal surface area on the same lung. Using the so-called geometrical method on the same five normals Weibel (1963) obtained results the mean of which was 95·7 per cent. of those given above obtained by the method of mean linear intercept. Our results (Hicken *et al.*, 1966) on our five normals give a mean for the geometrical method of 91·1 per cent. of the mean linear intercept method. With the third method, the method of linear dimensions, Weibel's results gave a mean of 98·2 per cent. of the mean by the method of mean linear intercept and our results gave a mean of 94·4 per cent. of our results by the mean linear intercept method.

The methods developed by Weibel (1963) for estimating the total number of alveoli also provide consistent results. He made estimates on the same five normals using his geometrical method and obtained a mean of 295×10^6 alveoli. We (Hicken *et al.*, 1966) have used the same methods and in our five normals obtained a mean of $266{\cdot}6 \times 10^6$ alveoli. We also estimated the total number of alveoli in the same five normals by using the method of linear dimensions and obtained a mean of 295×10^6, 109·8 per cent. of the mean obtained by the geometrical method.

In emphysema the air spaces in the respiratory system in which gaseous exchange takes place are abnormally enlarged so that we must consider now the normal anatomical arrangement of the 300×10^6 alveoli and the approximately 80 m^2 of internal surface they provide and also how they are reached by a complex branching system beginning with a single tube, the trachea.

The quantitative data on the pattern of branching and on the total number of branches at any level is scanty and not entirely consistent. Weibel (1963) considers that the terminal bronchiole, that is the lowest branch of the respiratory tree not to bear alveoli, is the 16th branching, counting the main bronchus as branch 1. Lynne Reid (1967) in her description of the branching uses a different system of numbering. She stresses the slight variations in branching in different areas of the lung. However, converting her figures to the numbering system of Weibel, she considers that the terminal bronchiole may be the 17th to 19th branch.

Of course the character and size of the air passages alter as they branch. The first branches are lined by columnar ciliated epithelium. There is in the wall a complete ring of cartilage and mucous glands lie both internal and external to this cartilage (Fig. 1). These bronchi with the wall completely supported by cartilage are called *large bronchi* to distinguish them from the *small bronchi* the walls of which have only an incomplete ring of cartilage which gets progressively less in amount as the bronchi get smaller. Ultimately the cartilage disappears and the air passage is then called a *bronchiole*. Its wall consists of fibrous and elastic tissue and smooth muscle (Fig. 2). The mucous glands disappear with the cartilage until in the bronchioles no mucous glands are present. Mucus at this level is secreted by goblet cells in the lining epithelium.

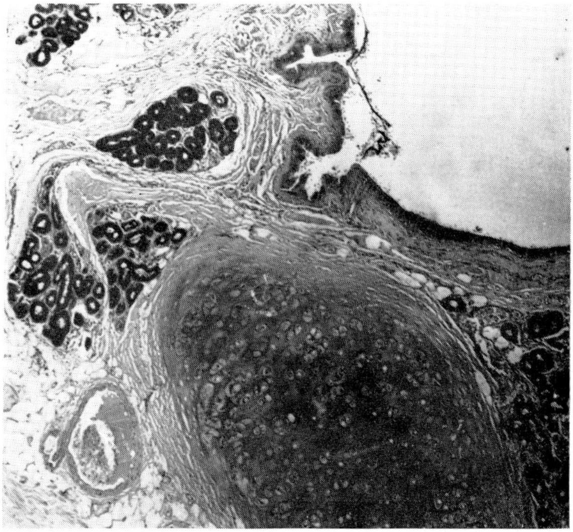

FIG. 1. Wall of large bronchus. Lumen, upper right. Mucous glands in wall extending outwards between cartilage plates. P.A.S. ×35.

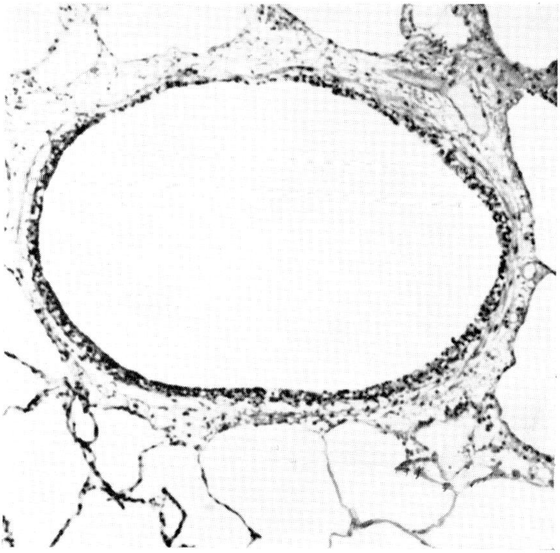

FIG. 2. Bronchiole from lung fixed inflated by formalin steam hence its smooth outline. There is no cartilage in its wall. P.A.S. ×150.

[To face page 4

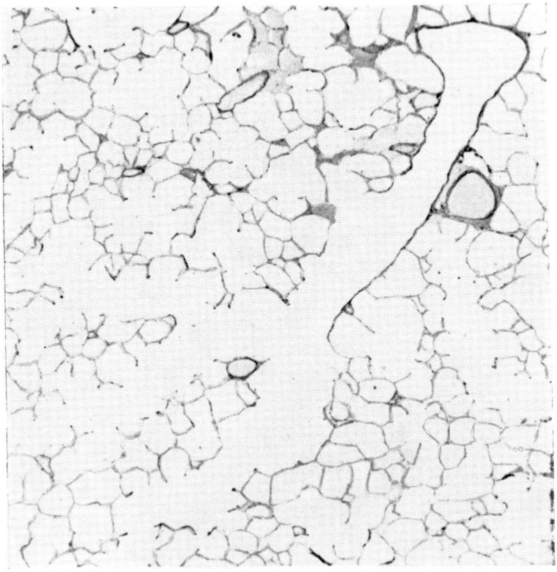

FIG. 3. Terminal bronchiole and respiratory bronchioles. Terminal bronchiole cut almost transversely in upper right corner. First order respiratory bronchiole running obliquely downwards from it and giving rise to second order respiratory bronchioles and alveolar duct. Elastic and van Gieson ×30.

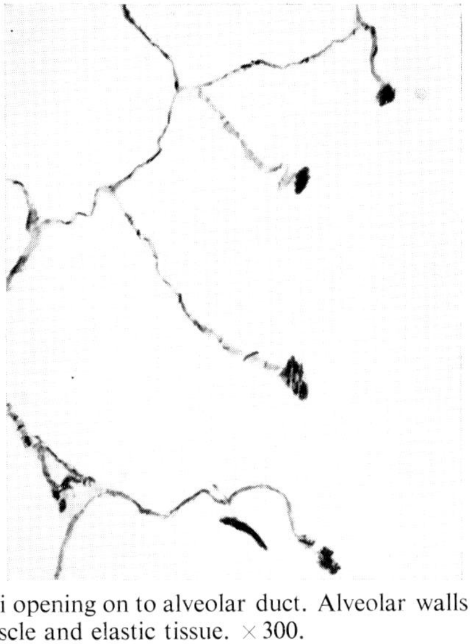

FIG. 4. Alveoli opening on to alveolar duct. Alveolar walls end in knobs of smooth muscle and elastic tissue. ×300.

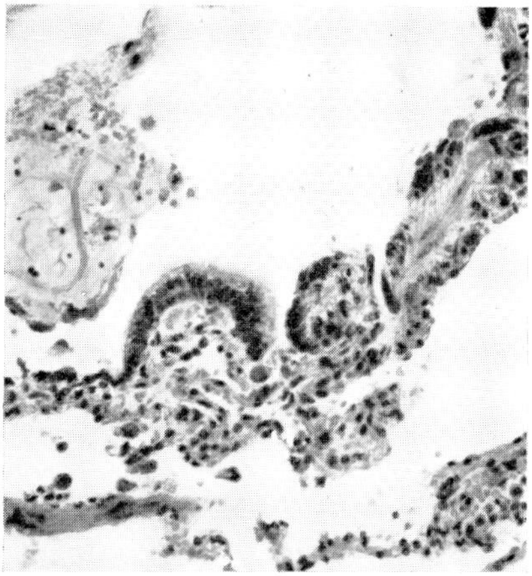

FIG. 5. Lambert's bronchiole-alveolar communications. Bronchiolar lumen upper half of picture. Two communications run downwards through the wall of the bronchiole. Haematoxylin and eosin ×150.

The last bronchiole not to bear alveoli is the terminal bronchiole (Fig. 3). Beyond this we come to the zone where gaseous exchange takes place. The first alveoli encountered are in the walls of the respiratory bronchioles (Fig. 3), the branches of the terminal bronchioles. There is some disagreement as to the numbers of branchings made by the respiratory bronchioles, in fact it probably varies, and the commonest number of branches made is probably three. With each branching the number of alveoli present in the wall of the respiratory bronchiole increases. The walls of the alveoli along the edge of the respiratory bronchioles end in what appear, in sections, as little knobs of smooth muscle and elastic tissue (Fig. 4). In fact, considered in three dimensions the mouths of the alveoli are circular openings, ringed by smooth muscle in the walls of the respiratory bronchioles. The presence of smooth muscle constitutes another landmark as the most distal air passage in which smooth muscle is found is the alveolar duct. There is only one order of alveolar ducts, beyond this are the atria and alveoli.

Two terms in relation to the arrangement of the terminal airways must be defined as they are used in some classifications of emphysema. The term *acinus* as in *panacinar emphysema* consists of that part of the lung formed by the branching of a single terminal bronchiole. It consists therefore of the respiratory bronchioles arising from a single terminal bronchiole with their alveolar ducts and alveoli. The *lobule* as in *centrilobular emphysema* consists of that portion of lung parenchyma demarcated by the lobular septa of fibrous tissue. It is variable in size and may consist of three, four or five acini.

Obviously great changes take place in the number and size of the various air passages in their branching course from the trachea to the alveoli. Some idea of the change is given by Weibel's (1963) estimates based on the assumption of regular dichotomous branching. According to this at the trachea the total cross-sectional area is 2·54 sq. cm. There are 65,500 terminal bronchi with a total cross-sectional area of 180 sq. cm.

In addition to this branching pattern there are other communications linking air sacs and air passages at different levels. The best known of these are the pores in the alveolar septa, Kohn's pores, that join adjacent alveoli. These must be quite numerous as they are readily seen in conditions where there is a fibrinous exudate in the alveoli as then strands of fibrin may be seen passing through them.

A more recently described communication is that between terminal or respiratory bronchioles, and an adjacent alveolus (Fig. 5). Although as yet no physiological significance has been attached to these structures they must be of some importance. They are present in great numbers. In her original description of them Margaret Lambert (1955) gives a drawing of a reconstruction from serial sections in which an average of 7 bronchiole-alveolar communications are present per respiratory or terminal bronchiole. Taking Weibel's (1963) estimate of the total number of terminal and respiratory bronchioles as 982,000 gives a total of 6,874,000 bronchiole-alveolar communications.

LUNG ARCHITECTURE IN EMPHYSEMA

A. G. HEPPLESTON

LUNG function studies, expressed in terms of ventilation, perfusion and diffusion, refer either to the whole organ or to a part such as a lobe but do not yet distinguish particular forms of emphysema. Radiologically emphysema is characterised by an excess of air in the lung, cardiovascular changes and the presence of bullae (Simon, 1964), but these features too are not specific for given types of the disorder. Different forms of emphysema may, however, be recognised by their architectural features and microanatomical studies are of further value in that they raise pathogenetic possibilities and may assist the analysis of physiological disturbance.

THE MORPHOLOGICAL APPROACH

The pathology of emphysema has been studied in two main ways. A commonly adopted method, recently exemplified by Reid (1967), aims to establish a clinicopathological correlation by examining lungs from subjects who died from emphysema (with or without other lung conditions) and who in life were investigated radiologically and physiologically. Such material represents an end-state and its anatomical value tends to be limited because different disease processes may well be obscured by extensive disruptive changes sometimes of a secondary nature. The object of the second approach (Heppleston, 1953 ; Heppleston & Leopold, 1961) is to study from an early stage the evolution of the anatomical changes in the different forms of emphysema, that is before non-specific disruptive and inflammatory changes supervene. For this purpose material is required from subjects without clinical manifestations referable to the chest as well as from individuals whose disordered lung function was investigated during life.

Comparisons of size require a standardised technique of specimen preparation and for this purpose each lung should ideally be preserved in its resting expiratory position, using a method such as Hartung (1960 ; 1963) adopted. Fluid fixation by uncontrolled intrabronchial infusion is open to the objection that the size of the specimen may be influenced by its compliance, thus tending to exaggerate the volume of emphysematous lungs. Because expansion of the lungs is limited by the thoracic cage, the total lung capacity does not conspicuously change in most forms of emphysema (Hartung, 1962 ; 1963 ; 1964). Hence fixation in a position corresponding to full inspiration by intrabronchial injection of fluid at constant pressure (Heard, 1960) tends to minimise differences between emphysematous and normal lungs that should become more apparent by preservation as nearly as possible in the resting expiratory position in order to reflect changes in the functional residual capacity. Dunnill (1962 *b*) and Hartung (1962) are also opposed to pressure fixation where more exact size comparisons are required. Formalin steam fixation under negative pressure, designed to expand the lung to approximately $\frac{3}{4}$ total capacity (Weibel & Vidone, 1961), is not so susceptible to control as Hartung's method when precise quantitation is sought. To obtain a three-dimensional concept of lung structure in emphysema long series of sections have been employed, though for these qualitative studies precise control of fixation was not attempted.

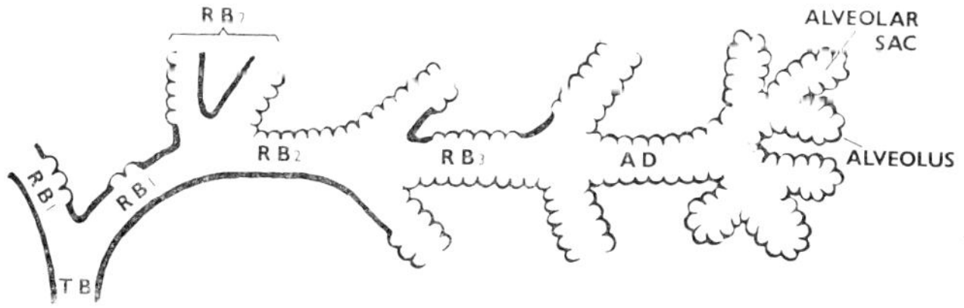

FIG. 1. The usual arrangement of the normal lung acinus.

TB — terminal bronchiole
RB1, 2, 3 — respiratory bronchioles
AD — alveolar duct

Although the branching pattern of the respiratory portion of the bronchiolar tree is subject to some variation, the usual arrangement is indicated in Figure 1. (Heppleston, 1953). The most distal order of non-respiratory bronchiole, *i.e.* the terminal bronchiole, commonly gives rise to three successive orders of respiratory bronchiole, which bear increasing numbers of alveoli as they proceed distally. The last order of respiratory bronchiole leads to the single order of alveolar duct which is completely lined by alveoli and which terminates in the alveolar sacs surrounded by alveoli. The respiratory territory dependent upon a terminal bronchiole is generally recognised as the lung acinus.

DEFINITION

Emphysema is a term meaning inflation and the earliest attempt at an anatomical definition in regard to the lung was made by Laennec (1819). He stated that emphysema represented an exaggeration of the natural configuration in which air vesicles were much increased in size but not necessarily uniformly. Large spaces were probably produced through rupture of the intermediate partitions between air cells but sometimes they appeared to arise by simple enlargement of a single vesicle. Modern knowledge of the pulmonary architecture demanded a more explicit definition of the term emphysema. This necessity arose in establishing the micro-anatomy of focal emphysema, when Heppleston (1953) showed that emphysematous enlargement of air spaces might affect any segment or group of segments of the bronchial tree in which haemo-respiratory gaseous exchange occurred. In other words chronic pulmonary emphysema represents a persistent enlargement of respiratory bronchioles, alveolar ducts or alveolar sacs as well as of their associated alveoli. This basis was accepted by Leopold and Gough (1957) and forms the non-controversial element of subsequent definitions (Ciba Symposium, 1959 ; Amer. Thorac. Soc., 1962).

CLASSIFICATION

The presence or absence of airways obstruction, judged pathologically by failure of the isolated emphysematous lung to deflate as does a normal lung, has been proposed as the primary basis of classification (Reid, 1967). Combining functional impairment and structural state in this way encounters the difficulty that forms of emphysema which, it is claimed, do not exhibit airways obstruction may do so when sufficiently severe (Pratt *et al.*, 1961 ; Hartung & Einbrodt, 1965), because lung tension is then so reduced that air is ‘ trapped ’ and breach of alveolar walls renders the condition ‘ irreversible ’. Conversely, widespread pan-acinar emphysema (v.i.), classified by Reid in the group with airways obstruction, may not show this feature in its earlier stages (Pratt *et al.*, 1962).

Laennec appreciated that both dilatation and destruction contribute to the genesis of emphysema. A destructive element is readily recognised should there be an interruption in the continuity of the walls of respiratory air passages or alveoli. On the other hand atrophy of the walls of affected spaces is a likely consequence of their persistent enlargement and may be regarded as a degree of destruction short of a breach in continuity. The term destruction, emphasised by the American Thoracic Society (1962), thus carries a dual meaning and so forms an unsatisfactory basis for the primary differentiation of the various types of emphysema. It must also be stressed that destruction of pulmonary elements is often a later, secondary manifestation of non-specific type which obscures the original form of the emphysematous change. A breach in the walls of alveoli or respiratory bronchioles will therefore be indicated by the term disruptive emphysema in a purely descriptive sense.

Three-dimensional studies show that emphysematous enlargement may affect predominantly certain segments or a combination of segments of the bronchiolar tree whilst leaving others unaffected at least initially. Moreover, in some forms of emphysema other changes of a characteristic nature coexist. The morphological classification of chronic pulmonary emphysema here adopted (Table 1) thus rests on the distribution of the enlargement as seen

Table 1. *Classification of chronic pulmonary emphysema according to the airways mainly affected*

1. *Respiratory bronchioles*
   (a) Focal emphysema due to dust
   (b) Centrilobular emphysema
2. *Alveolar sacs and alveolar ducts*
   Distal-acinar emphysema
3. *Alveolar sacs, alveolar ducts and respiratory bronchioles*
   Pan-acinar emphysema
4. *Irregular*
   (*a*) Scar emphysema
      (*i*) Coarse scarring
      (*ii*) Fine scarring, mature or incipient (chronic bronchiolo-alveolitis)
   (*b*) Linear emphysema
   (*c*) Bullae

in the earlier phases of development, disruption being indicated as a separate feature. Attention will be concentrated on the principal anatomical varieties of emphysema.

Focal emphysema

Focal emphysema and centrilobular emphysema constitute the two distinct types of emphysema which involve only respiratory bronchioles.

Industrial exposure to dusts with a low or negligible content of free silica leads to the development of a form of pneumoconiosis typically seen in coal workers but not restricted to them or even to work underground. A mild degree of this form of simple pneumoconiosis may be seen in town dwellers who have had no occupational exposure to dust.

Numerous, discrete foci of dust widely scattered throughout the lung characterise simple pneumoconiosis as found for instance in coal workers. Three positive features identify these dust foci and distinguish them from silicotic nodules (Heppleston, 1947) : a large amount of dust, a relatively small amount of fibrous tissue, and commonly enlarged air spaces in and around the dust aggregates. Serial section studies (Heppleston, 1953) show, firstly, that the dust accumulates preferentially around the three orders of respiratory bronchioles, especially the middle one, and, secondly, that these three orders of respiratory bronchioles often undergo dilatation to constitute the enlarged air spaces described as focal emphysema (Fig. 2). Three negative features may also be emphasised : there is

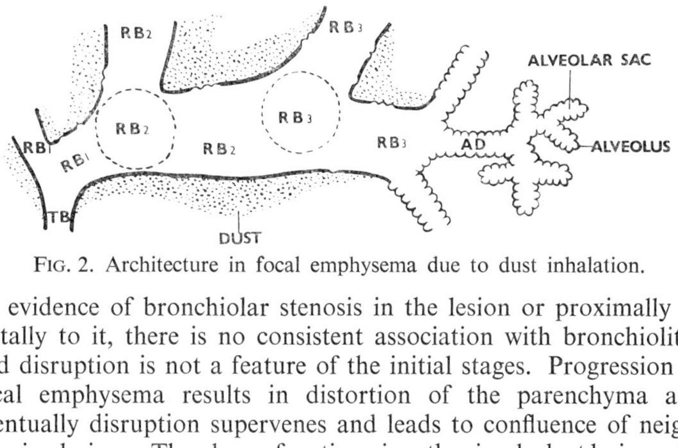

FIG. 2. Architecture in focal emphysema due to dust inhalation.

no evidence of bronchiolar stenosis in the lesion or proximally or distally to it, there is no consistent association with bronchiolitis, and disruption is not a feature of the initial stages. Progression of focal emphysema results in distortion of the parenchyma and eventually disruption supervenes and leads to confluence of neighbouring lesions. The plane of section gives the simple dust lesion with focal emphysema various appearances, but cinephotography of serial sections reveals the essential continuity of the dilated airways and their regular relationship to the aggregated dust (Heppleston, 1955).[1]

The factors which appear to be involved in the production of focal emphysema are indicated in Figure 3. (Heppleston, 1954).

[1] At this point a cine-film was shown.

Inspiratory expansion of the vesicular tissue immediately around the respiratory bronchioles is prevented by consolidation with dust-laden phagocytes enmeshed by relatively little fibrous tissue. The inspiratory traction that would have been expended on the consolidated alveoli presumably augments the pull exerted directly on the respiratory bronchioles. In the presence of focal emphysema, bronchiolar smooth muscle incarcerated in the dust focus becomes atrophic and may even disappear. Conversely advanced focal emphysema has not been found where smooth muscle is well preserved in dust lesions. Eventually it seems that expiratory contraction and shortening of the respiratory bronchioles is reduced or even abolished. Both the inspiratory and expiratory movements of the bronchioles may thus be affected and the disturbances summate to produce the permanent dilatation known as focal emphysema.

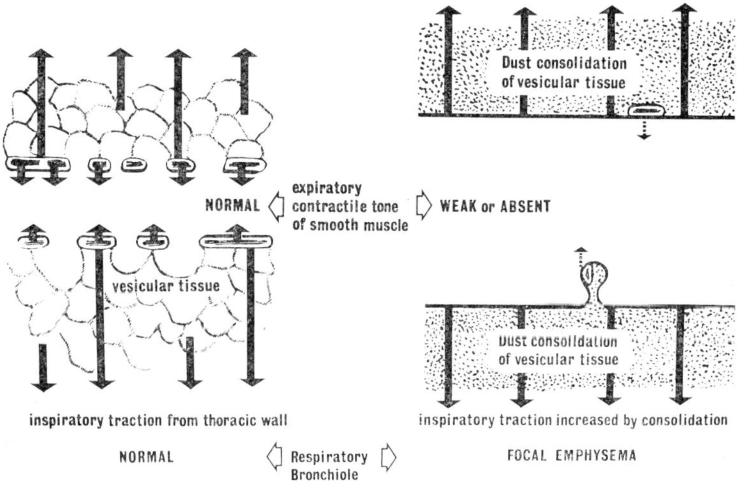

FIG. 3. Interpretation of the mechanism of focal emphysema due to dusts with a low content of free silica.

Centrilobular emphysema

This variety is characterised by enlarged air spaces grouped more or less centrally in lung lobules, which may otherwise appear normal (Leopold & Gough, 1957). Histologically two identifying features are encountered in early as well as in developed lesions, namely disruption and inflammation. Architecturally the enlarged spaces represent loss of alveolar tissue through disruption of adjacent respiratory bronchioles, especially the more distal orders (Fig. 4). A centrilobular lesion may thus replace the territory formerly occupied by two or more sequences of respiratory bronchioles. Chronic inflammation of bronchiolar walls is a constant concomitant of centrilobular emphysema. The distal non-respiratory and/or proximal respiratory bronchiole are so affected that they connect with the emphysematous spaces in the form of a fibrosed parent bronchiole. Less severe and more variable inflammatory changes also occur amongst the disrupted structures remaining in the spaces. The histological features suggest

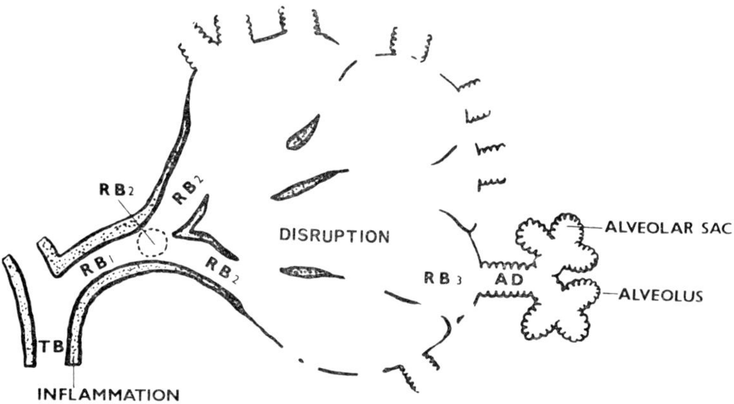

FIG. 4. Architecture in centrilobular emphysema.

that the primary change is a respiratory and terminal bronchiolitis which apparently leads to disruption of the more delicate distal segments and to fibrosis of the more resistant proximal segments. Chronic inflammation of parent bronchioles suggests that they become rigid structures unable to dilate or elongate during inspiration. Inspiratory traction is therefore likely to aggravate the disruption of distal respiratory bronchioles.

Two further features must be mentioned. Firstly, luminal stenosis is not a constant finding in parent bronchioles. Some may be narrowed though not obliterated, but others have a lumen of normal calibre, whilst still others may even be dilated. Bronchiolar calibre and severity of emphysema thus do not correspond and it may be concluded that bronchiolar stenosis as such is not likely to determine the emphysematous state. Secondly, centrilobular emphysema is not confined to individuals exposed to an occupational dust hazard.

Alveolar ducts leading distally from the emphysematous spaces may be of normal size, although distal-acinar emphysema may be present as well.

Distal-acinar and pan-acinar emphysema

Although these varieties may be confined to certain areas or even lobules, the whole of both lungs is commonly affected. The air spaces become visible to the naked eye but the enlargement is not always uniform. Serial-section studies showed that the basic anatomical pattern of the alveolar tissue is not altered at first. In *distal-acinar emphysema* (Fig. 5) the respiratory bronchioles are

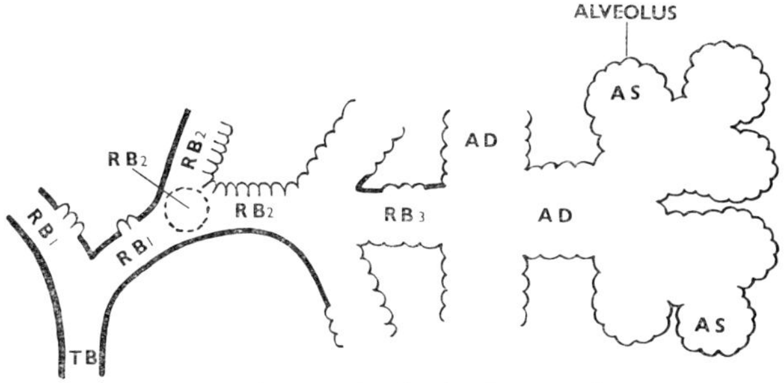

FIG. 5. Architecture in distal-acinar emphysema.

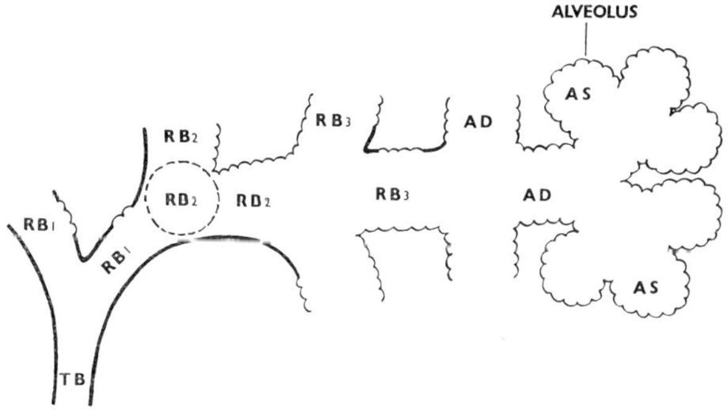

FIG. 6. Architecture in pan-acinar emphysema.

usually normal in calibre, though the third order may be a little enlarged. Dilatation characteristically affects alveolar ducts and alveolar sacs and the enlargement tends to occur at the expense of the associated alveoli many of which become shallower and wider (Heppleston, 1953). The existence of distal-acinar emphysema has been confirmed by Thurlbeck (1963).

The distal order of respiratory bronchiole may, as already mentioned, be enlarged along with alveolar ducts and sacs, but proximal respiratory bronchioles may also become involved, when the term *pan-acinar* is applied (Fig. 6). The appearances suggest that respiratory bronchioles are involved after alveolar sacs and ducts, and hence it seems that the pan-acinar change may sometimes represent an extension of the distal form.

Chronic inflammatory changes are inconstant in the bronchiolar tree of subjects with distal- or pan-acinar emphysema and non-inflammatory factors are evidently involved. Anatomical obstruction of air passages is not a common feature, and lack of an obvious cause has led to the use of the term primary emphysema for these forms. In clinical emphysema the thorax tends to adopt a position of partial inspiration, a state to which the anatomical changes of distal- and pan-acinar emphysema in particular approximate. Enlargement of the lung has often been attributed to defective elastic tissue, but evidence has been adduced throwing doubt on the importance of elastic tissue in expiratory recoil of the lung (Heppleston, 1954). Pierce and Ebert (1965) suggested that the elastic behaviour of the lung depends not on axial elongation of elastic fibres but upon unfolding of the ductal helices, and they considered collagen to be more important than elastin in maintaining the structural integrity of the lung. These authors also point out that emphysematous lungs possess normal amounts of collagen and elastin. As an alternative possibility it seems that the natural variations in the amount of smooth muscle in the bronchial tree (Heppleston, 1954) might underlie acinar emphysema. Recoil of the lung on expiration is influenced by surface forces and by the contractile tone of smooth muscle. Deficiency of the bronchial and bronchiolar muscle might, over a period of many years, lead to fixation of the thorax in a position of partial inspiration. Conversely where bronchiolar smooth muscle is hypertrophic, as in asthma, emphysema is rarely found (Williams & Leopold, 1959).

The distribution of the anatomical changes supports the idea of a muscular factor in pathogenesis. Because alveolar sacs lack smooth muscle they would be expected to reflect a weakened expiratory movement before alveolar ducts and respiratory bronchioles which possess muscle in amounts which tend to increase proximally. It is thus possible to account for the lack of emphysematous change in second and first order respiratory bronchioles in some cases. If, however, all the orders of respiratory bronchiole and the alveolar duct were particularly deficient in smooth muscle, the emphysema could have a pan-acinar distribution from the inception. It is worth examining whether in pan-acinar emphysema the bronchial tree has a somewhat underdeveloped pattern of branching that requires the respiratory segments to occupy relatively more space in the thorax as postnatal growth occurs. A uniform pattern of emphysema, affecting most respiratory segments of the bronchiolar tree *ab initio*, may also develop in otherwise healthy lung after lobectomy or pneumonectomy.

A further alternative is that the thoracic cage may become fixed in the inspiratory position because of skeletal changes and that enlargement of the lungs and atrophy of muscle in the air passages occurred as a consequence. Barrel deformity of the chest, often considered an accompaniment of emphysema, may however occur independently of pulmonary change (Pierce & Ebert, 1958).

Irregular emphysema

In this category are placed forms of emphysema showing haphazard involvement of respiratory bronchioles, alveolar ducts or alveolar sacs. Irregular emphysema is often associated with pulmonary *scars* or areas of inflammatory fibrosis that involve bronchioles as well as parenchyma. A scar may be enveloped by emphysematous air passages and spaces belonging to more than one acinus and involving different segments of each.

Scars may be coarse when large areas of lung are fibrosed, as in tuberculosis or complicated pneumoconiosis. On the other hand fine fibrosis, often widely distributed, may result from the organisation of a bronchopneumonic exudate or from a chronic inflammatory process which takes the form of an active bronchiolo-alveolitis. Inflammatory disruption may affect alveolar walls from an early stage and bronchioles may become fibrosed, stenosed or even obliterated ; bronchiolar and alveolar changes are, however, not necessarily of comparable severity. Scars prevent expansion of the affected lung, so that enlargement of adjacent air spaces may result not only from primary disruption but also from inspiratory overstretching of neighbouring lung tissue, aggravated by contraction of fibrous tissue. Three-dimensional studies of fine scarring with irregular emphysema (Heppleston, 1956) suggest that bronchiolar stenosis as such is not a major factor in the genesis of the emphysema, since spaces communicate with patent or with narrowed airways. Fine fibrosis with irregular emphysema may differ from centrilobular emphysema only in that the inflammatory change of the latter is for some reason less severe and more restricted in its initial distribution.

Irregular emphysema may be confined to a zone immediately adjacent to septa, bronchi and arteries as well as just beneath the pleura, the remaining lung tissue showing little if any deviation from normal. This *linear* form of irregular emphysema is not usually of a severity that suggests clinical importance. It is generally disruptive in nature and slight fibrosis may be associated, some spaces being enclosed by thin fibrous walls and thus resembling a cystic state. The fibrous component suggests an inflammatory origin, and the process may be thus localised because restricted inspiratory expansion of vesicular tissue abutting on relatively rigid components impedes resolution of exudate.

The term *bulla* refers to air-containing spaces large enough to have overrun acini. Bullae may possess an epithelial lining over part of their surface and are sometimes associated with fibrosis of varying degree. Air passages from different levels of the bronchiolar tree open into them and the communications may be quite patent or be stenosed, whilst in some instances the orifice appears to be valvular when the space tends to become rounded. Bullae may occur in association with some other form of emphysema, of which they may represent an extreme stage, but they are also found as isolated lesions often on the lung surface and sometimes of large size. A sharp distinction between bullae and cysts may not be possible (Heppleston & Leopold, 1961).

COMMENTS

Coexistence of different types of emphysema

Workers exposed to coal and similar dust hazards do not invariably develop focal emphysema and they may be affected with any of the other varieties. Emphysema involving respiratory bronchioles evidently cannot assume focal and centrilobular forms in the same acinus, although in one lung centrilobular emphysema may affect some acini and focal emphysema others. The dilated respiratory bronchioles of focal emphysema are enveloped by cylinders of dust enmeshed in fine fibrous tissue, and hence may be able to resist the disruptive effects of a subsequent bronchiolitis. Conversely, the existence of alveolar disruption and bronchiolar distortion in centrilobular emphysema or the fine form of scar emphysema precludes dust collection and the development of focal emphysema in the usual manner. For the same reason the development of true focal emphysema is likely to be prevented if the causative factors of the centrilobular or scar (fine) and the focal forms operate simultaneously. Air pollution by particulate matter, whether specifically occupational or merely urban, will lead to a variable degree of pigmentation in relation to the parent bronchiole and the walls of spaces in centrilobular emphysema. The architecture, however, remains essentially that of the disruptive centrilobular form with no indication of the dilatation pattern of focal emphysema. In the nonindustrial population true focal emphysema is customarily only minor in degree and larger spaces are likely to represent the centrilobular form. Failure to employ serial sections has repeatedly led to confusion between the two forms of emphysema affecting respiratory bronchioles. Since distal-acinar and focal emphysema affect different anatomical sections of the airway they may coexist and, likewise, centrilobular and distal-acinar forms may also occur together. Scar emphysema (coarse or fine) may be associated with any other form, though in different parts of a given lung.

The pathogenesis of emphysema

Knowledge of pathogenesis is incomplete and present ideas may well need modification, but, so far as is possible, primary and secondary factors should be distinguished in terms that imply processes rather than morphological states. The *primary factors* already mentioned in relation to individual types are assembled in Table 2.

Table 2. *Summary of factors which may be involved in the pathogenesis of emphysema*

PRIMARY FACTORS	
Distal- and pan-acinar	Deficiency of smooth muscle in the bronchial tree. Abnormalities of the thoracic cage
Focal (dust)	Immobilisation of alveolar tissue Atrophy of muscle in RBs
Centrilobular	Chronic bronchiolitis (RBs) with anatomical disruption Immobilisation of lung tissue Contraction of fibrous tissue
Irregular	Inflammatory disruption Immobilisation of lung tissue Contraction of scars, coarse or fine
SECONDARY FACTORS	
Disruption	As a consequence of atrophy
Lung tension	Effect of loss
Distribution	Influence of anatomical and physiological differences between upper and lower zones.

Widespread distal-acinar or pan-acinar emphysema may depend upon deficiency of muscle in the bronchial tree or possibly abnormalities of the thoracic cage leading to fixation of the thorax in a position of partial inspiration. Focal emphysema is probably determined by immobilisation of alveolar structures and atrophy of smooth muscle in respiratory bronchioles. In centrilobular and in various forms of irregular emphysema anatomical disruption, often inflammatory, is a primary event, but immobilisation of lung tissue, usually by fibrosis, also contributes and the overstretching so induced will be aggravated by contraction of fibrous tissue. The effect of inspiratory movement is evidently a common factor in the genesis of several varieties of emphysema.

The severity of a particular type of emphysema may increase either because the primary factor(s) continues to operate or because secondary factors not specific to any one form of emphysema come into play. Disruption characterises centrilobular and scar emphysema from an early stage, but although not a primary feature of focal or acinar emphysema anatomical disruption may eventually supervene. In the focal type disruption mainly affects alveolar walls around dust accumulations, whilst in the acinar form a gradual atrophy of alveolar walls evidently leads to a reduction of the capillary network and at first gives rise to the small, rounded holes on which a number of investigators have commented. A breach in structural continuity presumably disturbs the local lung tension and it seems that an affected space will continue to enlarge until the tension of its walls balances that in surrounding lung. Atmospheric pressure transmitted through the airways suffices for the development of such spaces, the size of which will increase further if tension in the surrounding lung is reduced as by acinar emphysema. Dayman's (1951 ; 1956) suggestion that anatomical disruption leads to loss of lung tension and the development in intrathoracic airways of an expiratory check-valve mechanism is borne out by pathological findings. This phenomenon represents in effect an exaggeration of the normal expiratory relaxation of air passages and stresses that in emphysema the increased resistance to expiratory air-flow is a result and not a cause of the anatomical changes.

Irrespective of their type, emphysematous lesions are often more severe in the upper than in the lower parts of the lung. The upper zone is known to be less well ventilated and perfused than the lower. Radioactive gas studies (West & Dollery, 1960; Ball *et al.*, 1962) reveal a lower ventilation in the upper parts of the lung and this may be related to larger alveolar size, if the results from dogs (Glazier *et al.*, 1966) can be applied to man. According to Dock (1946 ; 1954) the pulmonary arterial flow is relatively diminished in the upper third of the lung in the erect adult. Using radioactive xenon, Hughes, Glazier and West (1967) have lately extended this observation and demonstrated diminished alveolar perfusion in the upper parts of the lung at functional residual capacity or total lung capacity. Accordingly it is possible that fewer of the humoral and cellular elements involved in the inflammatory reaction will reach the upper zones and that disposal of micro-organisms or their products will be less effective. Emphysematous disruption may thus become more severe in the upper part because of relative hypoxia or reduced defence against inflammatory agents, or, if the situation in man parallels that in the dog, from a greater tendency to capillary obliteration associated with increased alveolar size. A greater inspiratory tension is probably experienced at the periphery of the lung because, in addition to the traction needed for its own expansion, this zone transmits that required to expand the central part, thus offering a possible explanation for the greater severity of disruption often seen at the periphery of the lung.

ACKNOWLEDGMENTS

Figures 1 and 2 are reproduced in modified form from Heppleston (1953) and Figure 3 from Heppleston (1954) by courtesy of the Editor of the Journal of Pathology and Bacteriology. Figures 4 and 5 are reproduced from Heppleston and Leopold (1961) by courtesy of the Editor of the American Journal of Medicine.

MORPHOMETRY OF THE HUMAN LUNG IN HEALTH AND DISEASE

M. S. DUNNILL

INTRODUCTION

THE brief inviting us to speak here instructed us to survey the problems, fit in available data and indicate lines of progress. Measurement in histology has been a relatively neglected subject until quite recently and even now it is only feeling its way gingerly down a dimly lit tunnel. I propose first to give a very brief outline of the quantitative anatomy of the normal lung and then to discuss some of the problems arising in lungs taken from patients suffering from chronic non-specific lung disease.

THE NORMAL LUNG

The quantitative anatomy of the lung has been described by Weibel (1963) from a detailed study of five normal lungs. The lung is divided into two main anatomical zones. The first is the conducting zone, which is concerned with the transport of gas and blood to and from the second, or respiratory, zone where gaseous exchange between the blood in the alveolar capillaries and the gas in the alveoli takes place. In between these two zones is a small but important transition zone.

The conducting zone consists of the pulmonary arterial and venous systems and the bronchi. The latter constitute an irregularly dichotomous branching system of airways, commencing with the trachea whose average diameter is 1·8 cm. and ending 16 generations later with the terminal bronchioles whose average diameter is $5{\cdot}4.10^{-2}$ cm. The 17th to 19th generations, the respiratory bronchioles (average diameter $4{\cdot}6.10^{-2}$ cm.) and the 20th to 23rd generations, the alveolar ducts and sacs (average diameter $4{\cdot}2.10^{-2}$ cm.) constitute the transition zone. In this region the elements of the conducting and respiratory zones are intimately mixed as alveoli are found in the walls of the respiratory bronchioles, alveolar ducts and air sacs.

The respiratory zone contains the alveoli and alveolar capillaries. The mean number of alveoli in the normal human adult lung was calculated by Weibel and Gomez (1962) to be $296{\cdot}10^{6}$ ($\pm 13{\cdot}10^{6}$), using an elegant method they devised for estimating the numbers of structures in a volume from counting the number of transections of the structures in a thin histological section. The full complement of alveoli is not present at birth but is achieved by the age of 8 years. (Dunnill, 1962 *a*). In the normal lung each alveolus has a shape approximating to a truncated cone surmounted by a cone. The average diameter is 250 μ, a fact which was determined as long ago as 1731 by Stephen Hales. The total alveolar surface area is approximately 75 sq. m. in the adult but varies with (1) the size and age of the individual and (2) the state of inflation of the lung.

Recently West and his colleagues (Glazier *et al.*, 1966), using a freezing technique on greyhounds with the lungs *in situ*, have demonstrated a regional variation in alveolar volume, the volume of the alveoli in the dependent, or lower, regions being smaller than in the upper portions of the lung. The size and shape of the alveoli may change during various phases of the respiratory cycle. While there may be little or no change during quiet breathing at rest, the anatomical changes which occur during deep inspiration and expiration are the subject of some argument. Macklin (1929) considered that during deep inspiration the main increase in volume took place in the alveolar ducts and that the alveoli underwent little or no stretching but merely became ' shallower and wider at the mouth when the tube into which they open dilated '. Storey and Staub (1962) on the other hand, using a rapid freezing technique on the lungs of living cats, concluded that the alveoli increased in size. Dunnill (1967), using greyhound lungs fixed and inflated at different pressures, showed that, at higher lung volumes, the greater the degree of inflation the greater the alveolar surface area, S, and that the relationship follows the form : $S = K.V^{2/3}$ where V is the alveolar volume and K is a constant. The percentage of the lung volume occupied by the alveoli rises with an increase in lung inflation and the percentage volume of the ducts shows a corresponding fall. The increase in alveolar surface area might well account for the findings of McGraith and Thomson (1959), who showed that there was little change in diffusing capacity from near residual volume to mid-capacity, but an increase at higher lung volumes.

In man, and in mammals generally, there is a close relationship between alveolar surface area and body surface area, which is itself related to oxygen consumption. Tenney and Remmers (1963) have demonstrated this in a variety of species and Dunnill (1962 *a*) has shown a similar relationship in children.

Weibel (1963) has made extensive studies of the alveolar capillary network and has demonstrated that it has a hexagonal pattern in the alveolar wall. In the adult lung the total capillary surface area is closely related to the corresponding alveolar surface area, being approximately 75 sq. m. The total capillary volume varies between 150 and 200 ml.

There is little work on the pulmonary blood vessels corresponding to Weibel's analysis of the airways, and this is a field for further research. It promises to be difficult because the method and mode of branching of the vessels is much more irregular than that of the airways, small tributaries and side branches being given off both the pulmonary arteries and veins at irregular intervals.

CHRONIC NONSPECIFIC LUNG DISEASE

Any attempt at understanding form and function in the diseased human lung necessitates collection of quantitative anatomical data and comparison with the normal morphometry. This is a particular need in a field where clinicians are making numerous complex measurements.

Chronic bronchitis

The actual definition of disease is best accomplished in quantitative terms and this is well illustrated by the problem of chronic bronchitis. The credit for showing that this disease represents a quantitative anatomical difference from the normal belongs to Reid (1960). She measured the ratio of the thickness of the mucous gland layer, as it lies between cartilage and epithelium, to the thickness of the bronchial wall at the same point, that is, from the basement membrane of the epithelium to the inner aspect of the perichondrium. The measurement is made at a point where the cartilage and mucous membrane are parallel. This is the Reid Index. She also employed a method of acinar counting ; the total number of acini, complete or incomplete, in a high power microscopic field were counted. This method has presented certain difficulties. In many bronchi it is not easy to find many suitable areas where the cartilage is parallel to the mucous membrane. The exact point at which the measurement is made is to a certain extent arbitrary and from examination of a histological section of a bronchus (Fig. 2) it is at once apparent that a certain amount of bias must enter into the selection of the point at which the measurements are made. In any one bronchus Reid took the average of at least two measurements, and occasionally of as many as six.

The Reid method has the great advantage that it is independent of any need to define the adventitia of the bronchus. This can be difficult unless the bronchi which are to be measured are selected with care. Restrepo and Heard (1963 *a*) overcame this difficulty by concentrating on transverse sections of the bronchus to the basal segments of the lower lobe and the bronchus to the inferior segment of the lingula. They projected 5 μ thick sections of the bronchi onto a white card and traced the inner edge of the mucosa, the outer limit of the fibrous wall and the outlines of the mucous glands and cartilage. The tracings of the glands were cut out, as were the tracings of the cartilage and the rest of the wall. All these collections of tracings were weighed and the weights are proportional to the areas of the various structures in the sections. This is an adaptation of the method used by Charles Darwin in some of his geological researches, and it is extremely accurate. It has the advantage that the gland tissue outside and between the cartilage is sampled as well as that internal to the cartilage. The disadvantage of the method is that it is tedious and time-consuming.

In a further valuable paper Restrepo and Heard (1963 *b*) studied the distribution of the mucous glands in both normal and bronchitic subjects. Altogether they sampled 36 sites in each bronchial tree and showed that the absolute quantity of gland tissue differed significantly at any given site in normal subjects. The variation, as might be expected, was greater in bronchitis. We have carried out similar experiments in Oxford using the technique of point counting (Hennig, 1958 ; Dunnill, 1962 *b*), which can be adapted to this problem. It combines the advantages of both methods. It is simple and rapid to count 500 points, using a Zeiss I integrating eyepiece, spread over a transverse section of the entire bronchial wall. All structures in the bronchial wall are sampled. Providing a constant bronchus is examined, this method gives a good indication of the quantity of mucous gland tissue and comparative studies are possible. It is important to establish what variation exists in the mucous gland content within a bronchus and between bronchi in a lung. It can be shown that there is a difference in the proportion of mucous gland tissue between bronchi in the same lung which is significant at the 1 in 1,000 level (Table 1). There is thus a considerable sampling

Table 1. *Test for homogeneity of mucous gland content of bronchi*

Bronchus	Hits on mucous glands	Non hits on mucous glands	Percentage mucous glands
1	82	418	16·4
2	93	407	18·6
3	83	417	16·6
4	93	407	18·6
5	68	432	13·6
6	104	396	20·8
7	77	423	15·4
8	74	426	14·8
9	106	394	21·2
10	98	402	19·6
11	83	417	16·6
12	101	399	20·2
13	110	390	22·0
14	112	388	22·4
15	114	386	22·8
16	96	404	19·2
17	113	387	22·6
18	149	351	29·8

Mean 19·5 ± 6·77

$\chi^2 = 76{\cdot}86$ $\quad$ $P < 0{\cdot}001$

Table 2. *Test for homogeneity of mucous gland content within bronchi*

Bronchus	No. of sections	Degrees of freedom	χ^2	P	Total No. of points counted
1	3	2	0·50	> 0·05	1500
2	3	2	1·67	> 0·05	1500
3	3	2	0·38	> 0·05	1500

difficulty to be overcome. The variation in sections taken from the same bronchus over a short distance is not significant (Table 2). It would seem that in any study it would be wise to concentrate on a few named constant bronchi and to obtain a mean value. The bronchi to the inferior segment of the lingula and to the basal segments of the lower lobe would appear to be suitable for this purpose.

Restrepo and Heard (1963 *a*) and Thurlbeck and Angus (1964) both found a considerable overlap between normals and bronchitics, and the latter authors showed that in a series of random necropsies the distribution curve for the Reid Index approached a Gaussian shape. In fact the situation with regard to the definition of chronic bronchitis is exactly comparable to that in hypertension (Pickering, 1961) and osteoporosis (Dunnill *et al.*, 1967). The concept that there is a certain value for the volume of mucous gland tissue in the bronchus above which the diagnosis of chronic bronchitis can be made and below which it is not present is an erroneous one. It is important to collect a large amount of data from the population, preferably using autopsies on accident cases, to establish a distribution curve for the mucous gland content of given bronchi. When assessing a specific case it is better to quote a value for the proportion of gland tissue in the bronchial wall than to state dogmatically that the mucous glands are normal or hypertrophied.

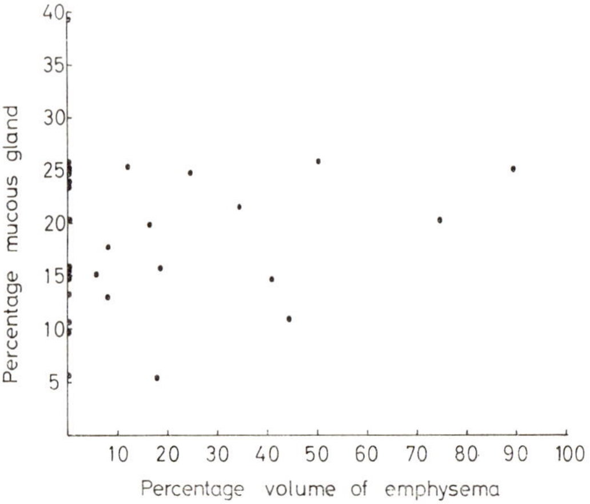

FIG. 1. The percentage mucous gland content of the bronchi plotted against the percentage volume of emphysema, in 27 cases of chronic obstructive airway disease, showing that there is no simple relationship.

Relationship between chronic bronchitis and emphysema. The quantitative assessment of the mucous glands in the bronchial wall is essential if the relationship between chronic bronchitis and emphysema is to be determined. It is usually assumed that chronic bronchitis and emphysema are related, but remarkably little work has been done to substantiate this view. Thurlbeck and Angus (1963)

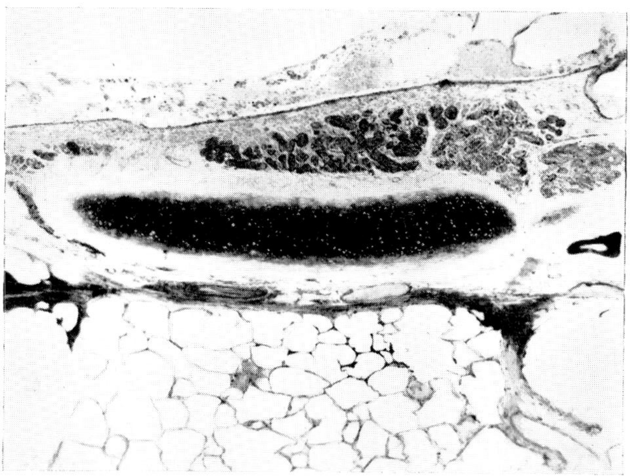

FIG. 2. Section of part of a bronchial wall showing the variable thickness of the mucous gland layer lying between the perichondrum and the mucosa. P.A.S. ×20.

[*To face page* 24

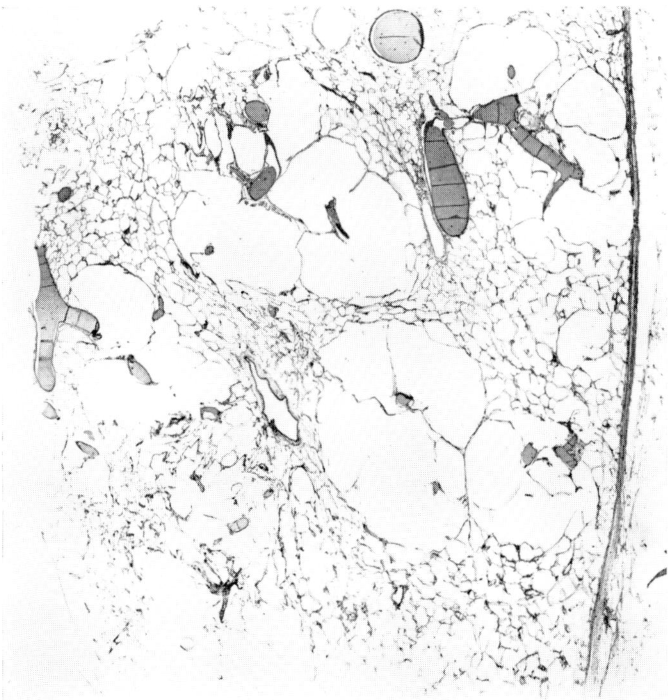

FIG. 3. Photomicrograph of case of extensive centrilobular emphysema which exhibited marked right ventricular hypertrophy. Pulmonary artery injected H and E $\times 5$.

investigated this problem, using the Reid Index on the bronchi and a grading method for assessing the emphysema, and showed that, in general, the more severe the emphysema the higher the Reid Index. It was noted though that chronic bronchitis was present in 20 per cent. of patients without destructive emphysema, and also that some patients with emphysema had no chronic bronchitis. These findings are endorsed in Figure 1, where the percentage volume of emphysema is plotted against the proportion of mucous glands in the bronchial wall. It can be seen that there are several cases with a high mucous gland content in the bronchi and no emphysema. Furthermore, some cases with a large volume of emphysema have only a small mucous gland volume. In any consideration of these findings it must be remembered that some workers (Kourilsky *et al.*, 1960) have reported gland atrophy in the later stages of chronic bronchitis. It is possible that gland hypertrophy represents only one stage in the natural history of the disease.

Chronic bronchitis and right ventricular hypertrophy

Chronic bronchitis without emphysema can be a severe and fatal disease causing cor pulmonale (Hentel *et al.*, 1963). Millard and

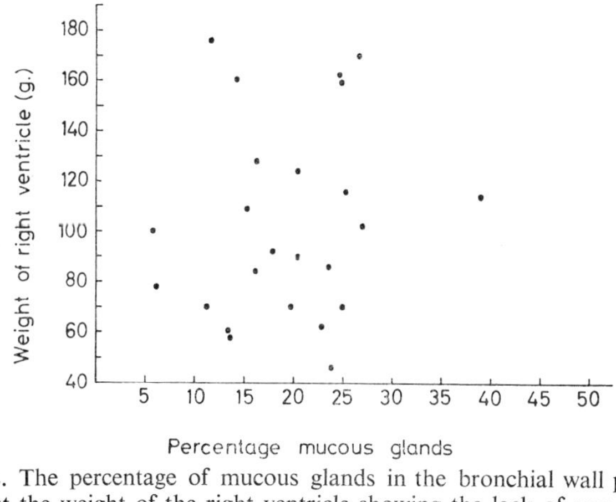

FIG. 4. The percentage of mucous glands in the bronchial wall plotted against the weight of the right ventricle showing the lack of any simple correlation.

Reid (1967) have concluded that bronchial mucous gland hypertrophy is related to right ventricular hypertrophy. Once again the relationship is by no means a simple one. Right ventricular hypertrophy is best assessed by weighing the separated right ventricular wall without the septum and comparing it with the weight of the separated left ventricle with the septum (Marshall, 1961 ; Fulton, 1953). As there are many causes of right ventricular hypertrophy apart from chronic nonspecific lung disease, and patients with chronic bronchitis are usually from the older age group and may suffer in addition from hypertension and ischaemic heart disease, assessment of the degree of right ventricular hypertrophy may be difficult. In Figure 4, the right ventricular weight is plotted against the mucous gland content of the bronchial wall and it can be seen that there is no simple relationship. There is a closer relationship between the ratio of left ventricular to right ventricular weight and the mucous glands, as shown in Figure 5. The relationship

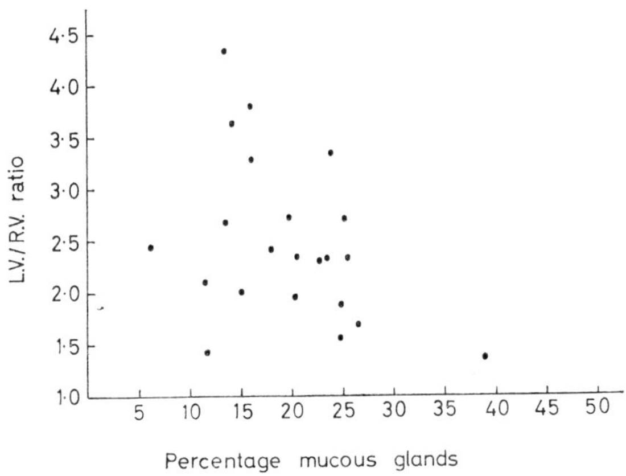

FIG 5. The ratio of the left ventricular weight to the right ventricular weight plotted against the percentage mucous gland content of the bronchial wall.

may not be a simple one but the work of Mitchell *et al.* (1966) has established that the clinical manifestations of severe mucous gland hyperplasia are hypoxia, pulmonary hypertension and right heart failure.

Emphysema

In measuring the changes in the lung parenchyma both macroscopic and microscopic analysis are needed. It is important to assess (1) the volume and distribution of diseased tissue, (2) the number of normal alveoli, (3) the alveolar surface area, and, although this will not be dealt with here, (4) the size and distribution of the pulmonary blood vessels.

On the gross specimen of fixed lung it is possible to measure the volume of emphysematous tissue using the point counting method

(Dunnill, 1962 *b* ; Anderson & Dunnill, 1965). This is best performed in lungs fixed by the formol steam method but can be carried out on lungs fixed with liquid formalin. It has been known for some time that there is no direct relationship between the volume of

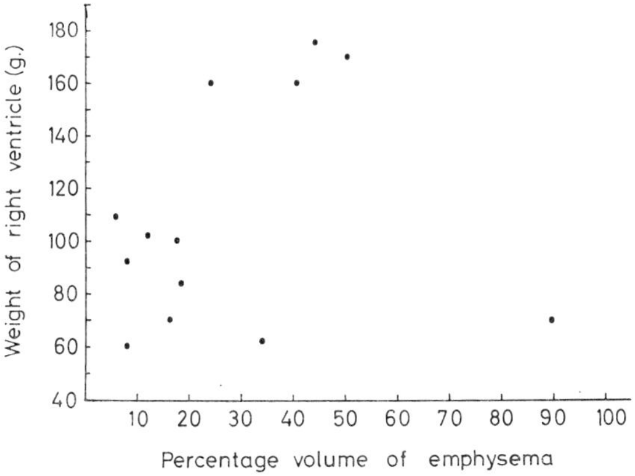

FIG. 6. Illustrating that there is no simple relationship between the weight of the right ventricle and the percentage volume of emphysema.

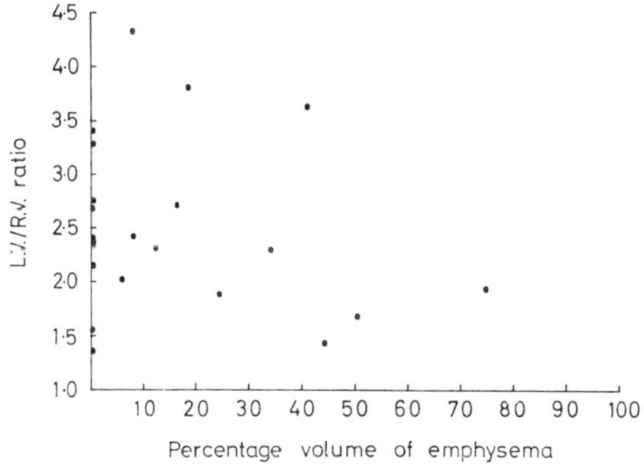

FIG. 7. Illustrating that the ratio of the left ventricular weight to the right ventricular weight is not directly related to the percentage volume of emphysema.

emphysematous tissue and clinical findings or between the volume of emphysematous tissue and right ventricular hypertrophy (Cromie, 1961 ; Dunnill, 1961). This is shown in Figures 6 and 7. It is apparent that any attempt to elucidate relationships must take into account the other factors involved and in particular the changes in the bronchi. However, in the lung parenchyma merely measuring the volume of diseased tissue will not suffice and some measure of its distribution is needed. For this reason the point counting method has been modified in an attempt to assess the distribution of disease in a quantitative manner. A coordinate grid has been used with the points placed 1 cm. apart. The grid is drawn on transparent plastic material and is placed on slices of fixed lung which are 1 cm. thick. Thus in effect this is a three dimensional grid with points placed at the corners of cubes of side 1 cm. The position of each point, that is, its coordinates, and whether it lies in normal lung parenchyma, conducting tissue or emphysematous tissue is noted. From the practical standpoint, considerable care has to be taken in orientating the slices. Two fixed points are obtained for each slice by passing parallel markers, placed in a plane at right angles to the plane in which the slices are cut, through the fixed lung before it is sliced. It is hoped that the type of information obtained by this method, which can be readily analysed by a computer, may eventually be of more value in the assessment of disease than expressing the results in terms of the anatomical form of emphysema.

It is possible, by means of careful sampling techniques in emphysematous lungs (Dunnill, 1964) to obtain values for the number of alveoli (Weibel & Gomez, 1962) and the area of the air-tissue interface (Campbell & Tomkeieff, 1952). The volume proportions of the alveoli, ducts, emphysematous spaces, tissue and vessels can be estimated using the point counting technique on histological sections. Emphysematous lungs assessed in this way fall into fairly well-defined groups corresponding to the recognised anatomical types of the disease, though frequently there is some mixing of the anatomical varieties.

Table 3. *Bullous disease of the lung*

Case number	1	2	3
Volume proportions of normal parenchyma :			
Alveolar air	66·3	62·6	60·8
Duct air	22·1	25·2	27·5
Tissue	9·9	10·2	9·5
Vessels	1·7	2·0	2·2
Number of alveoli (10^6)	280	296	284

The data on Cases 1 and 2 were given in a previous paper (Dunnill, 1965)

Bullous disease of the lung. Various varieties of this condition have been described by Reid (1967) but the cases referred to here are those in which the bullae are situated in the subpleural regions and the underlying lung parenchyma is essentially normal. In life the normal parenchyma is compressed by the bullae, which act to a large extent as space occupying lesions. When fixed by the formalin steam method the parenchyma can expand to its normal volume. If it is then sampled and analysed the volume proportions of the alveoli, ducts, tissue and vessels are found to be normal and in addition the number of alveoli are within normal limits (Table 3).

Centrilobular emphysema. In this condition, first described by Leopold and Gough in 1957, and referred to by Reid (1966) as centri-acinar emphysema, the respiratory bronchioles are damaged in a selective manner. Presumably as a result of an inflammatory reaction, the walls of the respiratory bronchioles, together with a variable number of surrounding alveoli, are damaged or destroyed and dilated spaces form in the centre of the acinus. As between two and five acini make up the secondary lobule, the lesions also appear to be centrilobular and hence the semantic confusion. Clinically these cases may have relatively normal lung volumes, absent or minimal radiological changes of emphysema in the lungs, but quite often, though not invariably, they have right heart failure.

Pure cases of this disease have a characteristic morphometric pattern (Table 4). The volume of the lung is normal or only slightly raised. The volume of diseased tissue when measured on the gross fixed lung may be relatively small, often of the order of 20 per cent. The volume proportions of the parenchyma often differ little from those in the normal lung, apart from the intervention of the centrilobular space which may account for between 10 and 30 per cent. of the parenchymal volume. The number of alveoli is reduced, but not markedly so, and the surface area of the air-tissue interface shows only a moderate reduction, say to 60 sq. m.

There has been some argument as to whether this disease is of any significance and it has been suggested that it only gives rise to cor pulmonale when associated with chronic bronchitis. Chronic bronchitis undoubtedly can be a serious complicating factor but the disease can also cause cor pulmonale on its own. The case illustrated in Figure 2 had a right ventricular weight of 176 g. and a left ventricle weighing 250 g., which by any standards represents right ventricular hypertrophy. Death was due to cor pulmonale and yet the mucous gland content of the bronchial wall was only 11·7 per cent., which is a relatively low value and could not be classified as chronic bronchitis.

Table 4. *Centrilobular emphysema*

Case number	1	2	3	4	5	6	7	8
Total lung volume (ml.)	6340	6550	6760	7000	4825	6350	6390	9135
Volume proportions of parenchyma :								
Alveolar air	56·1	55·5	50·8	48·5	40·8	42·5	52·3	34·9
Duct air	24·1	17·6	18·4	16·9	15·3	14·8	18·2	12·8
Centrilobular space	11·6	14·4	18·6	22·9	30·5	30·2	16·4	41·0
Tissue	7·1	11·2	11·0	9·6	11·5	10·4	11·3	9·4
Vessels	1·1	1·3	1·2	2·1	1·9	2·1	1·8	1·9
Number of alveoli (10^6)	300	213	250	230	100	152	248	130
Area of air tissue interface (sq. cm.)	66	68	69	68	40	51	67	61

The strategic position of the centrilobular spaces, placed as they are in the transition zone between the conducting airways and the regions of gas exchange in the alveoli, must allow them to interfere with normal ventilation and play some part in causing hypoxia. Admittedly there is no straightforward relationship between the total volume of the emphysematous spaces and the weight of the right ventricle, but in this connection the distribution of the disease may be of paramount importance (Dunnill, 1965) and this is a problem for further investigations using the modified point counting technique described earlier.

Panacinar destructive emphysema. In this condition the entire acinus, and usually the entire secondary lobule, is involved in the disease with complete disorganisation of the normal architecture. The alveoli are replaced by air spaces of irregular size and shape. The condition is quite distinct from centrilobular emphysema, where a ring of normal alveolar tissue, often very small, surrounds the centrilobular space. These patients tend to have clinical chronic obstructive lung disease, are diagnosed as having emphysema radiologically and seldom have right ventricular hypertrophy.

On pathological examination the lung volume is much larger than in patients with centrilobular emphysema. Using the point counting method on the gross lung, it is found that the volume of the emphysematous tissue is frequently very large and may account for almost the entire volume of the lung parenchyma and this is confirmed in the histological analysis of the volume proportions. The number of alveoli is greatly reduced and frequently falls below 100.10^6. The surface area of the air-tissue inter-face per unit volume of lung is very greatly reduced but, due to the increase in the total lung volume, the total surface area may still be quite high and of the order of 45 sq. m. (Table 5).

Table 5. *Panacinar destructive emphysema*
(Mean values in 10 cases)

Lung volume (ml.)	8000
Volume proportions of parenchyma :	
Alveoli	31
Ducts	12
Abnormal spaces	47
Tissue	8
Vessels	2
Number of alveoli (10^6)	96
Mean linear intercept (10^{-2} cm.)	5·981
Area of air-tissue interface (sq. m.)	49 (61 sq. cm./ml.)

CONCLUSION

There is no easy answer to the morphological relationships between the heart, pulmonary blood vessels, bronchi and lung parenchyma in chronic non-specific lung disease. There is a very great need for careful collection of quantitative anatomical data which will enable multiple correlation techniques to be employed. Many cases of emphysema are of mixed anatomical types and so the intensive study of pure cases, particularly if they have been the subject of cardiopulmonary investigation during life, is likely to be of great value in elucidating the role of individual lesions in the disease process. Nevertheless, it must be borne in mind that we may have concentrated too much in the past on the anatomical minutiae of whether any given case represented a variety of centrilobular, panacinar, paraseptal, cicatricial or some other form of emphysema. Instead perhaps more fruitful results might be obtained if we studied the size and distribution of abnormal air spaces in the lung together with the quantitiative changes in the bronchi, blood vessels and heart.

SUMMARY

A brief outline is given of the quantitative anatomy of the normal lung. It is emphasised that the shape and dimensions of the structures in the lung parenchyma are not static but change with the respiratory cycle and with posture.

The problem of the diagnosis of chronic bronchitis has been discussed and reasons are given for preferring the point counting to other methods for assessing the mucous gland content of the bronchi. There appears to be no direct simple relationship between the mucous gland content of the bronchi and the volume of emphysema in the lung, or the degree of right ventricular hypertrophy.

A method for estimating the volume and distribution of the abnormal air spaces in the lungs has been briefly described. The main morphometric features of bullous disease of the lung, centrilobular emphysema and panacinar emphysema are given.

Finally it is suggested that, although exhaustive studies of pure cases of the various anatomical types of emphysema are of value, concentration on the measurement of the size and distribution of abnormal air spaces in the lung, together with assessment of the quantitative changes in the bronchi, blood vessels and heart may yield equally, or even more useful results.

DISCUSSION OF SESSION ONE

Dr Fletcher. Professor Heppleston, destruction and disruption seem to be very similar terms ; the difference between the two was not quite clear.

Professor Heppleston. I use the term ' disruption ' to mean actual breach of continuity in the walls of respiratory bronchioles or alveoli. I suggest that the term ' destruction ' should be avoided because it has a dual meaning, which includes not only disruption but also atrophy, a degree of destruction short of breach in continuity.

Dr Mead. You spoke of the muscle being important in the elastic recoil. I wondered what was the basis for that view.

Professor Heppleston. I took human tracheas and tested their extensibility before and after dissecting off the mucous membrane containing the elastic network. The mucous membrane with the elastic tissue was little if at all extensible and did not recoil, whereas the trachea retracted equally before and after removal of the mucosa. This suggested that elastic tissue might not be of major importance in pulmonary recoil and that some other element may be involved.

Dr Mead. How does this relate to the recoil of the parenchyma of the lung and the influence of smooth muscle on this ?

Professor Heppleston. The ' geodesic ' disposition of the muscle of bronchioles and small bronchi implies that on muscular contraction the airways will be narrowed and shortened. At the same time the associated alveoli will be reduced in volume and their orifices onto respiratory bronchioles and alveolar ducts diminished.

Dr Mead. What is the evidence that it actually functions in this way ?

Professor Heppleston. I have always assumed that smooth muscle, wherever it is found, exercises a contractile tone. Because of its anatomical distribution the effect on the bronchiolar tree would be to narrow and shorten it, an action which Nadel's physiological studies support.

Dr Mead. Would that influence the overall elastic recoil of the parenchyma ?

Professor Heppleton. The smooth muscle extends to the distal end of alveolar ducts.

Dr Macklem. We have some evidence on that. If by pharmacologic means you alter the smooth muscles in the living lung, by and large, you do precious little to its static pressure/volume characteristics. You can give atropine and create a change in airways resistance and produce no measurable change in static recoil. I think that

Nadel *et al.*, (1964) were the first to show that when you constrict the smooth muscle at the alveolar duct and respiratory bronchiole level you do indeed get an increase in elastic recoil, but if you dilate the smooth muscle as much as possible, either by excising the lung and therefore taking all nervous influence away, or by giving any form of bronchodilator, there is no loss of elastic recoil. The static pressure/volume characteristics remain the same.

Professor Heppleston. The experimental evidence to which Dr Macklem refers indicates that contraction of smooth muscle at the respiratory bronchiole—alveolar duct level is concerned in pulmonary recoil, from which it may be deduced that recoil will be adversely affected if smooth muscle is deficient. If in man the muscle of smaller bronchi and conducting bronchioles is deficient, as well as that of respiratory bronchioles and alveolar ducts, recoil may be so impaired as to increase the functional residual capacity and lead to the architectural state of acinar emphysema. Under such conditions the pharmacological response of animals to smooth muscle dilators may not be relevant.

Dr Strang. I think I understood Dr Mead to say that he didn't think any part of the muscle in the lung could affect the compliance. Yet claims have been made that certain kinds of bronchoconstrictor agents will in fact reduce the volume of the lung.

Dr Mead. I was thinking principally of the influence of decreased smooth muscle tone and the striking fact that when you produce such changes you can't, in normal individuals, show any change in static recoil.

Dr Macklem. Dr Woolcock and I have been giving propranolol to block the adrenergic fibres in dogs and found that there was a constriction of the peripheral airways and an increase in the elastic recoil properties of the lung. We gave propranolol to two human subjects and also found small changes in the elastic recoil properties of the lung with an increase in airway resistance. I don't know where the increase was, but I presume it was in the small airways.

Chairman. Did you find it aggravated asthma ?

Dr Mead. As regards asthma, there's some experimental evidence that during attacks, patients with asthma may actually have, not an increased tendency for the lung to recoil at a given lung volume such as one might expect, but a decreased tendency, and this is in the opposite direction from the changes just spoken of. This is an influence of smooth muscle on elastic retraction and a very mystifying one.

Chairman. How does one separate the effect of increased tone of muscle fibres from oedema or stiffening of tissues due to altered capillary permeability, or even to the forming of a layer of mucus on the internal surface?

Dr Macklem. Well, it's very difficult to do that, although the time relationships may help. In the experiments we have done on vagal stimulation, in a matter of 2 or 3 seconds you get an increase in resistance of the peripheral airways and changes in the elastic recoil properties, which disappear immediately when you take off the stimulus.

Dr Heath. Professor Heppleston, in his paper this morning, made it apparent that he believes that focal and centrilobular emphysema are two very distinct variants of the disease. He believes, moreover, that the centrilobular form is associated with chronic bronchiolitis. On the other hand, Dr Lynne Reid in a recent report is quoted as saying that symptomless centriacinar emphysema is present in 50 to 60 per cent. of people who die from non-respiratory disease. It could be thought of as a normal anatomical variant. Moreover, in her recently published book (Reid, 1967) she has a chapter labelled ' Centriacinar Emphysema ' and in brackets beneath, ' Synonymous with Centrilobular or Focal Emphysema '. So clearly she thinks that centrilobular and focal emphysema are the same thing and can best be termed Centriacinar. Would you care to comment on that, Professor Heppleston?

Professor Heppleston. In considering the distinction between focal and centrilobular emphysema, as well as the occurrence of asymptomatic centrilobular emphysema in the non-industrial population, I think the main source of confusion lies in the incidental association of dust pigmentation. In the normal urban population focal dust pigmentation is frequent and a proportion of such people show mild dilation of the respiratory bronchioles in every way comparable to the early lesions of coalworkers. Early centrilobular emphysema, with the characteristic microanatomy, may also be an incidental finding and some pigment may occur irregularly in the fibrosed bronchioles and at the margin of the emphysematous spaces, but the disposition of the dust is not that associated with focal emphysema. If serial section studies are made of the early and the more developed lesions, then there is an anatomical as well as a histological distinction between focal and centrilobular emphysema, as Dr Leopold and I found. The term centriacinar obscures this difference.

Dr Heath. Dr Brewer and I have been using a method of inflating and fixing lungs by formalin steam and I must say that, during the past 4 years using this technique, we have had almost insuperable difficulty in distinguishing centrilobular and focal emphysema.

Professor Heppleston. I appreciate the difficulty of doing this solely on gross appearances or on random histological sections, but the distinction can be made by three-dimensional studies.

Dr Reid. In the figures Dr Heath has attributed to me, I was quoting the work of Snyder and Brodie at Chicago (Snyder *et al.*, 1962) who used dried lungs and reported an incidence of centrilobular emphysema of between 50 and 60 per cent. in patients who had come to autopsy having had, so far as was known, no lung disease, no lung symptoms and normal X-ray. We do not find such a high figure as that ; we find it somewhere between 10 and 15 per cent. When we come to consider centrilobular and focal emphysema, I would agree with Dr Heath about the difficulty in distinguishing these two. However, I feel we should be careful to use these terms simply as a convenient form of morbid anatomical shorthand. They are a good way to describe the lesions you are looking at ; I don't think we should use them, as it were, to interpret what we think the disease is. For this reason, I use the term centriacinar as synomymous with centrilobular or focal ; both of these are centriacinar rather than peri- or panacinar lesions.

It is possible to distinguish two types on the grounds of their being either atrophic, when the original architecture remains intact, or destructive, where there is an interruption of lung substance. Each of these should be further sub-divided as to whether or not there is pigment present. In parenthesis may I say that I recognise four mechanisms producing large air spaces : hypoplasia, atrophy, over-inflation or destruction. I think the only way I can pick up centriacinar destruction on macroscopic examination of the cut surface of lung, is by whether or not there is an empty hole. In the atrophic form, one can pick up thin strands of lung through the ' hole ' even in section. Once there is a real ulceration with retraction of surrounding lung you pick up holes in the lung of maybe half of three-quarters of a centimetre with an absolutely flattened wall. I think it is desirable that in the first place we should try to recognise the different anatomical types by naked eye examination. Certainly, at the level at which we want to examine lung in relation to disease, the naked eye examination is still satisfactory.

Dr Leopold. May I make one comment on this ? I've had the advantage of working in two very different communities. First, in Cardiff where the air pollution has been small ; nevertheless, I have seen the lungs of persons living in that atmosphere which show mild degrees of focal emphysema and, of course, centrilobular emphysema too. I also worked for a while in Leeds where even the ordinary person's lung is dirty and focal emphysema is, therefore, not uncommon. I agree the amount of carbon material in the lungs makes a considerable difference to the ease with which one can distinguish centrilobular and focal emphysema without resorting to histological methods of examination.

Dr Fletcher. I should like to comment on Snyder's study. I think it was an excellent one but there is a great danger of assuming that people who have no history of respiratory disease according to their case-notes, have no respiratory abnormalities. When you go out into the population and start measuring ventilatory capacity on large numbers of people, you find people with gross impairment of function but absolutely no symptoms. We need, somehow or other, to obtain autopsies on a large number of people who have had adequate physiological studies done during life. We did attempt to do it by trying to get measurements of ventilatory capacity on patients with fatal disease, such as carcinoma of the stomach, or leukaemia. We found after a short study that at Hammersmith nearly all such patients had grossly abnormal ventilatory function. It seems very difficult to find people who you know are going to die who really have normal lungs.

The other point I'd like to make is that if focal emphysema and centrilobular emphysema are different and focal emphysema is induced by dust, in a mining population there should be a gross excess of total emphysema. If you could get some sort of random sample, *e.g.* from accident cases, and if centrilobular emphysema is a normal variant, then they would have the normal amount of centrilobular emphysema and, added to that, they'd have their focal emphysema, so there should be a gross excess. This might be one way of approaching the problem.

Dr Thurlbeck. With reference to Dr Dunnill's paper, as I understand it, the point count method of assessing emphysema doesn't correlate with right ventricular hypertrophy, doesn't correlate with the point count of mucous glands and the point count of mucous glands doesn't correlate with right ventricular hypertrophy either. I must also point out one other lack of correlation which he has reported (Dunnill, 1965) ; that's between surface area and the point count method.

There are some real difficulties with the point count method of measuring emphysema and I should like to draw attention to some of them. To begin with, the point count method of measuring emphysema is a subjective method. The mere fact that one is now counting points rather than assessing the whole lung doesn't make it an objective method. Every time you look at a point you are making a subjective judgment as to whether emphysema is present or not. The next point—the crux of the matter with the point count—is that the two common types of emphysema, centrilobular emphysema (CLE) and panlobular emphysema (PLE), affect the measurements entirely differently. CLE affects a small portion of the lobule, PLE involves the whole of it. So PLE gives you big numbers, and CLE small ones. Furthermore, the point count does not distinguish between mild and severe PLE, in so far as both mild and severe PLE involve 100 per cent. of the lobule. My final point is that, at least in our hands, the method maximises inter-observer error. This is because the mild grade of PLE is extremely difficult to recognise with precision. The point count method gives a high number for PLE if you recognise mild grade PLE. If you disregard this, you get zero. So you may get variations from a hundred to nothing from the same lung looked at by different observers.

Dr West. I'd like to refer to a further source of error in some of these morphometric techniques. We now have considerable evidence that the shape of the lung changes when it is reinflated outside the chest. This means that in order to obtain valid measurements of alveolar size, it is necessary to fix the lung *in situ.* Dr Glazier and his colleagues (1966) in our laboratories have accomplished this by freezing anaesthetized dogs intact and then removing pieces of lung at various levels. This work is referred to in my formal paper where it can be seen that the alveoli at the apex of the vertical (head up) lung may be four times larger than the alveoli at the base, which is the most dependent part. The smallest alveoli were always found in the most dependent parts of the lung. The reason for these differences in alveolar size is apparently to do with the way the lung is supported inside the chest. It follows that measurements of alveolar size made on lungs inflated outside the chest will not give a true picture of the state of the lungs *in situ.*

Dr Dunnill. I think this is very important and indicates that any sampling for histology must be very carefully considered. I'd very much like to repeat Dr West's experiment on a human, if only it were possible !

Dr Cumming. We were very impressed with the importance of finding out whether, in the human, this alveolar size gradient occurs or not. We considered various ways of freezing humans intact, and rejected all of them for the obvious reasons, but we did come up with a possible alternative. We were able to construct, in life, a model of the visceral pleura to the right dimensions and the right shape using X-rays in various projections and measuring the curvature of the chest. This model was formed from transparent plastic, and its volume was the volume of the FRC plus the lung tissue. We then took the lungs from a man who died of gastric carcinoma and had relatively normal lungs, and blew them up by external pressure until they just filled this box nicely, fixing one lung in the vertical position with the apex upwards and the other lung we fixed upside down and put the apex downwards. We fixed them with the gaseous technique advocated by Weibel and Vidone (1961) and we came out with the result that the alveolar size was uniform throughout no matter which way the lungs were fixed. This in no way denies what Dr West says, but does raise a very important point about the validity of the method of fixation. This is steam and formalin—a gaseous technique where gas density exerts almost no distending force. If you consider for a moment what happens if one blows steam into a lung from an autopsy specimen at 20° C—for the first few minutes the steam will condense and fix the alveoli with liquid. This is then a liquid fixation technique and under these conditions one expects to find the alveoli the same size and I think that is perhaps the explanation.

A Questioner. Could I ask Dr Dunnill what his upper limits of normal are for right and left ventricular hypertrophy ?

Dr Dunnill. There isn't any easy answer to this because insufficient cases taken from the population as a whole—accident cases and so on—have been analysed. My definition of right ventricular hypertrophy is based on a ratio of the weight of the left ventricle to the weight of the right. The normal range, given by Fulton (1953), is 2·3 to 3·3 and below that is right ventricular hypertrophy. The actual isolated weight of the right ventricle is a more debatable thing but personally I think about 70 G would be thought a normal value and for the left ventricle, about 200 G.

Dr Bates. I'd like to ask Professor Heppleston whether he's done serial sections across and down the typical small lesion of early centrilobular emphysema, and if he can tell me how the ventilation of the alveoli around that area of destruction is in fact achieved.

Professor Heppleston. The centrilobular lesion represents respiratory bronchioles that have been disrupted and that have fused together to form a communal space ; from such lesions, or many of them, substantially normal alveolar ducts proceed into the alveolar sacs.

Dr Bates. And the alveoli around the hole are essentially normal ?

Professor Heppleston. They appear so.

Dr Cumming. My paper includes an illustration (Fig. 2) which helps to make this point. It shows a three-dimensional cast of a terminal ventilatory unit containing a centrilobular space. The terminal bronchiole can be seen entering a large, smooth, dilated space with four exit holes from which emerge four branches of third order respiratory bronchioles. You can see the fairly normal-looking alveolar sacs and ducts coming off this space. It's rather like an in-series dead space.

Dr Leopold. The picture is one which I can easily understand, having examined such material by serial section techniques. I think it should be said that some alveolar ducts and sacs that emerge from the central spaces are not in very direct connection with the space ; they may be folded back, lying at an angle instead of lying radially, in which circumstance, one could imagine the point of communication being one of impeded flow.

Dr Filley. May I raise an objection to the use of the unmodified word ' flow '? This word has very important implications, of course, and represents one reason why this conference was held. We have been asked to try and make sense of Structure and Function and Dr Bates has put his finger on an important issue in this regard. To start with, it was a bit unfair of Dr Bates to ask Professor Heppleston how a lung unit is ventilated, because this is a physiological not a pathological question. Secondly, there are all kinds of implications in the word ' ventilation '. This is probably not the time to define them, but rather to call attention to the fact that it is easy to use such a word as ' flow ' too loosely. The question really should be not so much : how does the air flow into an air space ? but ultimately : how do gas molecules traverse this space ?

Professor Stuart-Harris. May I continue with this same issue by asking our pathologist colleagues if they have anything to offer us on the subject of obstruction to the airways ? I've never been entirely convinced by what they have to show us as the morbid anatomical equivalents to physiological changes. However, Dr Reid does use this question of the presence or absence of airways obstruction in her classification of emphysema so perhaps it's not entirely irrelevant to ask her how she does it.

Dr Reid. The most helpful approach to this problem at the moment is to take, as far as possible, individual patients of whom we can say : here we have as pure a lesion as it's possible to get, taking patients who die from the fatal complications of chronic bronchitis, or obstructive airways disease if you prefer, without any emphysema at all. Similarly, we want to gather together subjects in whom we find a given type of emphysema present without the complicating addition of chronic bronchitis. It's for this reason that, as Dr Fletcher has mentioned, we haven't got a satisfactory group of what I would call simple centriacinar lesions because mostly these patients don't die from this condition. We have to get them by going to post-mortems where there has been no suspicion of lung disease.

When we come, however, to the question of the aged lung, we can say that the typical finding is a panacinar emphysema. The individual holes are a millimetre or two in diameter and we know in these patients what the pattern of disturbed respiration can or may be. Then we turn to patients who have so-called primary emphysema and who come to post-mortem. These are the patients whom we know had no cough or sputum in life. In these patients we find a severe panacinar emphysema and it is in this group that I feel we can say : here are patients whom we know had airways obstruction in life but we know from anatomical examination they had no mucous gland hypertrophy and they have no goblet cell increase in the small airways. They have no peribronchiolar fibrosis, a decent airway right to the periphery, yet here we have evidence of airways obstruction during life. Presumably this is secondary to the atrophic changes in the peripheral parts of the lung and exemplifies the effect of the ' weakened spring ' as illustrated by Daymar (1951). This, then, is the main basis of our classification.

Finally, if we turn to the patient who has chronic bronchitis, we may find some anatomical traces of emphysema which in the first place we've got to regard as coincident with the bronchitis. Later we may consider those types that are caused by it. I put centriacinar emphysema into the benign group, but what I do not know is whether, in a patient with bronchitis and airways obstruction, this particular anatomical lesion contributes to his disability.

Dr Filley. Dr Reid, you mentioned that some emphysema is incidental to bronchitis and some is caused by it. Could you elaborate on that ?

Dr Reid. In the aged lung, for example, one commonly sees panacinar emphysema which is widespread throughout the lung. Many of our patients who have bronchitis die over the age of sixty and we will therefore expect to find a certain amount of panacinar emphysema of grade 2 type. I would regard this as being a coincident thing. I would regard many centriacinar lesions in the same light because we know they can occur in patients who haven't got chronic bronchitis : we know they can occur in people who have been down mines and those who haven't and therefore we may expect to find them coincident with the changes, structural and functional, of bronchitis.

Dr Filley. But then, on the other hand, is some emphysema caused by bronchitis ?

Dr Reid. An example of this is the ' obstruction ' emphysema caused by infective damage at the lung periphery seen not infrequently in these patients. Here one has evidence of the mechanism in the presence of micro-abscesses, to account for the irregular ulceration at the periphery. This type does not usually observe the anatomical niceties of the acinus.

Dr Fletcher. You are saying then, that damaged bronchi cause emphysema, therefore bronchitis causes emphysema. Could not the emphysema be encouraging the bronchitis ? Or could not the fact that a man has smoked cigarettes be encouraging both ? I think it's very important not to assume that association implies causation.

Dr Reid. These things also happen but I think the evidence is strong that as part of the infection in bronchioli, the alveoli may also be damaged, producing emphysema.

Dr Fletcher. And not the other way around ? You don't think emphysema can encourage infection ?

Dr Reid. I wouldn't say there is any evidence, really, for that view.

Professor Heppleston. I would agree with that interpretation. There are cases showing an active, and sometimes severe, chronic inflammation of the bronchioles with extension into the alveolar parenchyma which is undergoing disruption. In other areas of the same lungs the process has advanced to the state of fine scarring with disruptive emphysema of an irregular variety.

REFERENCES

AMERICAN THORACIC SOCIETY (1962). *Am. Rev. resp. Dis.* **85,** 762.

ANDERSON, J. A. & DUNNILL, M. S. (1965). *Thorax*, **20,** 462.

BALL, W. C., STEWART, P. B., NEWSHAM, L. G. S. & BATES, D. V. (1962). *J. clin. Invest.* **41,** 519.

CAMPBELL, H. & TOMKEIEFF, S. I. (1952). *Nature* (Lond.), **170,** 117.

CIBA SYMPOSIUM (1959). *Thorax*, **14,** 286.

CROMIE, J. B. (1961). *Amer. Rev. resp. Dis.* **84,** 657.

DAYMAN, H. (1951). *J. clin. Invest.* **30,** 1175.

DAYMAN, H. (1956). In *Pulmonary Emphysema*, p. 251, Ed. BARACH, A. L. & BICKERMAN, H. A. Baltimore: Williams and Wilkins.

DOCK, W. (1946). *Am. Rev. Tuberc. pulm. Dis.* **53,** 297.

DOCK, W. (1954). *Archs. intern. Med.* **94,** 700.

DUGUID, J. B., YOUNG, A., CAUNA, DZIDRA & LAMBERT, MARGARET (1964). *J. Path. Bact.* **88,** 405.

DUNNILL, M. S. (1961). *J. Clin. Path.* **14,** 246.

DUNNILL, M. S. (1962 *a*). *Thorax*, **17,** 329.

DUNNILL, M. S. (1962 *b*). *Thorax*, **17,** 320.

DUNNILL, M. S. (1964). *Thorax*, **19,** 443.

DUNNILL, M. S. (1965). *Med. thorac.* **22,** 261.

DUNNILL, M. S. (1967). *Nature* (Lond.). In press.

DUNNILL, M. S., ANDERSON, J. A. & WHITEHEAD, R. (1967). *J. path. Bact.* In press.

FULTON, R. M. (1953). *J. Med.* **22,** 43.

GLAZIER, J. B., HUGHES, J. M. B., MALONEY, J. E., PAIN, M. C. F. & WEST, J. B. (1966). *Lancet*, **2,** 203.

HALES, STEPHEN (1731). In *Vegetable Staticks: Analysis of Air.* p. 240. London

HARTUNG, W. (1960). *Zentbl. allg. Path. path. Anat.* **100,** 408.

HARTUNG, W. (1962). *Am. Rev. resp. Dis.* **85,** 287.

HARTUNG, W. (1963). *Ergeben. allg. Path. path. Anat.* **43,** 121.
HARTUNG, W. (1964). *Fortschr. Med.* **82,** 183.
HARTUNG, W. & EINBRODT, H. J. (1965). *Beitr. Silikosforsch. Sonderland* **6,** 379.
HEARD, B. E. (1960). *Am. Rev. resp. Dis.* **82,** 792.
HENNIG, A. (1958). *Zeiss-Werkz.* **6,** 78.
HENTEL, W., LONGFIELD, A. N., VINCENT, T. N., FILLEY, G. F. & MITCHELL R. S. (1963). *Rev. resp. Dis.* **87,** 216.
HEPPLESTON, A. G. (1947). *J. Path. Bact.* **59,** 453.
HEPPLESTON, A. G. (1953). *J. Path. Bact.* **66,** 235.
HEPPLESTON, A. G. (1954). *J. Path. Bact.* **67,** 51.
HEPPLESTON, A. G. (1955). *Lab. Invest.* **4,** 374.
HEPPLESTON, A. G. (1956). *Thorax,* **11,** 77.
HEPPLESTON, A. G. & LEOPOLD, J. G. (1961). *Am. J. Med.* **31,** 279.
HICKEN, P., BREWER, D. B., & HEATH, D. A. (1966). *J. Path. Bact.* **92,** 529.
KOURILSKY, R., DECROIX, G., VERLEY, J. M., MATOSSY, Y., HINGLAIS, J. C., PIERON, R. & BRILLE, D. (1960). *Bronches,* **10,** 76.
LAENNEC, R. T. H. (1819). In *De L'Auscultation Médiate,* vol. 1, p. 210. Paris : Brosson et Chaudé.
LAMBERT, MARGARET W. (1955). *J. Path. Bact.* **70,** 311.
LEOPOLD, J. G. & GOUGH, J. (1957). *Thorax,* **12,** 219.
LEOPOLD, J. G. & GOUGH, J. (1963). *Thorax,* **18,** 172.
MCGRAITH, M. W. & THOMSON, M. L. (1959). *J. Physiol.* (*Lond.*), **146,** 572.
MACKLIN, C. C. (1929). *Physiol. Rev.* **9,** 1.
MARSHALL, A. G. (1961). *J. clin. Path.* **14,** 578.
MILLARD, F. J. C. & REID, L. MCA. (1967). *Communication to the Thoracic Society.*
MITCHELL, R. S., RYAN, S. F., PETTY, T. L. & FILLEY, G. F. (1966). *Am. Rev. resp. Dis.* **93,** 720.
NADEL, J. A., COLEBATCH, H. J. H. & OLSEN, C. R. (1964). *J. appl. Physiol.* **19,** 387.
PIERCE, J. A. & EBERT, R. V. (1958). *Am. J. Med.* **25,** 13.
PIERCE, J. A. & EBERT, R. V. (1965). *Thorax,* **20,** 469.
PRATT, P. C., HAQUE, M. A. & KLUGH, G. A. (1961). *Am. Rev. resp. Dis.* **83,** 856.
PRATT, P. C., HAQUE, M. A. & KLUGH, G. A. (1962). *Lab. Invest.* **11,** 177.
REID, L. MCA. (1960). *Thorax,* **16,** 132.
REID, L. MCA. (1966). *Br. J. Dis. Chest.* **60,** 57.
REID, L. MCA. (1967). *The Pathology of Emphysema.* London : Lloyd Luke.
RESTREPO, G. & HEARD, B. E. (1963 *a*). *J. Path. Bact.* **85,** 305.
RESTREPO, G. & HEARD, B. E. (1963 *b*). *Thorax,* **18,** 334.
SIMON, G. (1964). *Clin. Radiol.* **15,** 293.
SNYDER, G. L., BRODY, J. S. & DOCTOR, L. (1962). *Am. Rev. resp. Dis.* **85,** 666.
STOREY, W. F. & STAUB, N. C. (1962). *J. appl. Physiol.* **17,** 391.
TENNEY, S. M. & REMMERS, J. E. (1963). *Nature* (Lond.), **197,** 54.
THURLBECK, W. M. (1963). *Thorax,* **18,** 59.
THURLBECK, W. M. & ANGUS, G. E. (1963). *Am. Rev. resp. Dis.* **87,** 815.
THURLBECK, W. M. & ANGUS, G. E. (1964). *Thorax,* **19,** 436.
WEIBEL, E. R. (1963). In *Morphometry of the Human Lung.* Berlin : Springer.
WEIBEL, E. R. & GOMEZ, D. M. (1962). *J. appl. Physiol.* **17,** 343.
WEIBEL, E. R. & VIDONE, R. A. (1961). *Am. Rev. resp. Dis.* **84,** 856.
WEST, J. B. & DOLLERY, C. T. (1960). *J. appl. Physiol.* **15,** 405.
WILLIAMS, D. A. & LEOPOLD, J. G. (1959). *Acta Allerg.* **14,** 83.

SESSION TWO

THE FACTORS DETERMINING GAS CONCENTRATIONS IN THE ALVEOLI AND THE ROLE OF REGIONAL AND STRATIFIED INHOMOGENEITY

Chairman W. MELVILLE ARNOTT

A MODEL OF LUNG ELASTICITY AND SOME OF ITS IMPLICATIONS

JERE MEAD

THE work I am going to describe has been done jointly with Dr T. Takishima and Dr David Leith from our Department.

Let me start out by saying that I know absolutely nothing about emphysema. That, at least, puts us on common ground. Let me also point out that all of my remarks, unless I qualify them, will have to do with static circumstances, that is, when no flow is taking place. I am going to talk about a model of lung elasticity. Morphologists have been very kind to physiologists for years in permitting them to deal with the lung in a very over-simplified way. For example, we have been able to get away with saying that all of the air spaces within the lung are subjected to the pressure difference from the airway to the pleural surface, as if pleural pressure somehow invaded the substance of the lung and surrounded the air spaces. But it is clear that the inside of one alveolus is really the outside of the next. To speak of an alveolus as being exposed to a pressure difference is certainly naive. The classical model, which assumes that all air spaces are subjected to transplumonary pressure, has been a very useful one, nevertheless. It has led to some very important information about the lung, concerning the distribution of ventilation, the stability of air spaces, the effects of gravity and the distribution of alveolar size. The classical model works pretty well, in short.

I would like to develop a different model. It behaves, in certain circumstances, like the classical one, and this may explain the latter's success—but at the same time, it behaves in a very different way in other circumstances, which I shall also develop. This model is based on an analysis of the balance of forces at walls within lungs. You pick a wall—any wall—and write down as best you can the balance of forces applied to it, and then see where this takes you.

Figure 1A shows such a wall. First of all, we need a convention for ' inside ' and ' outside ', and this is indicated. We also need to distinguish the direction of movement. We shall take outward motion as being in the plus direction and vice versa. The various sorts of forces applied to the wall are illustrated in Figures 1B, 1C, and 1D. First of all, any gas (or fluid) at the wall surfaces exerts pressure. Second, any tissue attachments exert forces with components at right angles to the wall. Finally, tension in the wall itself if the wall is curved, tend to displace it.

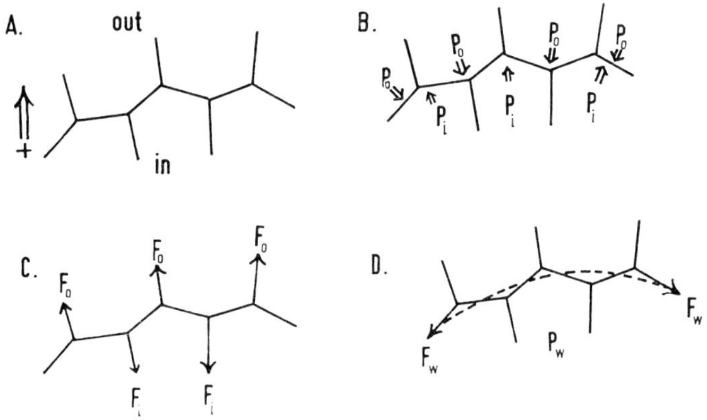

FIGS. 1A, 1B, 1C, 1D.

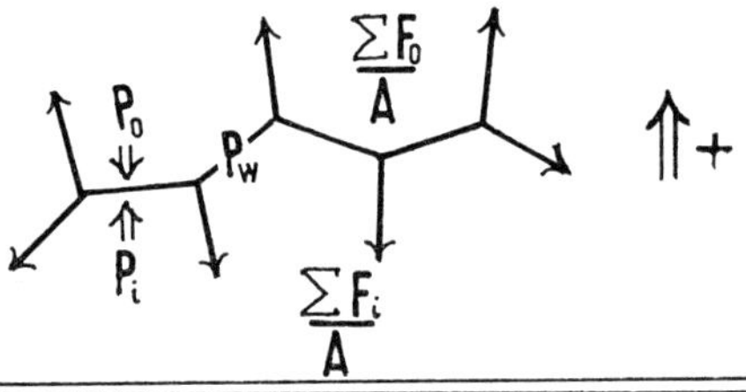

$$P_i - P_o + \frac{\Sigma F_o}{A} - \frac{\Sigma F_i}{A} - P_w = 0$$

FIG. 2

Now let us try to write an equation for the balance of forces operating at this wall, including all three sorts. First, we want to put the terms in the same dimensions. We have chosen to express everything in terms of pressure. To express the tissue forces operating at right angles to the wall in terms of pressure, we have summed them and distributed them on the area of that surface, so that they have the units of pressure. Similarly, we have expressed the tension in the wall in terms of the pressure differences that these tensions would produce. Under static conditions, these forces must be in equilibrium—that is, they must add up to zero, as shown in Figure 2. Each term has a sign which depends on its direction of action.

For example, any gas pressures outside tend to move the wall inward and are negative in sign, whereas tissues under tension attached to the outside tend to move the wall outward, and are positive in sign.

Next, we apply this equation to some specific ' walls ' in lungs. First of all, the wall at the pleural surface. The pressure outside is pleural pressure. The pressure inside is alveolar pressure. The pressure difference then is simply the pressure difference across the lung, or what we refer to as the static recoil pressure of the lung. There are no outward-acting tissue forces, so that term drops out. There are inward-acting forces. The gentle curvature of the major part of the pleural surface is such that you would expect, for the sorts of forces that develop within such a wall, that the pressure drop related to this curvature would be extremely small. I have chosen to say that it is approximately zero once we get out to a radius of curvature as big as this—some 500 times that of the alveoli. So this expression simplifies to the one shown in Figure 3. The static

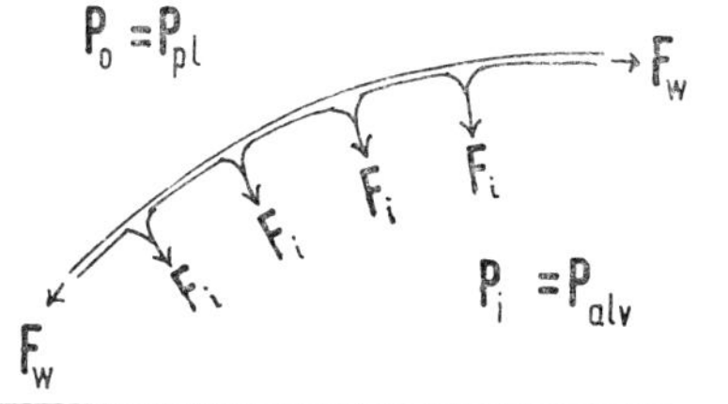

$$P_i - P_o + \frac{\sum F_o}{A} - \frac{\sum F_i}{A} - (P_w) = 0, \quad P_w \approx 0$$

$$P_{alv.} - P_{pl} \approx \frac{\sum F_i}{A}$$

FIG. 3

recoil pressure seems to be equally opposed by the inward-acting tissue forces applied at the pleural surface. So much for the pleural surface.

Now let us advance to the innermost surface and apply the same sorts of considerations (Figure 4). At an innermost wall, which might be at an alveolar septum, we have alveolar pressure outside and alveolar pressure inside ; accordingly, the first two terms cancel and drop out. There are outward-acting forces, but there are no inward-acting tissue forces other than those in the wall itself. So the term for inward-acting tissue forces drops out. The radius of curvature is such that the wall tension must certainly contribute substantially, and this term stays in. We see that, at this innermost wall, the pressure related to wall tension (which includes that from surface as well as tissue forces) is equally opposed by the outward-acting pressure exerted by outward-acting tissue forces.

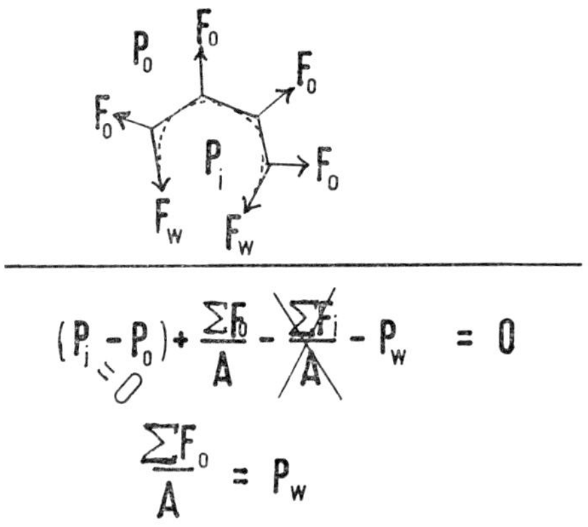

FIG. 4

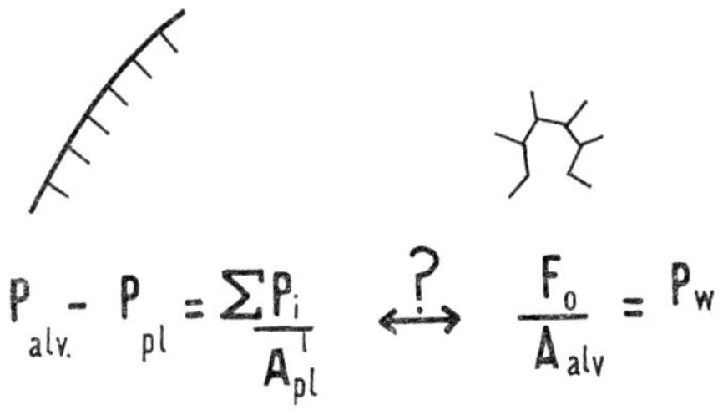

FIG. 5

Now let us see how the expressions at the outermost and innermost walls relate to one another (Fig. 5). At the outermost wall, the expanding force is simply transpulmonary pressure. At the innermost wall, the expanding force is totally supplied by tissue forces. To relate transpulmonary pressure to these tissue forces we need to know the relationship between the inward-acting tissue forces at the pleural surface and the outward-acting ones at the alveolar level. If they are the same, then we are, in effect, applying transpulmonary pressure at the alveolar level.

It is not unreasonable to think that in the normal lung the force per fibre or tissue structure, or whatever you will, might be on average much the same throughout the lung ; and that there might be, on the average, the same number of elements per unit area of attachment throughout the lung, as well. In which case, it would not matter which surface you went to, you would find the same density of stress. For such a lung, the inward-acting pressure exerted by tissue forces at the pleural surface would equal the outward-acting ones at the alveolar level, and we would indeed be permitted to speak of the alveoli as being effectively exposed to transpulmonary pressure. I suggest that this is the basis for the success of the classical model of lung elasticity.

But in abnormal lungs, all bets are off ! I am going to spend the rest of my time talking about departures that may take place from this ' ideal ', and the implications of these departures. I will be taking up two sorts of circumstances in which the lung would be expected to behave in a highly non-uniform way. First of all, the situation where, for some reason or other, there is some region in the lung which cannot be further inflated, but meanwhile, the lung around it is inflated. Here I will be speaking of a constant volume of a small portion of the lung and considering the implications of expansion of the rest of the lung on the forces applied to that region. I will jump immediately to an example. Think of the group of alveoli which are obstructed for some reason and have not expanded when you expand the rest of the lung. The question is : what is the effect of pressure distending these unexpanded elements ?

In the case of the classical model, when you think of all units being exposed to transpulmonary pressure, the situation is straightforward. The unit in question ' sees ' pleural pressure on the outside, so it ' sees ' as the distending pressure the same pressure as the rest of the lung.

But the pressure distending this region is solely that applied by traction from surrounding tissue, and, in this situation, we can predict that this is not the same as pleural pressure. In fact, the local distending pressure will be greater than that for the rest of the lung. After all, the tension in the outward-acting attachments will be, if anything, greater—but certainly not less, than that elsewhere—but, more important, the area on which these attachments operate will be *less* than that of corresponding areas elsewhere, and the effective distending pressure will be correspondingly greater. We can get a useful estimate of ' how much greater ' by assuming that the force per attachment is the same at the restricted surfaces as elsewhere and that the area of the region is proportional to the two-thirds power of its volume.

Let's see how this works out on a volume-pressure diagram. Volume in Figure 6 is relative to collapsed volume. A five-fold

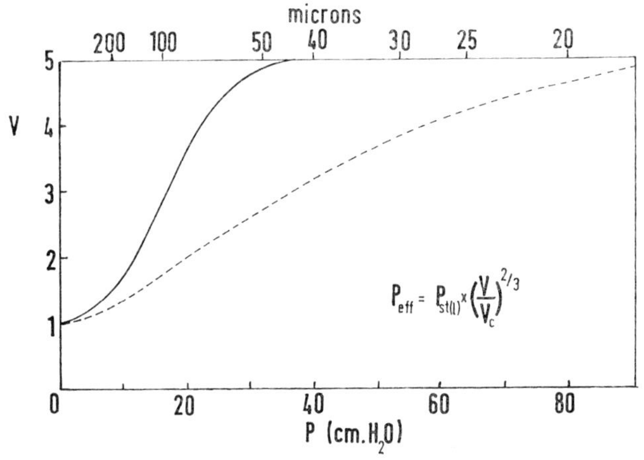

FIG. 6

increase in volume—a very substantial increase from the collapsed level—is equivalent to maximum inflation. The solid line is a standard sort of inflation curve such as one might obtain from almost any mammalian lung. In the 'classical' lung, this solid line describes the distending pressure ($P_{st(l)}$ *i.e.*, the static recoil pressure of the lung) for all elements operating in parallel, whether they be obstructed or not. But not in the present model. Consider a unit obstructed at its collapsed volume. The dashed line corresponds to our prediction. With a two-fold increase in volume the effective distending pressure, P_{eff}, is roughly twice, and up near the top more than three-fold transpulmonary pressure. Across the top of the Figure, I have indicated the diameters of structures that would open with a surface tension of 40 dynes per cm. at these various pressures. It is known that some small mammals (for example, the bat, mouse, and the shrew) have alveoli with diameters in the neighborhood of 30 μ. Could they be expanded in the classical lung? Now I do not think anyone knows, in fact, what sorts of pressures are required to expand fully the lungs of these species. It would be fun to find out. I think in mice, such pressures are not very large; perhaps about 30 cm. H_2O would do it. Is it possible that in these species, these very small structures are expanded on the basis of the mechanism we have been discussing?

The pressure inside a region held at constant volume while surrounding regions expand, should change equally with its surface pressure. This is so because the static pressure difference from the inside to the outside of a structure depends solely on the static properties of its walls and their configuration. At constant volume this pressure difference should also be constant and the pressure inside should change equally with that outside.

We have taken advantage of this in two sorts of experiments. In one experiment carried out by Macklem and Stigol (personal communication) pressures inside blood vessels were measured. In another, carried out by Takishima and myself (manuscript in preparation) airway obstruction was accomplished by wedging small catheters in airways and recording the pressures within them. In lungs of dogs and cats, collateral pathways prevented isolation of air spaces beyond, but in the lungs of cows and goats, there was little or no collateral flow beyond airways wedged with catheters 1·5 mm. in diameter, and successful measurements were possible. In both types of experiments, the pressures inside the obstructed structures, whether blood vessels or air spaces, changed more with inflation of the lung than transpulmonary pressure changed and by amounts which approximated predictions based on our model.

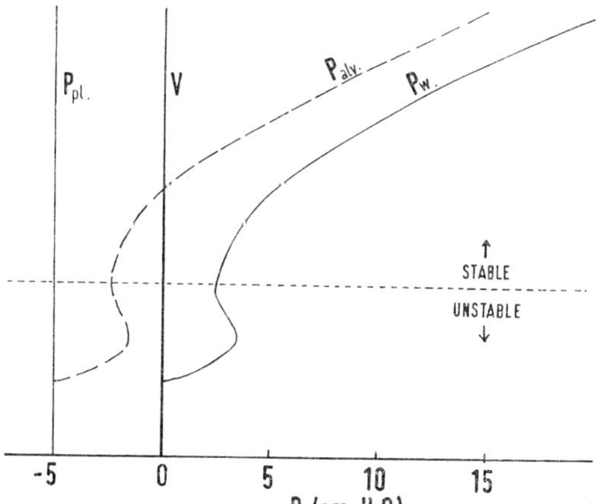

FIG. 7

We have considered what happens when a local region is restricted while the remainder of the lung expands. We need now to consider the opposite side of this coin, namely, the implications of local volume changes while the remainder of the lung remains at constant volume.

Figure 7 shows how alveolar pressure would change in an air space in which gas is forcefully removed by way of its conducting airway, while the remainder of the lung is continuously exposed to a constant pleural pressure of -5 cm. H_2O. For the classical model (Fig. 7) all air spaces would be exposed at their outside walls to pleural pressure, and alveolar pressure and volume would decrease together to reach complete collapse when alveolar pressure equalled pleural pressure or when the pressure difference from the inside to the outside equals zero. The sigmoid shape illustrates the effect of surface tension on this process. As volume decreased, a point would be reached when the unit would become unstable, and with further decrease in volume, surface forces would cause it to collapse and empty completely.

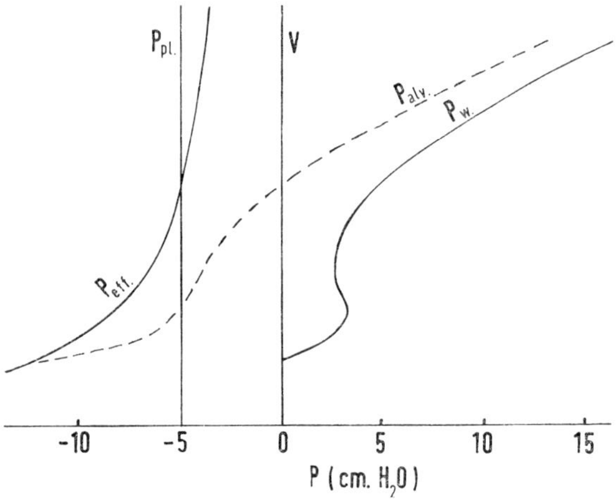

FIG. 8

In our model, (Fig. 8) the air spaces would not behave independently. As alveolar pressure decreased, and the unit grew smaller, the outward-acting forces would be concentrated on a smaller area and their pressure equivalent would be increased, even though pleural pressure remained the same. As a result, the unit would not be emptied when alveolar pressure equalled pleural pressure. Furthermore, the increasing tendency to resist volume decrease would oppose the influence of surface tension and prevent instability and collapse. Thus, the mechanism would have a stabilising influence.

But this same mechanism could have a deleterious influence as well. Consider what would happen if the airways were obstructed so that eventually, as gas uptake by the blood continued, the units became completely gas-free. For the classical lung pressure in the air spaces would be -5 cm. H_2O as they approached complete collapse. This would not be sufficiently negative in normal circumstances to produce capillary transudation and, accordingly, simple atelectasis would occur. If air spaces were interdependent, however, alveolar pressure would fall to levels where transudation would be produced, and the atelectasis would be accompanied by fluid filling. I suggest that this train of events is rare in normal adult lungs simply because, due to the presence of collateral pathways, complete obstruction of air spaces is rare. Indeed, we wonder if this may not be the major functional significance of collateral ventilation—namely, to reduce the likelihood that obstruction of small airways will lead to complete isolation of air spaces beyond. If the lung beyond an obstruction extends to the pleural surface, the pressure within would not fall below pleural pressure, as the lung beyond the obstruction became gas-free, and the threat of transudation would be averted. We suggest that this should be a feature common to all dry atelectasis—namely, that such regions should always extend to a pleural surface.

To sum up a bit, I have developed a model of lung elasticity which in the normal and uniformally inflated lung allows all distensible elements to behave as if they were essentially independent from one another and all exposed to transpulmonary pressure. When, however, a region is either bigger or smaller than those surrounding, the local distending pressures deviate from overall transpulmonary pressure and in such a direction as to oppose local changes. Thus our model is essentially a conservative one : it acts to hold distensible elements ' in line ' ; it assists in expansion of air spaces, but resists either their over-expansion or collapse. Functionally, individual regions within lungs are rendered, in effect, less compliant. This hastens their approach to a statically determined volume distribution under dynamic conditions, and renders the distribution of ventilation less sensitive to the distribution of airway resistance. But the mechanism has implications to pathology as well. I discussed the possibility that local amplification of stress may predispose to transudation. Presumably, stress-amplification of this sort could lead to other types of tissue disruption, and this probably bears looking into.

I am going to say one last word that just occurred to me before we started this afternoon. We physiologists can talk about the influence of stresses upon lung, and we can talk about their immediate effects, for example, in terms of pressure-volume curves done in a matter of seconds or minutes. I would suggest that pathologists, if they will make themselves think along similar lines about an organ which, from birth on, is subjected to stress and grows while stressed and repairs itself while stressed ; if they will apply the physiologists' concepts of mechanical events on a far longer time-scale—to matters of weeks and months and even years—a productive combination of physiologic considerations and pathological ones can be made.

INHOMOGENEITY OF VENTILATION IN NORMAL AND ABNORMAL LUNGS

GORDON CUMMING, KEITH HORSFIELD, J. GARETH JONES
and D. C. F. MUIR

INSPIRED gas is distributed in the lungs by the system of branching tubes which constitute the bronchial tree, and the laws of gas transport by mass movement are relevant to this distribution. The second stage in the ventilatory process is that of gas mixing, where the laws of gaseous diffusion are the relevant consideration. The understanding both of gas transport and gas mixing requires a knowledge of structure, and Figure 1. shows the structure of a terminal ventilatory unit with its terminal bronchiole, several generations of respiratory bronchioles and alveolar ducts. A human lung contains about 28,000 such ventilatory units and gas is distributed to them during inspiration by the branching system of the main airways ; such distribution is achieved by mass flow. Inequalities of mass flow result from the asymmetrical character of the bronchial tree (Horsfield & Cumming, 1967) and from gravitational forces acting upon the lung. Thus the time taken for a molecule of gas to arrive at its destination—the transit time—will differ throughout the lungs, so that anything which alters transit times will produce regional inhomogeneity.

As gas molecules reach the terminal ventilatory unit their forward velocity diminishes progressively as the area of cross section of the air passages increases. In this structure then, the major force affecting molecular movement towards the periphery changes from mass flow to gaseous diffusion.

During a normal inspirate the anatomical level at which the inspired gas and the residual gas have their boundary is about the first order alveolar duct, from which interface there remains a distance of about 2 mm. to be covered for gas mixing to be complete.

Figure 2 shows a terminal ventilatory unit in which there is

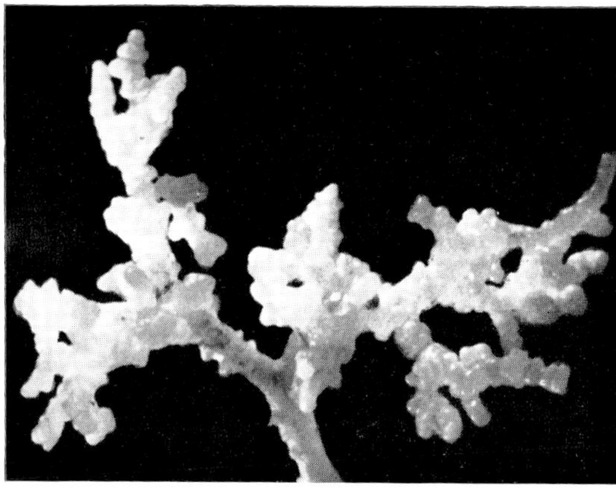

FIG. 1 Resin cast of a normal terminal ventilatory unit. The beginning of the branching system is the terminal bronchiole.

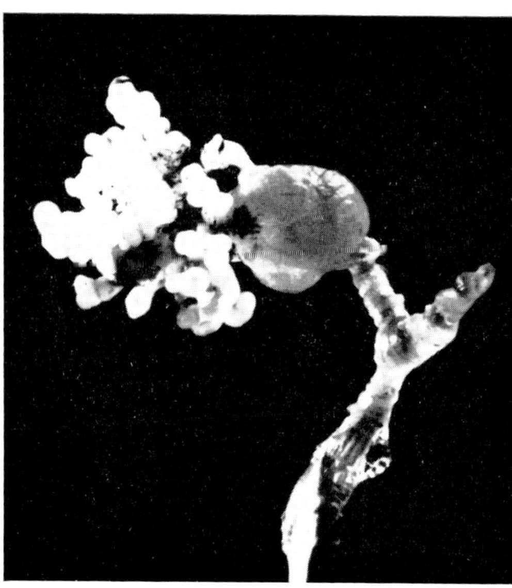

FIG. 2 A terminal ventilatory unit with a dilatation replacing the first and second order respiratory bronchioles—centrilobular emphysema.

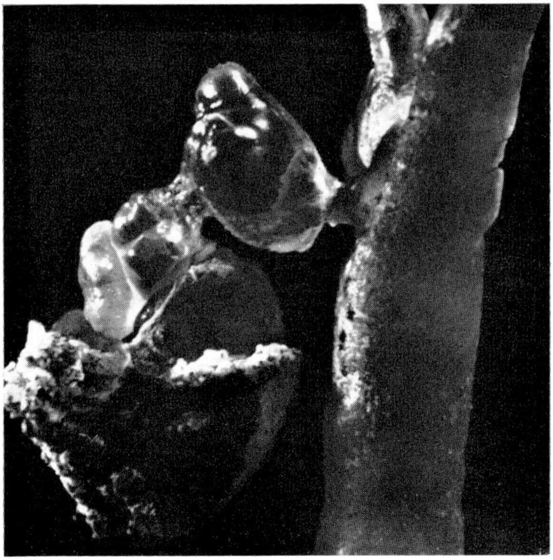

FIG. 3. Showing complete destruction of airways architecture—panacinar emphysema.

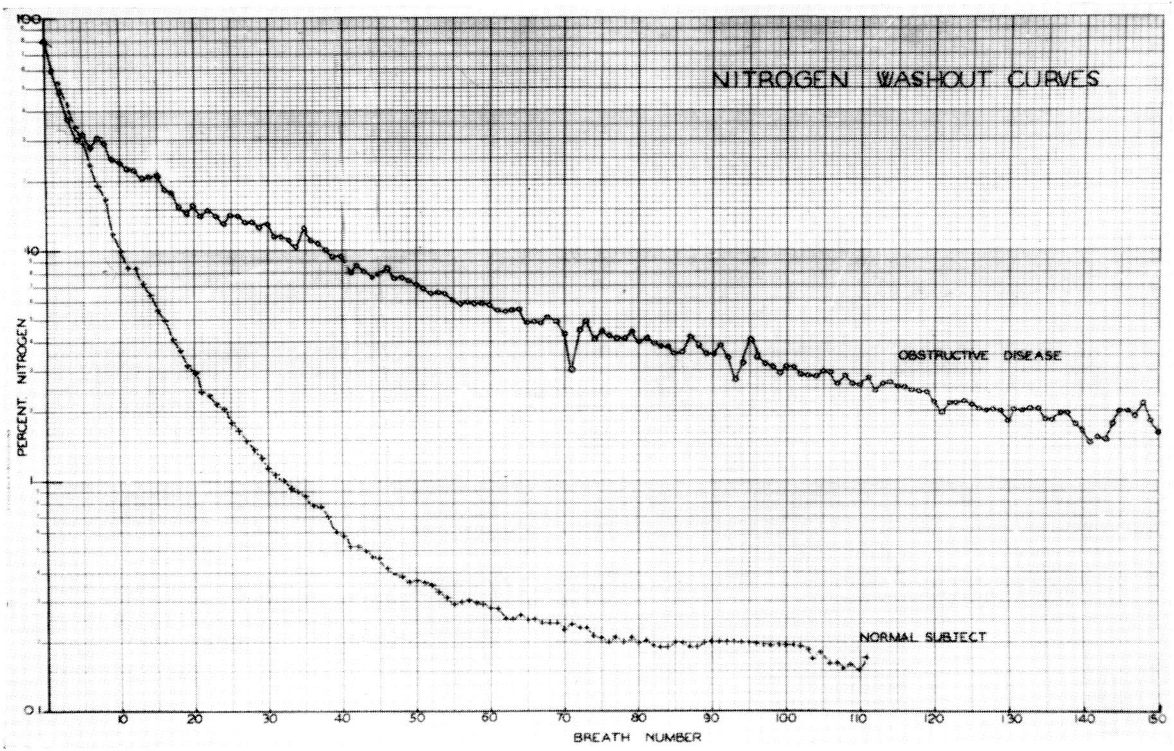

FIG. 4. Nitrogen washout curves, plotting end tidal nitrogen concentration against breath number, using a semi-logarithmic plot.

disruption of the first and second order respiratory bronchioles with the formation of a dilated space. This is an example of centrilobular emphysema (Horsfield *et al.*, 1966). The effect of such a structure on ventilatory efficiency can be estimated if a few assumptions are first made. The diameter of the dilatation is about 2 mm. and, if the assumption be made that one half of the ventilatory units are involved in the destructive process, this means that the total volume of all the dilatations is about 560 ml. To this must be added about 140 ml. of airways dead space, making a total of 700 ml.

An inspirate of 500 ml. into this sytem will bring the interface between inspired gas and residual gas somewhere within the dilatation. In order to mix with the gas in the exchange zone the inspirate must diffuse out of the dilatation and into the alveolar ducts, a distance of some 7 mm. with four constrictions in the pathway. Centrilobular emphysema thus presents a notable obstruction to diffusive gas mixing.

A similar diffiiculty in ventilation is encountered in panacinar emphysema, as shown in Figure 3. This shows a complex in-series dilatation with no normal alveolar structures remaining. The interface is established within the dilatation, and the linear distance over which diffusion must occur is again large, and may be over 10 mm. Thus gas mixing will be impaired in much the same way as in the case of centrilobular emphysema.

In order to assess the validity of the foregoing arguments it is of some importance to estimate the speed with which diffusion equilibrium is achieved. There is general agreement that gas mixing occurs by diffusion, but controversy about the rate of this process.

The historical development of ideas about this rate is of interest. When Krogh and Lindhard, (1917) noted that the carbon dioxide concentration of an expirate rose during expiration, they concluded that this was the result of sampling greater concentrations of the gas nearer to the alveoli—an example of stratified inhomogeneity due to slow diffusive mixing. This view held sway from the early part of the century until 1946 when Rauwerda, after making some calculations based upon lung dimensions, came to the conclusion that gas mixing was so rapid as to leave no detectable gradient of concentration under normal conditions. Thus the hypothesis of Krogh which had satisfactorily explained the genesis of the alveolar plateau was abandoned, to be replaced in 1952 by that of Otis *et al.*, based upon the time constant hypothesis.

More recently evidence has accumulated that diffusion is not so rapid as is currently believed (Georg *et al.*, 1965 ; Cumming *et al.*, 1966) and this is reinforced by the paper of Mead at this symposium suggesting that a recomputation of time constants in the lung makes this an unlikely cause of sequential emptying.

It is possible to investigate the speed of diffusion in the lungs by employing a mixture of gases with differing rates of diffusion, all other variables being maintained constant. If the diffusion coefficient is very small, such as in the case of an aerosol, then mixing between inspired gas and residual gas will be minimal, showing the dependence of gas mixing on gaseous diffusion (Altshule *et al.*, 1959 ; Muir, 1967). On a theoretical basis, Ficks diffusion equation can be solved for a mixture of two gases in a model of the lung, and the distribution of concentrations for the two gases may be predicted, together with its behaviour on breath holding. (Cumming *et al.*, 1967). Figure 5 shows the concentrations of neon and sulphur

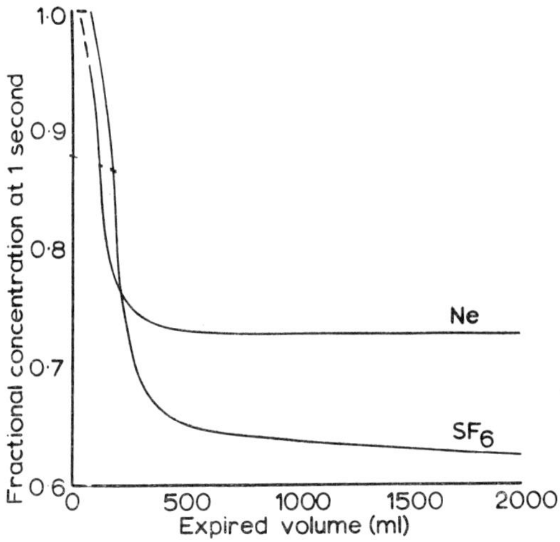

Fig. 5. Predicted concentrations of a mixture of Neon and Sulphur Hexafluoride after 1 sec. of diffusive mixing.

hexafluoride 1 second after the establishment of the interface. It will be seen that two different concentration gradients exist and that they cross over. If a second calculation is made, corresponding to breath holding for 5 seconds the results are as shown in Figure 6, with the differences between the two curves markedly diminished, the terminal concentrations of both gases being higher, and the curves less steep.

Having established the probable behaviour of a mixture of neon (Mol. wt. 20) and sulphur hexafluoride (Mol. wt. 146) when inspired into the lung, the results of an experiment in which a normal subject inspires the gas mixture may now be compared. Figure 7 shows a

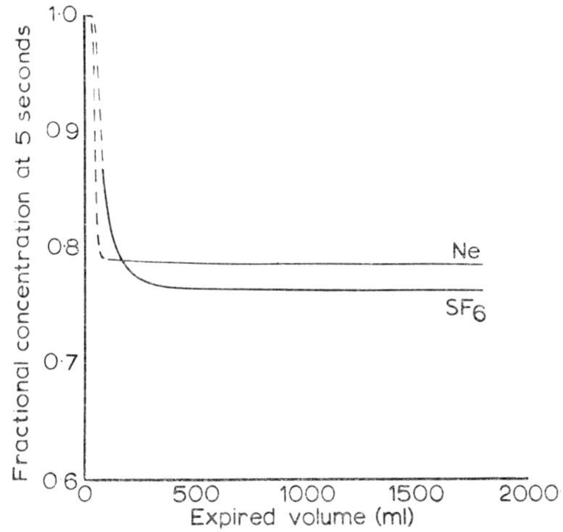

FIG. 6. The same as Figure 5 but after 5 secs mixing.

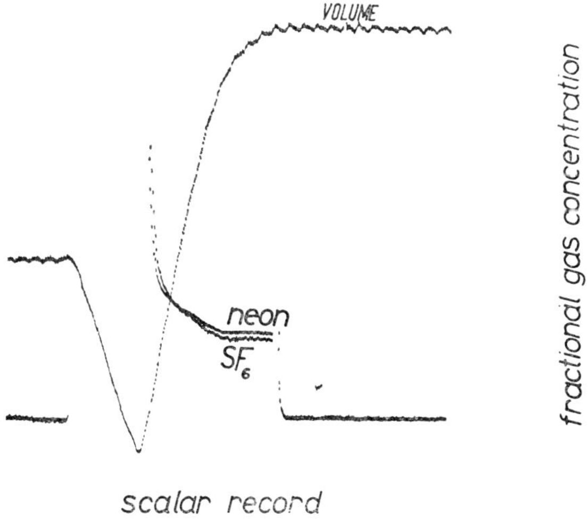

FIG. 7. Expired concentrations of Ne and SF_6 in a normal subject.

typical record from such an experiment and confirms the fact that two different alveolar plateaux are produced.

Figure 8 shows the average results from six normal subjects

inspiring the test gas from residual volume, functional residual capacity and 1 litre below total lung volume. Figures 9 and 10

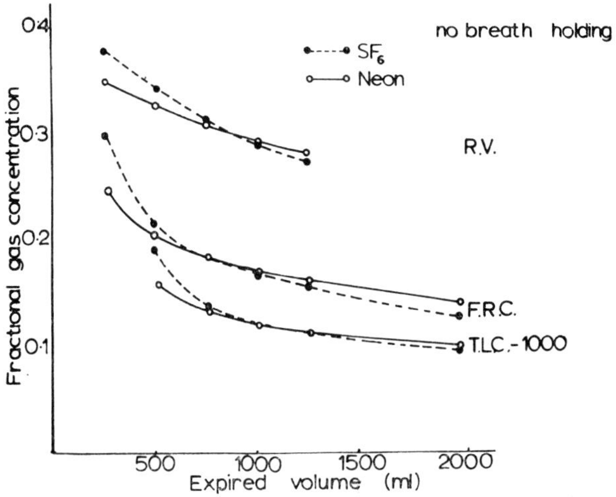

FIG. 8. Average results from six subjects made without breath holding using a mixture of Neon and SF_6 inspired at different lung volumes.

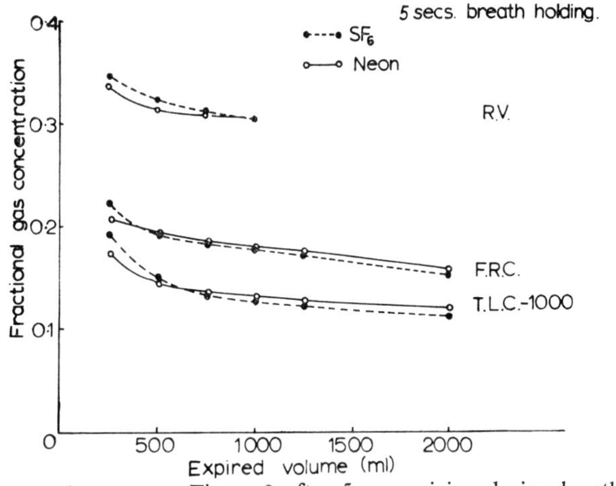

FIG. 9. The same as Figure 8 after 5 secs mixing during breath holding.

show the results after 5 and 30 sec. breath holding. These confirm the general predictions made from the geometrical model of the lung in that two different alveolar plateaux exist at every lung volume.

However the predictions about behaviour at residual volume are not entirely confirmed. The crossover point at FRC is to the left of that at TLC and by the same token that for RV should lie to the left again. As is seen in Figures 8 and 9, the crossover point at RV is moved further to the right than expected. On breath holding the crossover scarcely moves its position at RV whilst a marked shift to the left is seen at FRC and TLC. This evidence suggests that at residual volume in normal subjects there is an increased stratified inhomogeneity in the normal lung.

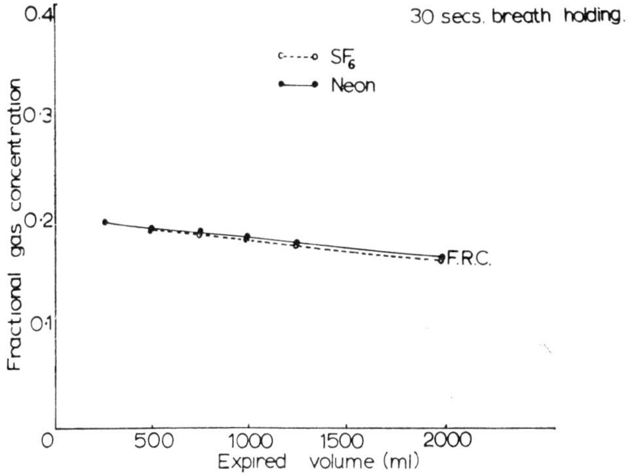

FIG. 10. As Figure 8 but after 30 secs breath holding.

Bronchitic patients, with a small expiratory reserve volume, ventilate as if they are at residual volume (Milic-Emili *et al.*, 1966 ; Young & Martin, 1966) ; studies with the mixed gas tracer in such patients confirm that the crossover point is shifted to the right, and is not demonstrable in some cases, when the gas concentrations entirely fail to meet.

Further evidence for incomplete gas mixing is obtainable by an entirely different technique, that of the lung nitrogen clearance curve. Figure 4 shows such a curve plotted in the usual way with the mixed expired nitrogen concentration on the ordinate with a logarithmic scale and the number of breaths along the abscissa, with a linear scale.

It is usual to interpret this curve in the following way. The latter part is regarded as being rectilinear, and the values of nitrogen represented by this line are subtracted from the original curve. The resulting curve is usually indistinguishable from a straight line, so that the curve is resolved into two straight lines. The physiological interpretation made from this manoeuvre is that the lung comprises two functional compartments with different ventilations, with complete gas mixing, and ventilated in parallel. The assumption that ventilation is in parallel is implicit in this method of analysis, but the authors who described the technique made no such assumption. Robertson *et al.*, (1950) suggested that the two compartments might be either in parallel or in series, but subsequent authors seem to have adopted the parallel situation and rejected the series one without, apparently, any good reason. It is now suggested that the series situation is once again considered in the interpretation of lung nitrogen clearance curve.

Figure 11 shows a simplified series compartment model, with a volume in the distal compartment of 3 litres and in the proximal

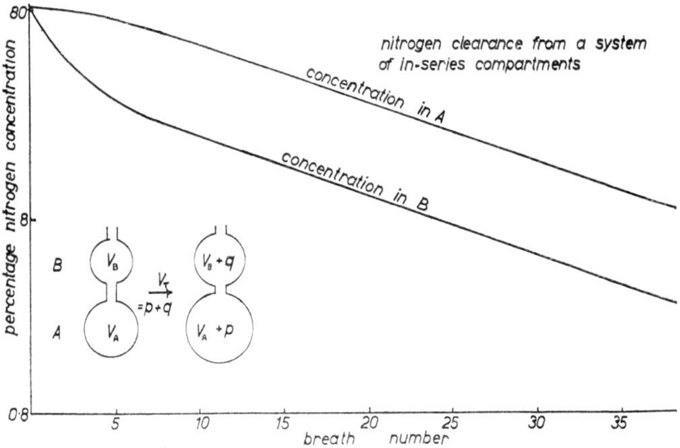

FIG. 11. The predicted washout of an in-series model V_A is 3 litres V_B is 2 litres and V_T 500 ml. The curves show the concentration in each of the chambers at any time during the washout process.

one of 2 litres. Assuming a tidal volume of 500 ml. and an equal compliance in the two compartments (a very gross assumption) it is possible to show what happens during the washout process using simple arithmetic, and this is shown in Figure 11. Consider now the nitrogen concentration during a single expirate at the middle of the curve. From zero nitrogen, concentration will rise steeply until the tidal volume of 500 ml. is expired, when it will be as shown by the lower curve. Continued expiration will result in a continued steep rise, limited only by the concentration in the distal compartment.

Furthermore this steep rise in the alveolar plateau should be the same at whatever point the curve is considered, after the first few breaths. These two points—the steepness of the alveolar plateau and its unchanging nature during the washout process—are strong evidence in favour of the in-series hypothesis. By contrast the parallel hypothesis would suggest that the alveolar plateau should be horizontal in the latter part of the washout process, and therefore that its slope would change as the process continues.

The use of the clearance curve for quantitative interpretations poses some difficulties, and it is possible to consider the same information in a slightly different manner.

Figure 12 shows a curve plotted not against breath number, but against turnover number. This means that for every increment in

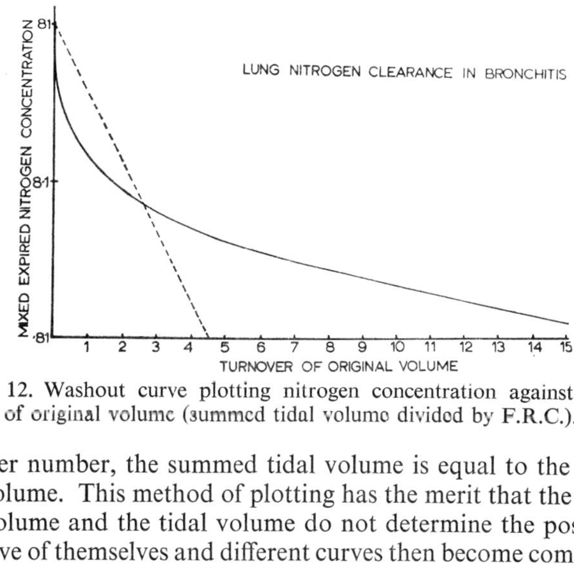

FIG. 12. Washout curve plotting nitrogen concentration against turnover of original volume (summed tidal volume divided by F.R.C.).

turnover number, the summed tidal volume is equal to the original lung volume. This method of plotting has the merit that the original lung volume and the tidal volume do not determine the position of the curve of themselves and different curves then become comparable. Furthermore it is possible to draw in the line (which is invariant) which would result if gas mixing were perfect, when every molecule of the tidal volume would be evenly distributed throughout the lung. The comparison between the normal subject and the bronchitic patient shows the difference between them, but is not much more helpful in giving information about the inefficiency of gas mixing.

The data may be regarded quite differently : in such a way that concentration of nitrogen is excluded as a variable. There are difficulties about using concentration, whether the correct value is end tidal, mixed expired, mean alveolar—or whatever. The available data which is measurable without equivocation comprises the tidal volume, and the volume of nitrogen which it contains. At the end of study, of appropriate length, it is possible to add up all the quantities of nitrogen in each breath to obtain the total volume originally present, making some corrections for tissue nitrogen and the amount left behind at the end of the study.

Given this information it is possible to construct a curve which shows the volume of nitrogen in 1 litre of lung volume at any instant during washout. This has been called the decay curve and it has some interesting properties (Cumming, 1967). If mixing and distribution are perfect, the line showing clearance of nitrogen is identical with the decay curve. If distribution is uniform on a regional basis, but mixing is impaired, a straight line decay curve will result but it will be displaced to the right. The ratio of intercepts on the abscissa of this decay curve and that showing perfect mixing is then a measure of the inefficiency of mixing which can be expressed as a percentage. This is illustrated in Figure 13.

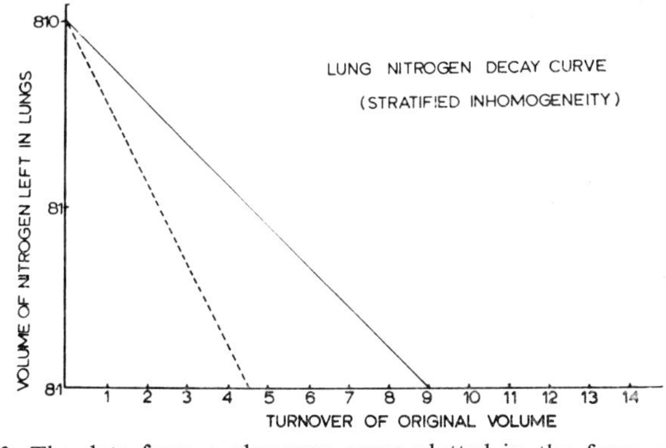

FIG. 13. The data from a clearance curve plotted in the form of the decay curve.

In the situation when regional distribution is non-uniform the decay curve becomes curved, so that the percentage inefficiency has contributions both from regional and stratified defects.

The rather tedious business of collecting and processing data has been done in the laboratory with an analogue computer and a paper tape punch out, followed by digital computation on the IBM 1440 or the KDF 9. Figure 14 shows the decay curves from three patients with bronchitis of varying severity, the hatched area shows the normal range and the straight line perfect mixing and distribution.

It will be seen that the three decay curves have as their major difference a displacement to the right, representing dominant stratified inhomogeneity. Assessment of their curvature poses a difficult problem which has not for the moment been solved. However a rough comparison may be made by moving the curves to the left so that they lie within the normal range at their lower end (at 8·1 per cent.). If the whole curve then lies within the hatched area the curvature is no greater than normal. In the 55 per cent. and the 33 per cent. curves the curvature was not increased but, in the worst case, the beginning showed a greater curvature.

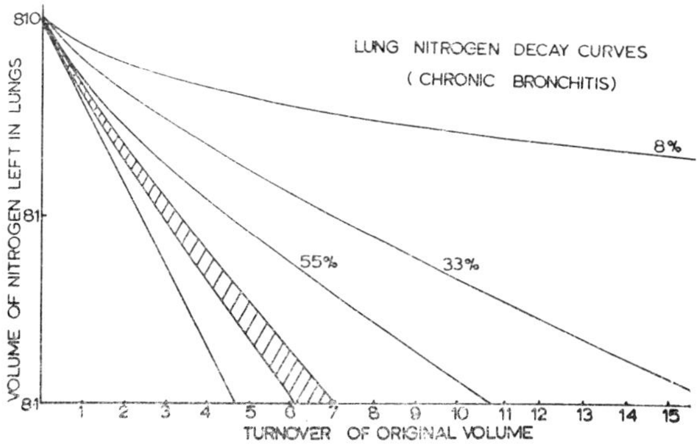

FIG. 14. Decay curves from patients with chronic bronchitis of varying severity. The hatched area indicates the normal range.

Thus from evidence of the single breath test and from the nitrogen washout, it would appear that gas mixing by diffusion is a time limited process, and that in bronchitis this time limitation is a dominant factor in impairing ventilatory efficiency.

ACKNOWLEDGMENTS

We are indebted to the editor of Respiration Physiology for permission to reproduce Figures 5, 6, 8, 9 and 10.

REGIONAL DISTRIBUTION OF PULMONARY VENTILATION[1]

J. MILIC-EMILI, J. A. M. HENDERSON, and K. KANEKO[2]

IN recent years knowledge of the regional ventilatory function of the lungs has advanced considerably, particularly as a result of studies using radioactive gases with scintillation counters externally over various lung regions. The radioactive-gas techniques used have been fully described in the literature (Ball *et al.*, 1962 ; West & Dollery, 1960 ; Milic-Emili *et al.*, 1966 ; Anthonison & Milic-Emili, 1966). This review is essentially limited to (1) a description of the regional ventilatory function of normal lungs, as studied using radioactive xenon (^{133}Xe), and (2) a discussion of the factors which determine regional distribution of gas within the lungs.

REGIONAL SUBDIVISIONS OF LUNG VOLUME

Traditionally, any account of the overall ventilatory function of the lungs starts with a description of the total lung capacity (TLC) and its subdivisions. Accordingly, it seems logical that our account of the *regional* ventilatory function of the lungs should start with a description of the *regional* subdivisions of lung volume. One of the methods most commonly used to measure over-all subdivisions of lung volume, *i.e.*, the helium method, is based on the gas-dilution principle. Our measurements of the regional subdivisions of lung volume also were based on the gas-dilution principle, but we used ^{133}Xe (Milic-Emili *et al.*, 1966) instead of helium. The measurements made on a normal, seated man are depicted in Figure 1. It is apparent that at the end of both a normal expiration (FRC) and a maximal expiration (RV) the lung units (' alveoli ') in the apical lung regions are more expanded than are corresponding units in the basilar lung zones, *i.e.*, the regional FRC and the regional RV are relatively greater in the upper zones of the lungs. These differences in expansion are caused chiefly by differences in pleural pressure down the lung (Wood *et al.*, 1963). In upright man there is a ' gradient ' in

[1] Supported by The John A. Hartford Foundation of the U.S.A., and the Medical Research Council of Canada.

[2] Present address : Department of Anesthesiology, Children's Hospital of Los Angeles, Calif., U.S.A.

pleural pressure down the lung, with the more negative values towards the apex (Krueger *et al.*, 1961 ; Milic-Emili *et al.*, 1964 ; Turner, 1962). Although its nature is not well understood, the

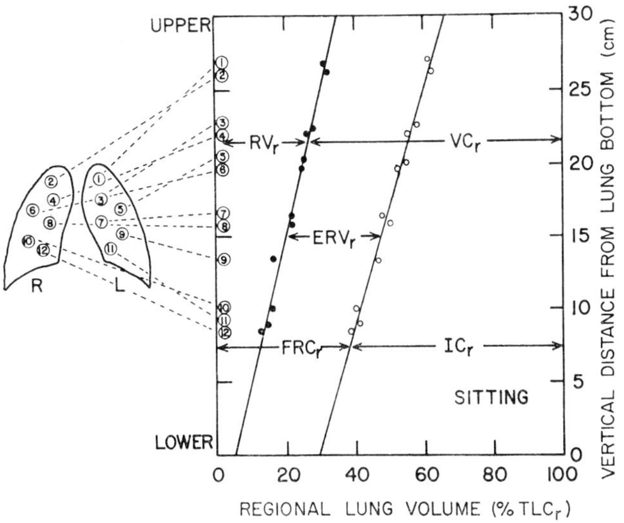

FIG. 1. Sub divisions of regional lung volume in a normal seated subject. Filled and open circles represent results recorded at residual volume (RV) and functional residual capacity (FRC), respectively, by scintillation counters placed externally. Schematic position of scintillation counters in relation to the lungs is shown. *Ordinate:* vertical distance from lung bottom (in cm.). *Abscissa:* regional lung volume expressed as a percentage of the volume of each region at full inspiration, *i.e.*, percentage of regional total lung capacity (% TLC_r). RV_r = regional residual volume; FRC_r = regional functional residual capacity; IC_r = regional inspiratory capacity; ERV_r = regional expiratory reserve volume; VC_r = regional vital capacity.

gradient appears to be gravity-dependent, *i.e.*, related to the weight of the lungs. Figure 2 shows how the gradient in pleural pressure, combined with the elastic properties of the lungs (which are assumed to be uniform), can account for the differences in lung expansion observed in radioactive-gas studies.[1] At full inspiration (TLC) all

[1] For simplicity, it is assumed that pleural pressure increases at a rate of 0·25 cm. H_2O/cm. down the lung ; thus, in a lung with a vertical length of 30 cm. the total difference in pleural pressure from lung top to bottom amounts to 7·5 cm. H_2O. In reality, the ‘ gradient ’ in pleural pressure appears to be more pronounced in upper than in dependent lung zones (3, 8).

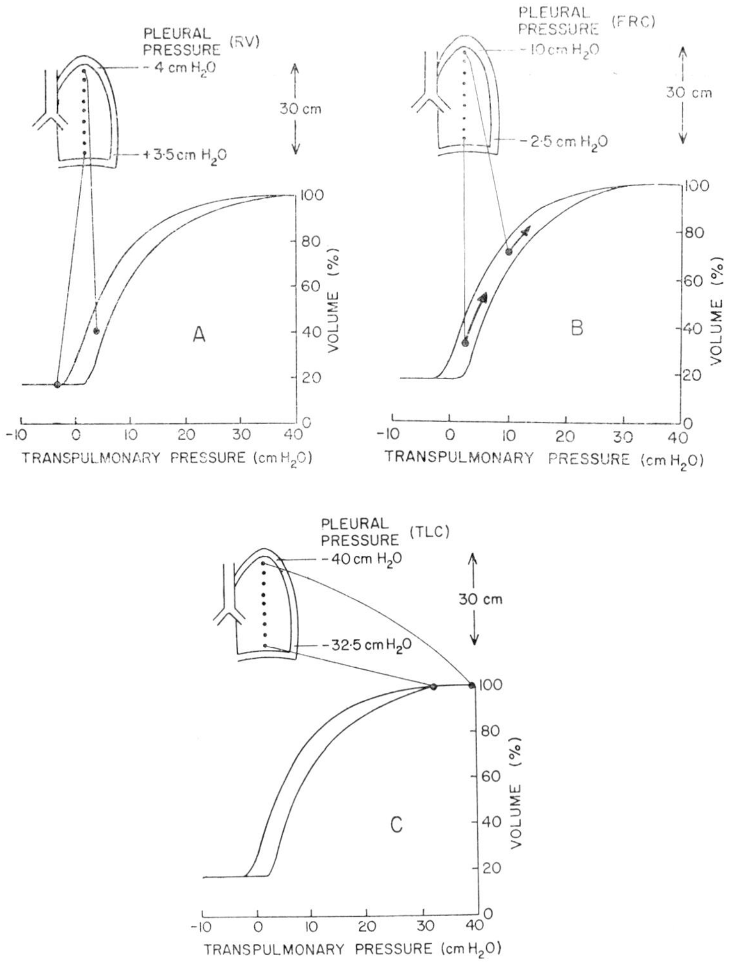

FIG. 2 Effect of the 'gradient' of pleural pressure on the distribution of gas within the lungs. The pressure is assumed to increase at a constant rate of 0·25 cm. H_2O/cm. vertically. The elastic properties of the lungs, as expressed by the S-shaped static volume–pressure curves in the lower part of each panel, are assumed to be uniform throughout the lungs. Pleural pressures at the apex and base, at three lung volumes (RV, FRC, and TLC), are shown in the upper part of each panel. In *C*, at full inspiration (TLC), all lung regions are expanded virtually uniformly, despite the pleural pressure differences down the lungs. By contrast, at RV and FRC (*A* and *B*, respectively), the pleural pressure 'gradient' results in a greater volume in upper than in lower lung zones.

lung regions are expanded almost uniformly, despite the vertical gradient in pleural pressure (Fig. 2 C).[1] This is because, near full inflation, the slope of the static volume–pressure curve of the lungs is nearly flat, with the result that the relatively small differences in pleural pressure down the lungs do not cause appreciable differences in regional lung expansion. As lung volume decreases below TLC the lung regions operate on a progressively steeper part of their static volume–pressure curve, so that the vertical gradient in pleural pressure causes marked differences in expansion down the lung. Indeed, at both RV and FRC the apical lung units are more expanded than those near the lung base (Fig. 2 A and B). This behaviour is reflected in the results obtained during radioactive-gas studies.

It is not known whether the gradient in pleural pressure down the lungs accounts entirely for the distribution of gas within the lungs under all conditions although, clearly, it is responsible for the relatively uniform distribution of gas between lung apex and base in man in the supine position (Bryan *et al.*, 1964 ; Kaneko *et al.*, 1966), in which position the pleural pressure differences between apex and base largely disappear. In the supine position, however, these differences occur between the upper (frontal) and dependent (dorsal) aspects of the lungs and are accompanied, not surprisingly, by differences in expansion between the frontal and dorsal parts of the lungs. Similar results are obtained in the prone position as well as in lateral decubitus. In all of these postures, the upper lung regions (which are always exposed to more negative pleural pressure) tend to be more expanded than the lower lung zones. It should be noted that the pleural pressure 'gradient' and the resulting differences in lung expansion tend always to occur vertically, *i.e.*, in the direction of gravity.

In the past, systematic regional differences in expansion were not recorded in the numerous reported morphological studies of the lungs. In most cases the lungs had been inflated outside the chest before fixation and, therefore, measurements did not reflect the state of the lungs inside the chest. Recently, however, Glazier *et al.*, (1966), who froze dog lungs *in situ* and measured alveolar size with morphometric techniques, demonstrated regional differences in alveolar expansion which agreed, at least qualitatively, with results obtained using ^{133}Xe.

[1] Figures 2 and 3 are shown in the diagrammatic form suggested by West (1965).

RELATIONSHIPS BETWEEN REGIONAL AND OVER-ALL LUNG VOLUME

A better understanding of the regional distribution of gas in the lungs can be gained by measuring regional lung volumes at different degrees of over-all lung inflation, encompassing the entire range of vital capacity (VC). Such measurements, in a normal seated subject, are shown in Figure 3, in which regional volumes obtaining at

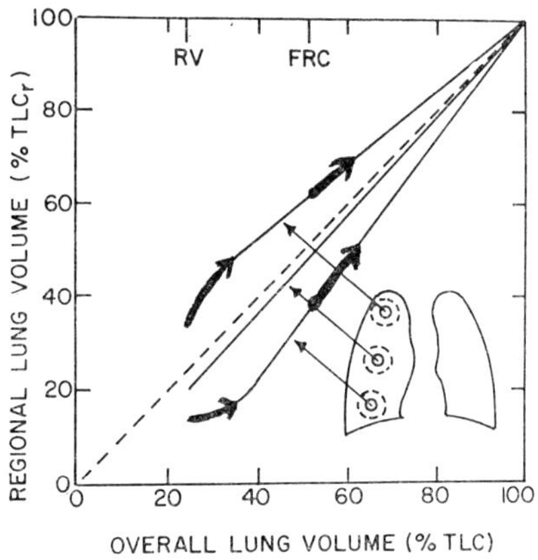

FIG. 3. Relationship between regional and over-all lung volume in a normal seated subject. The three regions are 5, 15 and 25 cm. vertically from the top of the lungs. *Ordinate:* regional lung volume (% TLC_r). *Abscissa:* over-all lung volume (% TLC). Over-all RV and FRC also are indicated. Note that when a tidal breath is taken from FRC the ventilation is greater in lower than in upper lung zones, as indicated by arrows. When a corresponding breath is taken from RV, ventilation is reversed, *i.e.*, greater in upper lung zones.

three different vertical levels of the lungs are plotted against over-all lung volume. If the alveoli of all lung regions had expanded uniformly, the volume of each region of the lung (expressed as a percentage of regional TLC) should be always the same as the over-all lung volume (expressed as a percentage of TLC ; *i.e.*, the relationship between regional and over-all lung volumes should be given by the line of identity (slope $=1$), which is shown as a broken line. Clearly this is not the case : the alveoli in the upper lung regions appear to be relatively more expanded than those in the lower zones, at all lung volumes except full inspiration.

REGIONAL DISTRIBUTION OF VENTILATION

The slopes of the curves in Figures 3 indicate the rate of filling (or *ventilation*) of the alveoli in the various lung regions in relation to volume changes in the lungs as a whole. It is apparent that, at lung volumes above FRC, the proportion of inspired gas delivered to any lung region is substantially constant, as shown by the linear relationships between regional and over-all lung volumes. Thus, in this range of lung volumes the zones do not fill sequentially. However, the slope of the curves is always greater in dependent than in upper lung zones, indicating that the dependent alveoli receive relatively more of the inspired volume (or *ventilation*). In brief, these results indicate that, when a normal subject takes a breath from FRC, the ventilation *per alveolus* is greater in dependent than in upper lung regions, but that the relative distribution of ventilation is independent of the magnitude of the inspired volume, *i.e.*, the difference in ventilation between upper and dependent alveoli is proportionately the same whether the subject takes a resting tidal breath or a maximal inspiration. Speed of inspiration appears to have little effect on ventilation distribution, provided that the breath is taken from FRC or higher lung volumes (J.A.M. Henderson ; unpublished observations).

When breathing takes place at lung volumes lower than FRC, *i.e.*, near RV, the distribution pattern of ventilation is entirely different. Indeed, as shown in Figure 3, at lung volumes lower than FRC the slope of the relationships between regional and over-all lung volumes is steeper in upper than in dependent lung zones. In these circumstances, therefore, the ventilation distribution is reversed, alveoli in upper regions being better ventilated than those in dependent zones.

Again, these results can be explained by a combination of the vertical gradient in pleural pressure and of uniform elastic properties of the lungs. As shown in Figure 4 B, at FRC the lower lung regions operate on a steeper (more compliant) part of the static volume–pressure curve than the upper lung zones. As a result, during inspiration initiated from FRC the difference in compliance between the lower and the upper parts of the lungs favours greater tidal volumes in the lower zones.

At lung volumes below FRC the regional distribution of ventilation is further complicated by air-trapping. As lung volume approaches RV, the transpulmonary pressure in the dependent regions of the lungs actually exceeds airway pressure, causing air-trapping in these units. When a small breath is taken from RV the trapped units in the lower lung regions receive none of the inspired air until pleural pressure reaches a critical value. Under these conditions, inspired gas is delivered predominantly to upper lung regions (Fig. 4 A).

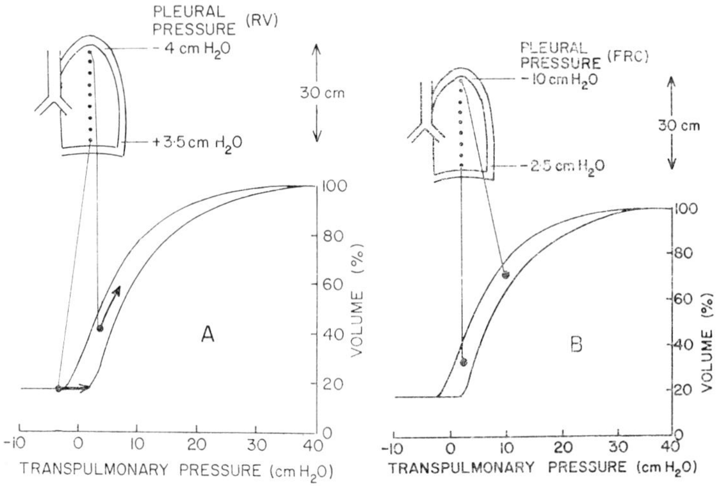

FIG. 4. Effect of pleural pressure 'gradient' on distribution of ventilation. *B:* At the beginning of a normal inspiration (FRC), the basilar lung regions operate on a steeper part of the compliance curve of the lungs than do apical lung zones. As a result, during tidal volume respiration the ventilation is greater in basilar lung regions, as shown by the arrows. *A:* By contrast, at residual volume (RV). pleural pressure at the lung base is positive (+3·5 cm. H_2O), and as a result the lower alveoli are not ventilated, because of airway closure (air-trapping). Under these conditions the lung apex is better ventilated than the base.

In summary, in the range of lung volumes at which breathing takes place under most physiological conditions, the alveoli of dependent lung zones ventilate more than the upper alveoli. This preferential distribution of ventilation to the lower lung zones is significant in relation to the efficiency of gas exchange within the lungs. Blood flow, also, normally is distributed preferentially to dependent lung zones ; thus, ventilation and blood flow are usually relatively well matched in normal, healthy lungs and, consequently, gas exchange is efficient.

At lung volumes approaching RV, ventilation is greater in upper than in dependent alveoli, a reversal which is of interest because in many physiological and pathological conditions the reduction in FRC at times may be large enough to produce a reversal in ventilation distribution. For example, obese subjects breathe at low lung volumes, because the increased abdominal mass tends to elevate the diaphragm and, hence, reduce the FRC. When the FRC is greatly reduced, one would predict a reversal in ventilation distribution. To test this hypothesis we studied the distribution of resting ventilation and pulmonary blood flow in obese subjects, using ^{133}Xe. The prediction was correct in that in many of these obese subjects the ventilation distribution was indeed reversed (Holley *et al.*, 1967) ; perfusion distribution, on the other hand, remained gravity-oriented, *i.e.*, chiefly to the lower lung zones. Thus, in many obese people there is marked ventilation/perfusion imbalance, a finding which may account for the arterial hypoxia frequently observed in obesity. This example illustrates that findings obtained in normal subjects may be applied to the investigation of clinical problems.

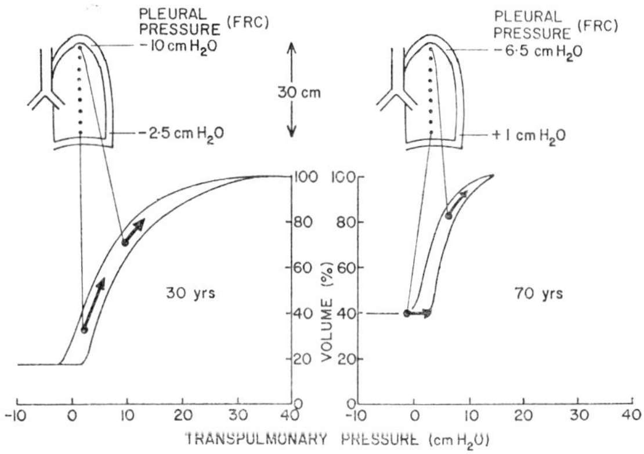

FIG. 5. Distribution of ventilation during quiet breathing in a young (*left*) and in an old (*right*) subject. In the old subject, at FRC the pleural pressure is positive at the lung base, causing airway collapse, so that ventilation is distributed preferentially to the upper zones (*see arrows*). Note the loss in elastic recoil of the lungs in the old subjects, *i.e.*, the static volume–pressure curve is displaced to the right.

Since the distribution of gas depends not only upon the gradient in pleural pressure but also upon the elastic properties of the lungs, any change in the latter must result in altered distribution of ventilation within the lungs. For example, it is well known that in old age there is loss of elastic recoil of the lungs : at any given lung volume, pleural pressure is less subatmospheric in elderly than in young subjects (Radford, 1964 *a*). Therefore, airways in the dependent lung units would be expected to close at higher lung volumes in older subjects. In fact there is reason to believe that in many people over the age of 65, the pleural pressure at the lung base may be positive even at FRC (Fig. 5); therefore it can be predicted that the airways in the dependent lung zones of these subjects are collapsed and cause reversal of ventilation distribution during quiet breathing. To test this hypothesis, using ^{133}Xe we measured the distribution of ventilation and pulmonary blood flow during quiet breathing in six subjects aged between 65 and 75 years (J. Holland and his colleagues, unpublished observations). As anticipated, some of these subjects had reversed ventilation distribution, *i.e.*, preferentially to the upper lung zones; by contrast, perfusion distribution was preferentially to dependent zones. Thus, some old people have marked impairment of regional ventilation/perfusion distribution, which may explain at least in part the reported increase in A–a oxygen differences with advancing age (Tenney & Miller, 1956).

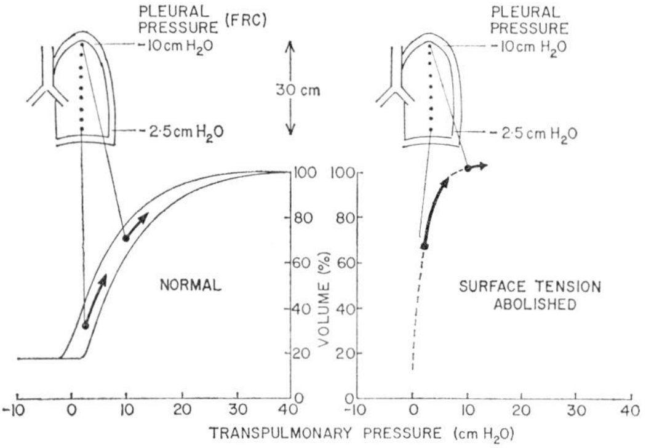

FIG. 6. Distribution of ventilation in a normal lung (*left*) and in a lung in which surface tension is abolished (*right*). The static volume–pressure curve on the right was obtained on saline-filled lungs. Note that when surface tension is absent the lung apex is almost fully expanded at a transpulmonary pressure of less than 10 cm. H_2O, so that, during inspiration (when there is further increase in transpulmonary pressure), ventilation at the apex is virtually nil.

This example indicates that changes in elastic-recoil properties of the lungs can result in severe alterations in ventilation distribution. In this connection it is of interest to review the importance of lung surface-tension phenomena in relation to the distribution of gas within the lungs. Part of the elastic recoil of the lungs is due to forces arising from the gas–liquid interface in the lung; when this interface is abolished (*e.g.*, in the saline-filled lung) the elastic recoil of the lung is reduced, more markedly at high than at low lung volumes (Fig. 6). This behaviour is due to the presence of surfactant, which has the remarkable property of lowering surface tension progressively as lung volume decreases, until at low lung volumes the surface tension is virtually abolished (Radford, 1964 *b*). As a result, the static volume–pressure curve of the air-filled lung normally is less steep (less compliant) than that of a liquid-filled lung, in which surface tension is abolished at all lung volumes. This phenomenon ensures adequate ventilation throughout the lungs, in that the static volume–pressure curve normally is sufficiently 'stiff' to accommodate the entire range of pleural pressures down the lung, while allowing all lung units to participate in ventilation (Fig. 6, *left*). On the contrary, if surfactant abolished surface tension at all lung volumes (so that the curve in the air-filled lung was similar to that in the fluid-filled lung), some alveoli would no longer participate in ventilation. Indeed, the static volume–pressure curve of lungs deprived of surface tension is too steep to accommodate the normal difference in pressure (about 7·5 cm. H_2O) between lung apex and base (Fig. 6, *right*). Thus, it appears that surfactant plays an important role also in relation to regional distribution of ventilation within the lungs.

Finally, since we live in 'the space age,' it is of interest to consider briefly the effects of increased acceleration on the distribution of gas in the lungs. During acceleration the 'gradient' in pleural pressure down the lungs increases, an effect which should result in increases in the differences in expansion of alveoli in the upper and lower lung zones. This chain of events due to increased acceleration was confirmed during ^{133}Xe studies by Bryan *et al.* (1966).

From this rather cursory review it is evident that significant contributions to our knowledge of regional lung function have been made by use of radioactive-gas techniques. In particular, they have established that gravity is a major factor in determining not only the distribution of pulmonary blood flow but also the distribution of pulmonary ventilation.

THE FLOW RESISTANCE OF CENTRAL AND PERIPHERAL AIRWAYS IN HUMAN LUNGS[1]

PETER T. MACKLEM, J. C. HOGG[2] and W. M. THURLBECK

INTRODUCTION

BOTH airway resistance and the distribution of ventilation are grossly abnormal in advanced chronic obstructive airway disease. We have studied human lungs obtained at necropsy to define some of the factors which govern airway resistance and ventilation distribution in normal lungs and how these factors may be deranged in chronic obstructive airway disease. In particular, we have studied the resistance of the small airways because it has been postulated that obstruction at this level may have an important effect on ventilation distribution with little effect on total pulmonary resistance (Macklem & Mead, 1967). We have also measured the resistance to collateral flow because, in emphysema particularly, this may be an important alternate pathway for ventilation when airways are obstructed. Finally, we have studied intact human subjects in order to see if the abnormalities that we could detect in the post mortem lungs could also be detected during life in the early stages of their illness. This is a preliminary communication that will be presented in detail elsewhere.

THE RESISTANCE OF CENTRAL AND PERIPHERAL AIRWAYS IN EXCISED HUMAN LUNGS

Recently the retrograde catheter technique was devised to measure pressure in small bronchi and thereby partition pulmonary resistance (Macklem & Mead, 1967).

The retrograde catheter is illustrated diagramatically in Figure 1. It is an ordinary piece of polyethylene tubing which is bell-shaped at one end. Instead of extending out the trachea, it passes through the wall of the bronchus in which it is measuring pressure and out through the pleural surface, leaving the central airways (between the catheter and the trachea) completely unobstructed.

[1] Supported in part by the James Picker Foundation on the recommendation of the Committee on Radiology, National Academy of Sciences, National Research Council (U.S.A.) and by grants from the Medical Research Council of Canada and John A. Hartford Foundation.

[2] Medical Research Council Research Fellow.

It is inserted in the following manner: a larger polyethylene catheter is advanced into the tracheobronchial tree until it is wedged. A piano wire is inserted into the wedged catheter past the wedged position and pushed through the wall of the bronchus, parenchyma, and pleural surface. The wedged catheter is then removed, leaving the wire extending both out through the trachea and the pleural surface. The end of the retrograde catheter without the bell is securely attached to the tracheal extension of the wire. The wire is then pulled at the pleural surface dragging the retrograde catheter into the lung until the bell, which is the widest part of the system, wedges in a bronchus. It then measures lateral bronchial pressure at the site of the bell.

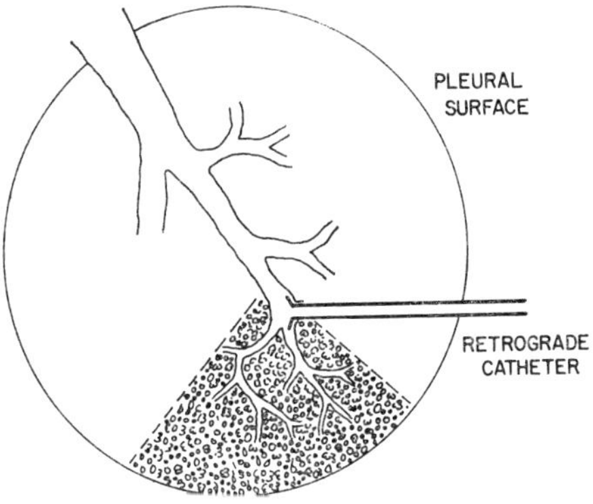

FIG. 1. Diagrammatic illustration of retrograde catheter.

By assuming that the pressure in the bronchus where the catheter is wedged is representative of the pressure in all other bronchi of a similar size, lower pulmonary resistance may be partitioned into two components. The central resistance Rc is made up of all airways from the trachea down to the airways of the same size as that in which the catheter is wedged. The peripheral resistance, Rp consists of the resistance from those airways to the alveoli plus the tissue viscous resistance.

The technique by which the pulmonary resistance is partitioned is shown in Figure 2. The lungs are enclosed in a plethysmograph from which volume is obtained. They are oscillated rapidly by a loud speaker powered by a variable frequency sine wave generator. A pneumotachograph placed between the loud speaker and the trachea measures flow. The loud speaker is in an enclosed chamber which is pressurized with air. The air leaks through the speaker cones and inflates the lungs to any desired transpulmonary pressure. The resistance is therefore partitioned at a variety of transpulmonary pressures. The pressure difference, as measured between the catheter and the pleural surface, contains an elastic component which is

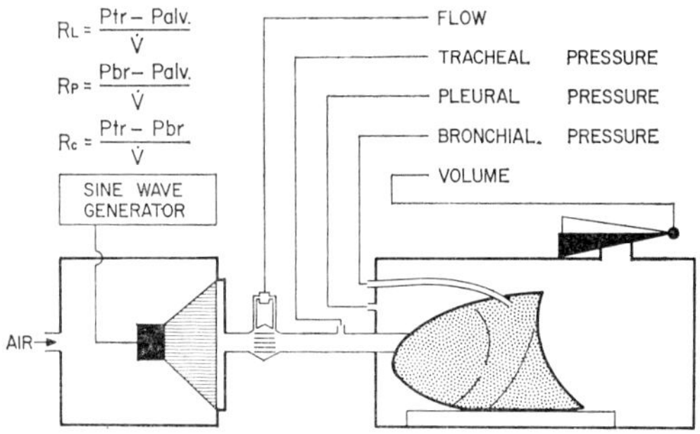

FIG. 2. Circuit diagram illustrating technique for partitioning pulmonary resistance, RL, into a peripheral component, Rp, and a central component, Rc. Ptr = tracheal pressure. Palv = alveolar pressure. Pbr = bronchial pressure. $\dot{V}$ = flow.

electrically subtracted either by a signal proportional to volume (Mead & Whittenberger, 1953) or acceleration (obtained by differentiating flow). The resultant is the difference between bronchial and alveolar pressure which is divided by flow to obtain Rp. Rc is the difference in pressure between the catheter tip and the trachea divided by flow. This pressure difference contains an inertial component which is also electrically subtracted. Pulmonary resistance, RL, is the sum of Rp and Rc. In these studies the bronchus in which the catheter was measuring pressure was identified either by bronchography or by cutting down on the catheter at postmortem. The internal diameter of the bronchus was generally 2–3 mm.

Results obtained from two catheters in a normal lung are shown in Figure 3. Rp obtained with a catheter in the 9th generation and the 12th generation (lobar bronchus equals generation 1) and RL are shown plotted against transpulmonary pressure. The whole lung section is in Figure 6. Rp is only a small component of RL particularly with the catheter in the 12th generation. Mean values ± 2 S.E. of nine catheters in four normal lungs are shown in Figure 4. Again Rp is a small percentage of RL. At a distending pressure of 5 cm. H_2O, Rp only averages about 0·2 cm. H_2O/lps.

Because Rp is a small component of RL, there can be considerable obstruction present in the peripheral airways which could markedly

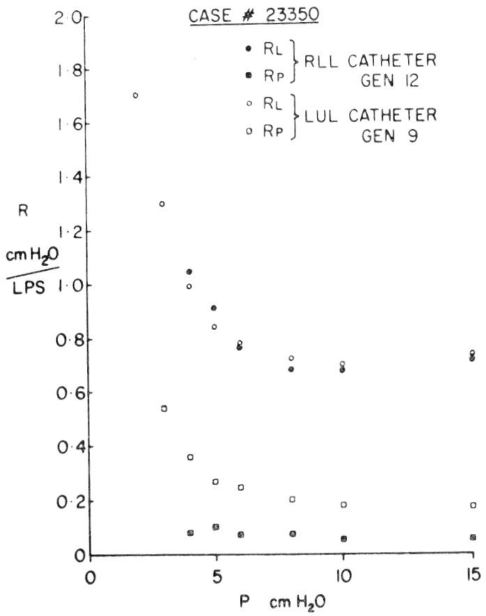

FIG. 3. RL and Rp at different transpulmonary pressures in a normal lung. Results obtained with one catheter in the 9th generation and another in the 12th generation are shown. Lobar bronchus = generation 1.

□ = Rp obtained with the catheter in the 9th generation.

■ = Rp obtained with the catheter in the 12th generation.

○ = RL obtained by adding Rp and Rc with the catheter in the 9th generation.

● = RL obtained by adding Rp and Rc with the catheter in the 12th generation.

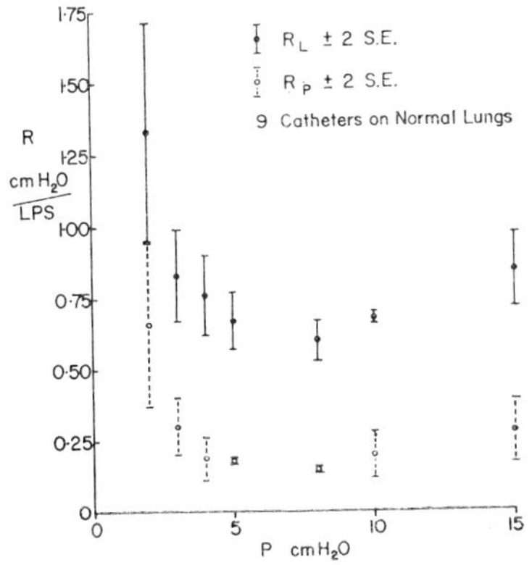

FIG. 4. Mean values ±2 S.E. of RL and Rp in 5 normal lungs.

influence ventilation distribution but would only have a minor effect on RL. As an extreme example, if one-half of the peripheral airways became obstructed in a randomly distributed manner, Rp would double. Because Rp is only 0·2 cm. H_2O/lps, RL would only increase by 0·2 cm H_2O/lps, an effect that would be difficult to measure with confidence. However, the airways to one-half of the lung would be blocked and the units peripheral to the obstruction could only be ventilated by collateral flow.

That such a situation may well occur at some stage of chronic obstructive lung disease is suggested by the results we obtained when he retrograde catheter technique was applied to lungs of patients

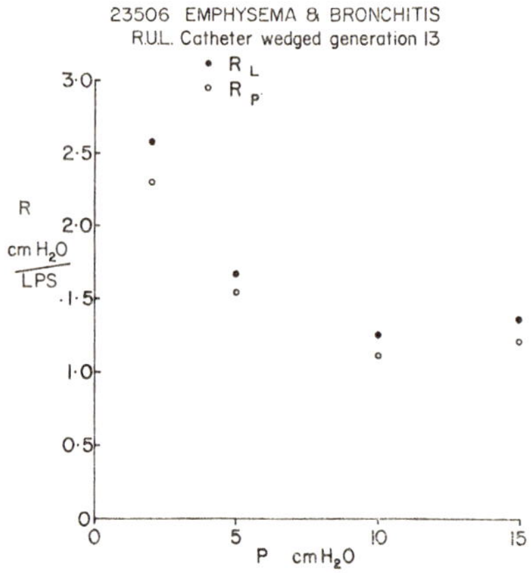

FIG. 5. RL and Rp at different transpulmonary pressures in the lungs of a patient dying with emphysema. The retrograde catheter was in the 13th generation.

● = RL ○ = Rp

Table 1. *Resistance at transpulmonary pressure of 5 cm. H_2O*

	Rp cm. H_2O/lps	Rc cm. H_2O/lps	$\frac{Rp}{RL} \times 100$
Normal mean ± 2 S.E.	0·18 ± 0·01	0·49 ± 0·09	27 ± 4
Emphysema + bronchitis	7·50	1·05	88
Emphysema + bronchitis	1·67	0·55	75
Emphysema + bronchitis	2·10	0·06	92
Emphysema + bronchitis	2·42	2·42	65
Bronchiectasis	3·00	0·62	83

Rp—peripheral resistance Rc—central resistance
RL—pulmonary resistance

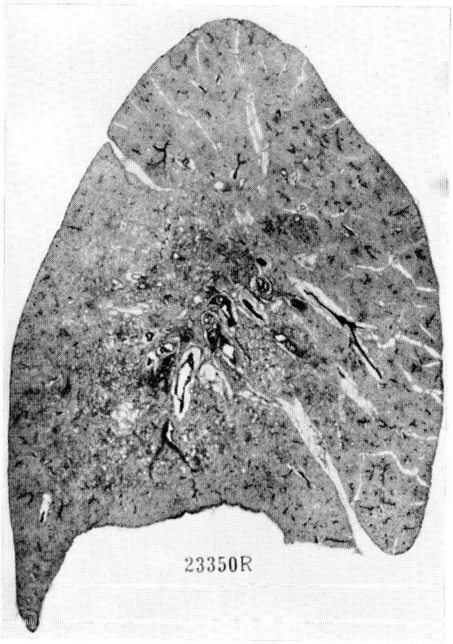

FIG. 6. Giant section of the lungs studied in Figure 3.

[*To face page* 80

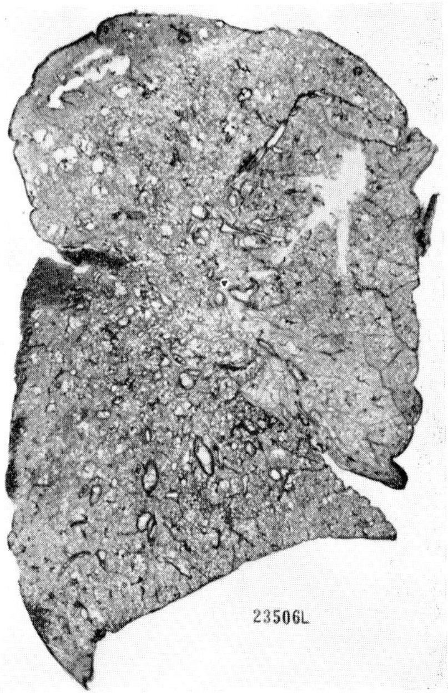

FIG. 7. Giant section of the lungs studied in Figure 5.

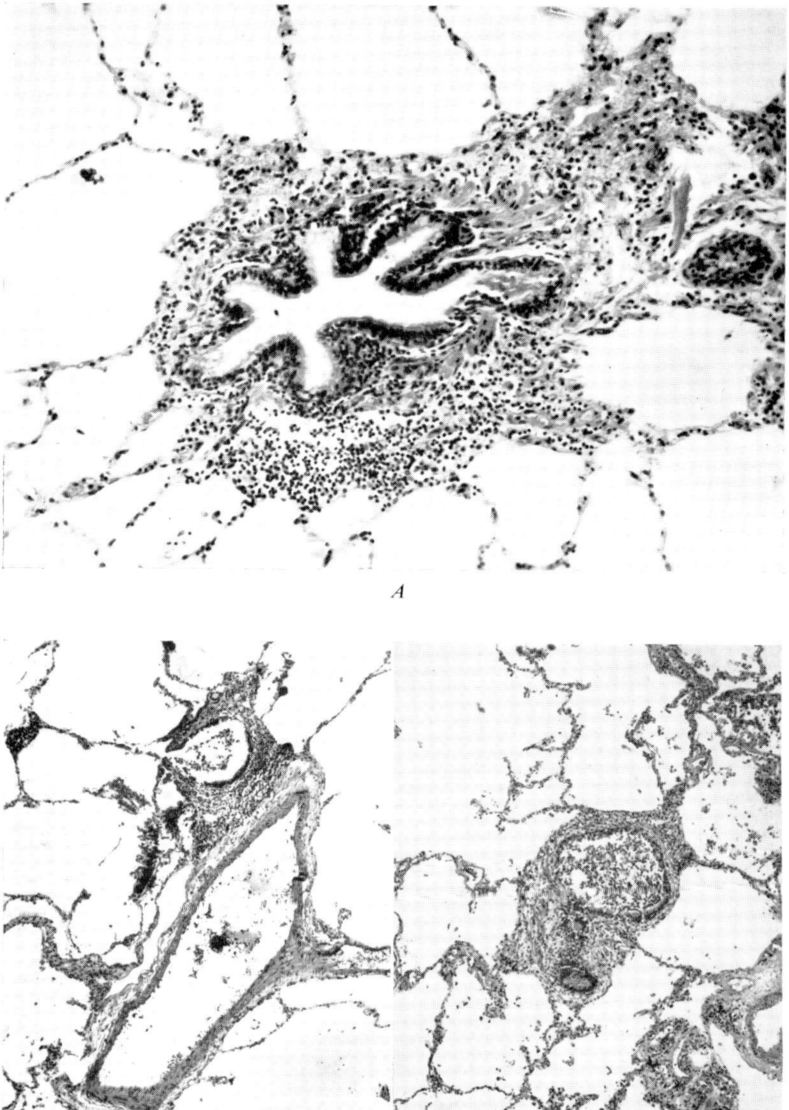

A

B *C*

FIG. 8. Examples of the morphology of small airway disease seen in lungs with an abnormally high Rp.
A. Peribronchiolar cellular infiltrate and infolding of bronchiolar walls.
B. Broncholar stenosis.
C. Mucus plug in bronchiole.

dying with emphysema and bronchitis. Figure 5 is a plot of RL and Rp at different transpulmonary pressures in the lungs of such a patient; Figure 7 is the whole lung section in this case. In this instance Rp which ranged between 1·2 and 2·3 cm. H_2O/lps made up most of RL. In Table 1, the measured values of Rp, Rc, and Rp as a percentage of RL are listed at a transpulmonary pressure of 5 cm. H_2O in the lungs of four patients dying of emphysema and one patient dying of bronchiectasis. The mean values ± 2 SE. for normal lung are also indicated. In every case Rp was markedly increased, ranging from 9 to 42 times the normal value comprising from 65 to 92 per cent. of RL. The values obtained for Rc scattered around the normal range. From these results it appears that the site of obstruction in obstructive lung disease is in airways smaller than about 2 mm. in diameter. It is not due to loss of elasticity because both normal and diseased lungs were studied at equal distending pressures. Neither is it due to a localised loss of alveolar support around bronchioles. If airways obstruction were due to this hypothetical situation, peribronchiolar pressure could approximate alveolar rather than pleural pressure (Hyatt & Flath, 1966). If this occurs, Rp will be low during inflation and high during deflation. We could detect no significant difference between the inflation and deflation slope of the pressure flow curve for the peripheral airways. In all cases, histological study of the lungs has indicated lesions in the small airways which explains the increase in Rp. These lesions are illustrated in Figure 8 *A*, showing a bronchiole with a marked peribronchiolar cellular infiltrate and considerable infolding of the bronchiolar wall (in spite of the fact that the lung was fixed in inflation). Figure 8 *B* is an example of a stenotic bronchiole (its lumen is considerably smaller than the neighbouring arteriole), while *C* shows a bronchiole containing a mucous plug. The small airway disease, therefore, appears to have three components, chronic inflammation, stenosis and mucous plugging. These lesions were clearly described several years ago by McLean (1958). He also stated that many small airways were completely obliterated—a suggestion which is supported by our investigations which indicate that the total number of peripheral airways may be decreased.

THE MEASUREMENT OF RESISTANCE TO COLLATERAL FLOW

When airways are completely obstructed the airspaces distal to the obstruction can only be ventilated via collateral channels. We have been unable to investigate this on a lobular basis, but have done so on a lobar and segmental basis. The technique by which this is done is shown in Figure 9. A Foley catheter is placed in the lower

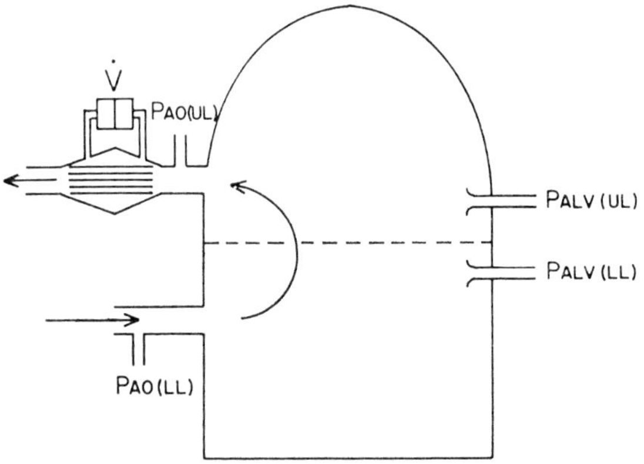

$$R_{LL} = \frac{P_{AO(LL)} - P_{ALV(LL)}}{\dot{V}}$$

$$R_{COL} = \frac{P_{ALV(LL)} - P_{ALV(UL)}}{\dot{V}}$$

$$R_{UL} = \frac{P_{ALV(UL)} - P_{AO(UL)}}{\dot{V}}$$

FIG. 9. Circuit diagram illustrating technique used to measure collateral flow resistance.

PAO (LL) = pressure in lower lobe bronchus
PALV (LL) = alveolar pressure in lower lobe
PALV (UL) = alveolar pressure in upper lobe
PAO (UL) = pressure in upper lobe bronchus
RLL = resistance of lower lobe airways
RUL = resistance of upper lobe airways
RCOL = resistance to collateral flow between upper and lower lobes
$\dot{V}$ = flow.

lobe bronchus and the balloon inflated. The upper lobe bronchus is left open to atmosphere through a pneumotachograph. A retrograde catheter is tied directly into the parenchyma of both the upper and lower lobes, through a small hole made in the pleural surface. The lower lobe is inflated via the Foley catheter, air leaks through collateral channels extending across an incomplete fissure and out the upper lobe airways. This collateral flow is measured by the pneumotachograph. The resistance of the lower lobe airways is the pressure difference between the tip of the Foley catheter and the lower lobe alveoli divided by the flow. The resistance of the collateral channels is the pressure difference between the lower and upper lobe alveoli divided by flow ; the resistance of the upper lobe airways is the pressure difference between the upper lobe alveoli and the atmosphere, divided by flow.

When this experiment is performed in normal lungs, the lower lobe inflates and flow is recorded from the upper lobe bronchus but the upper lobe remains completely deflated. Under the conditions of the experiment there is a virtually undetectable pressure difference along both upper and lower lobe airways whereas the pressure difference between the lobes is large. In emphysematous lungs, a quite different phenomenon is observed. When the lower lobe is inflated,

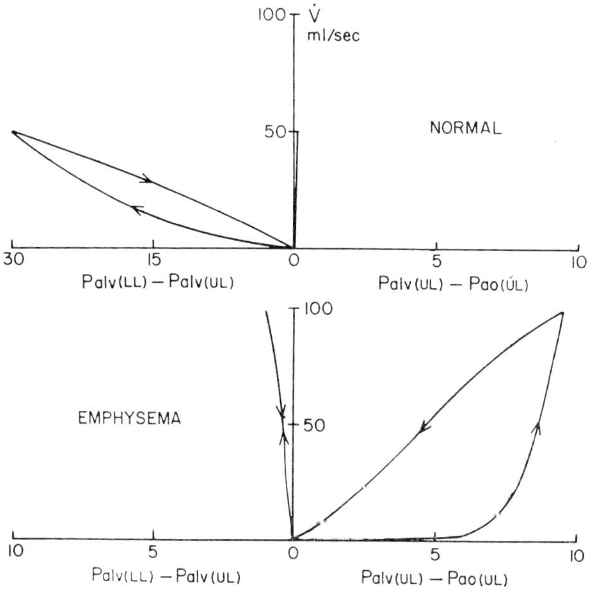

FIG. 10. Pressure-flow curves for collateral channels and upper lobe airways in a normal lung (upper panel) and an emphysematous lung (lower panel). The pressure-flow curves for the collateral channels are plotted to the left of the ordinate and for the upper lobe airways to the right of the ordinate. The symbols are the same as those used in Figure 9.

the upper lobe inflates also. Even though it appears to be fully inflated, in some instances no flow can be recorded from the upper lobe bronchus. In two such cases which we have observed, the airways to the upper lobe were completely obstructed and air easily entered the upper lobe via collateral channels.

Examples of the pressure-flow curves that we have obtained in a normal and an emphysematous lung are shown in Figure 10. The upper set of curves was obtained in the normal lung whereas the lower set was obtained in the lung with emphysema. The pressure-flow curves to the left of the ordinate are the pressure-flow relationships of the collateral channels. On the right of the ordinate are the pressure-flow curves for the upper lobe airways. In the normal lung the resistance of the collateral channels is large and at a flow rate of 50 ml./sec. it is 600 cm. H_2O/lps. Under the conditions of the experiment the resistance of the upper lobe airways was so small that it could not be accurately measured. In the emphysematous lung, the resistance of the collateral channels is much smaller than the normal and is also smaller than the resistance of the upper lobe airways. In fact, no air flowed out of the upper lobe until the upper lobe was distended to a pressure of 5 cm. H_2O. At this point flow started but even when the pressure in the upper lobe was 10 cm. H_2O, flow was only 100 ml./sec. At this value for flow the resistance of the collateral channels was 10 cm. H_2O/lps whereas it was 80 cm. H_2O/lps in the upper lobe airways.

Table 2. *Resistance to collateral flow*

	R coll. cm. H_2O/lps lower to upper lobe	R coll. cm. H_2O/lps basal to apical segment	Rul. cm. H_2O/lps
Normal	2000	560	0+
,,	200	400	0+
,,	–	80	0+*
,,	600	–	0+
,,	3000	–	0+
,,	150	–	0+
Emphysema	10	16	80
,,	20	–	10
,,	?	–	∞
,,	?	–	∞

R coll.—Resistance to collateral flow
Rul —Resistance of upper lobe airways
* —Resistance of apical segment airways
– —No measurement available

The structural abnormality responsible for this marked decrease in collateral flow resistance is shown in Figure 11. The fissure separating the apical segment of the lower lobe from the adjacent

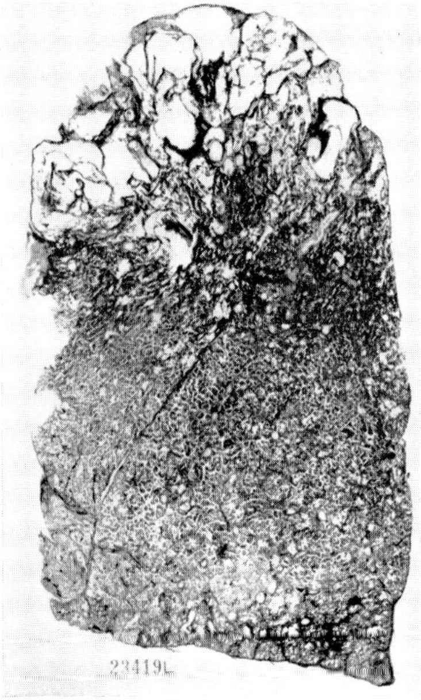

FIG. 11. Giant section of the emphysematous lung studied in Figure 10.

[*To face page* 84

upper lobe segment is incomplete and a loose network of destroyed parenchyma extends across it. These spaces are presumably the collateral channels and it is quite reasonable to expect that air would flow easily from one lobe to the next.

A summary of all the results obtained to date is shown in Table 2. Values for collateral flow resistance between lobes, and in some instances from the basal to apical segments of the lower lobe, are shown for both normal and emphysematous lungs. Also shown are the values for the resistance of the upper lobe airways. In the normal lungs the collateral flow resistance between lobe and between segments was, as might be expected, highly variable, ranging between 80 and 3,000 cm. H_2O/lps. However, in all instances it was much greater than the values obtained in emphysema.

The resistance of the normal upper lobe airways is designated as 0+. This is because the flow rates through them were so small, that almost no pressure differences could be measured. Quite clearly these airways have a finite value for resistance, but it is very small compared to the collateral flow resistance. The upper lobe airway resistances measured in emphysema are strikingly high. These measurements bear no simple relationship to total airway resistance, however, as we are measuring the resistance of less than a quarter of the total number of airways and in some instances we are measuring the resistance of airways which are more severely obstructed than the remaining ones.

The two instances where the upper lobe airway resistance is shown as infinite were the two cases in which the upper lobe inflated easily from the lower lobe, but no air flow was recorded from the upper lobe bronchus. Although no estimate could be made of collateral flow resistance, it is quite clear that it was considerably less than the resistance to flow through the upper lobe airways. Collateral flow resistance was less than upper lobe resistance in a *third* lung with emphysema. When collateral flow resistance falls to the extent that it is less than the airway resistance, ventilation of the parenchyma must be primarily via the collateral channels—a situation that is hardly conducive to efficient gas exchange. Although we do not think that the *in vitro* results of collateral flow resistance between lobes can be readily applied to the lung *in situ*, it does appear likely that *interlobular* collateral flow may play a very important role in ventilating emphysematous *lobules* whose airways are severely stenotic and plugged with mucus.

THE DETECTION OF SMALL AIRWAY DISEASE DURING LIFE

The obstruction to flow during quiet breathing in obstructive lung disease is clearly in the small airways. When the disease is advanced this is easy to detect. Can it be detected in the early stages? If it is true that there may be considerable obstruction in peripheral airways with little effect on RL and if static elastic properties of lungs remain normal, then there is no reason to suspect that

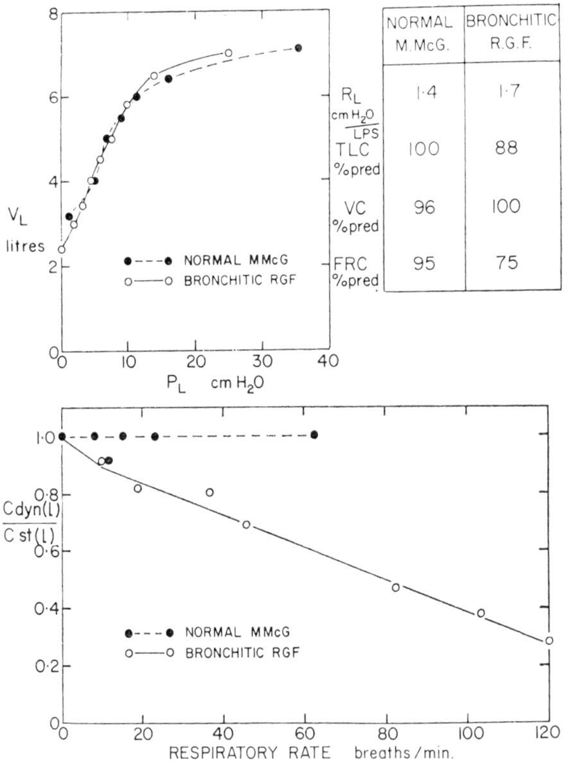

	NORMAL M.McG.	BRONCHITIC R.G.F.
RL cm H_2O/LPS	1·4	1·7
TLC %pred	100	88
VC %pred	96	100
FRC %pred	95	75

FIG. 12. Upper right: Pulmonary resistance and subdivision of lung volume in a normal subject, MMG, and a mild bronchitic, RGF. Upper left: Static pressure–volume curves in the two subjects.
Lower panel: Dynamic compliance, Cdyn(l), expressed as a fraction of static compliance, Cst(l), at different respiratory frequencies in the two subjects.

routine tests of lung function should be deranged. What other means are available to detect the abnormality? Anthonisen *et al.* have shown that bronchitics with almost normal maximal expiratory flow rates have grossly disturbed regional washout of ^{133}Xe. Their results are certainly compatible with small airway disease that affects ventilation distribution more than airway resistance. Figure 12 is an example of the results we, along with Dr Ann Woolcock, have obtained in studying the mechanical properties of the lungs in such patients. Subject RGF is a mild bronchitic who produces a small amount of sputum and who feels slightly dyspneic after two flights of stairs. He has never seen a physician for these complaints. The mechanical properties of his lungs are compared with a normal subject, MMG, who was approximately the same age and height. The panel at the upper left shows that the static deflation pressure–volume curves for both subjects are virtually identical. R_L in MMG was 1·4 cm. H_2O/lps, whereas it was 1·7 cm. H_2O/lps in RGF. Neither was hyperinflated. These results in both subjects are normal. However, when compliance is examined at different respiratory frequencies marked differences are observed. This is shown in the bottom panel. In the normal subject, MMG, there was no effect of frequency on compliance, but in the bronchitic, compliance was markedly frequency-dependent falling to less than 30 per cent. of the static value at a respiratory frequency of 120/min. These results are similar to others obtained in several mild bronchitics that we have studied. The theoretical basis for interpreting these results has been worked out in detail previously (Otis *et al.*, 1956). Compliance will be frequency-dependent if there are regional inequalities of elastic recoil or of airway resistance or both. If the static pressure–volume curve of the lung is within normal limits, marked frequency-dependence cannot be ascribed to inequalities of elastic recoil. The disease must therefore be located in the airways. If the obstruction were in central airways there should be a marked increase in airway resistance because these airways contribute over 70 per cent. of the total. Thus, when elasticity and airway resistance are normal yet compliance is frequency-dependent, it is difficult to imagine what morphologic abnormality could account for these findings other than obstruction in small airways.

It is likely, then, that considerable small airways obstruction can be present which will not result in abnormal routine lung function tests but will lead to unequal distribution of ventilation. It is only when the lung is stressed by increasing respiratory frequency that the obstruction becomes apparent. Alternatively, more sensitive tests of regional lung function using ^{133}Xe are able to detect the abnormality.

Whether or not other tests which measure ventilation distribution can do so is currently under investigation.

SUMMARY

On the basis of these studies it seems reasonable to conclude that :
1. In the early stages of chronic obstructive airway disease the distribution of ventilation is disturbed before there is much change in airway resistance.
2. This abnormality results from obstruction in small airways which do not normally contribute much to R_L.
3. In the end stage of chronic obstructive airway disease, the degree of obstruction in small airways is more severe than had previously been realised.
4. The small airway disease is due to chronic inflammation, stenosis and mucous plugging.
5. When emphysema co-exists with small airway disease, the ventilation of parenchyma subtended by severely obstructed airways may be predominantly by collateral channels.

ACKNOWLEDGEMENTS

We thank Miss N. J. Wilson for her expert technical assistance. Figures 1, 2, 3 and 4 are reproduced by kind permission of the editor of Journal of Applied Physiology.

DISCUSSION OF SESSION TWO

Dr Horsfield. References to the bronchial tree in some of our discussions today have implied that it is a symmetrical structure having the same number of divisions down and the same path length from the trachea to each terminal unit or acinus. However, the bronchial tree is, in fact, an asymmetrical structure (Fig. 1) with

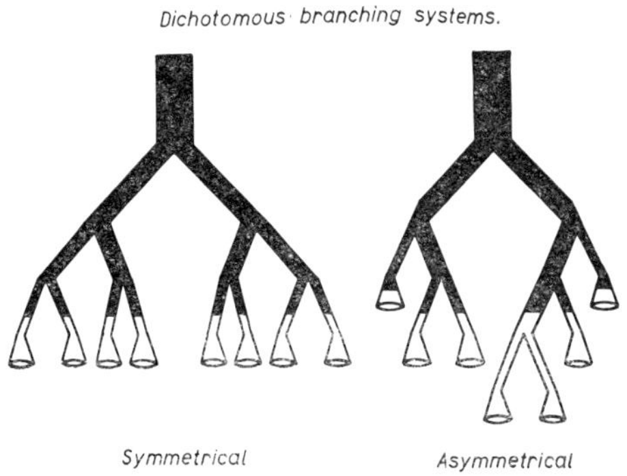

FIG. 1. Models of the bronchial tree. In the symmetrical model there is the same number of divisions between the carina and acini (represented as cones), and the pathways to the acini are all of the same length. In the asymmetrical model the number of divisions and the path lengths vary. An inspirate of a gas is represented in black. It has reached similar points in the branches of the symmetrical model, but in the asymmetrical model it is unequally distributed in the peripheral part of the tree.

a variation in the number of divisions down from the carina to the different acini. The range of divisions down, as ascertained from a study of a resin cast of a normal bronchial tree, is 8 to the nearest acinus and as many as 32 to the most distal acinus. So to talk in terms of divisions down is misleading and I think we must in future mention the specific diameters of the bronchi we are studying, because at 9 divisions down you can have anything from alveolar ducts to bronchi several millimetres in diameter. There is, in addition, quite a wide range of path lengths, from 7 cm. to the nearest acinus to about 24 cm. to the most distal acinus. Clearly this is going to have some effect on the distribution of ventilation because, if we take in a breath of gas (shown in black in Fig. 1), it will enter the most proximal acini long before it reaches the most distal ones.

To make an estimate of how this will affect the distribution of ventilation, we compute the transit time which is a function of the gas flow down the branch and its dimensions. To do this, we make certain assumptions which are not strictly correct, viz. that the gas flow is proportional to the volume of lung supplied by that branch, and that all areas of the lungs expand equally and synchronously. If we now measure every pathway down to every acinus (a total of approximately 10,000 branches) we can plot, in arbitrary units, the frequency distribution of the transit times from the carina to the various acini. We then find (Fig. 2) that the most proximal acini are reached after about 150 transit time units and the most distal after about 800.

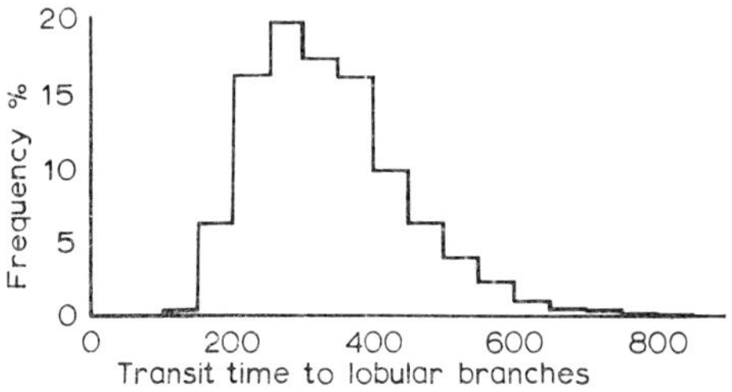

FIG. 2 The frequency distribution of computed transit times between the carina and the lobular branches. The calculations were based on measurements of a resin cast of the bronchial tree, the lobular branches being of 0·4 to 0·7 mm. diameter. Transit time is in arbitrary units.

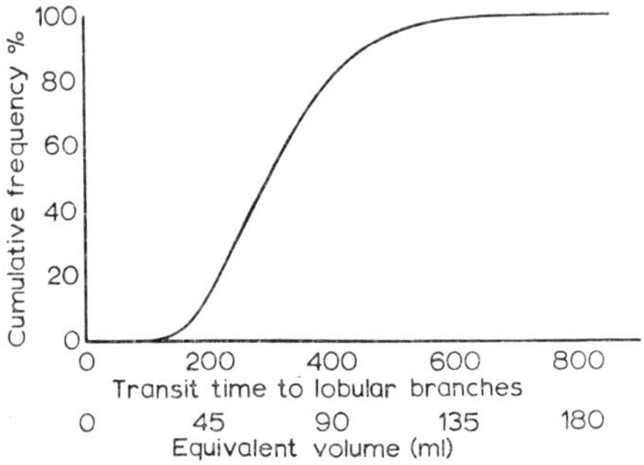

FIG. 3. A cumulative frequency plot of transit times from the same data as Figure 2. The volume equivalent of the transit times is also given on the x axis.

Next, we convert the transit times into inspired volumes. Figure 3 shows the same data as Figure 2 but plotted cumulatively and with the volumes equivalent to the transit times shown on the x-axis. If the gas front is situated initially at the carina and inspiration then proceeds, the front will reach the most proximal acini after 22 ml.

have been inspired and the most distal 170 ml. later in the inspirate. Thus the most proximal acini will receive more of the inspired gas, the distal ones less. If we inspired a litre of oxygen into a lung of 2,500 ml. FRC this will produce a range of 4 per cent. in the calculated alveolar concentrations of nitrogen.

Dr Muir. Dr Cumming has stressed the importance of molecular diffusion in the transport of gases in the airways of the lung. It was first shown by Altshuler *et al.* (1959) that inhaled aerosol particles with a low coefficient of diffusion did not mix with the alveolar air to the same extent as gases during steady state breathing. This effect can also be seen by comparing the distribution of 0·5 μ diameter particles in the exhaled air following a single inspiration of 600 ml. of aerosol, with that of an insoluble gas such as Argon following a single inspiration of 600 ml. of the gas. (Fig. 4). The shape of the two curves is completely different and the end-exhaled air is virtually free of particles. It can be concluded from this result that the transport of gases in the alveolar region of the lung depends on molecular diffusion.

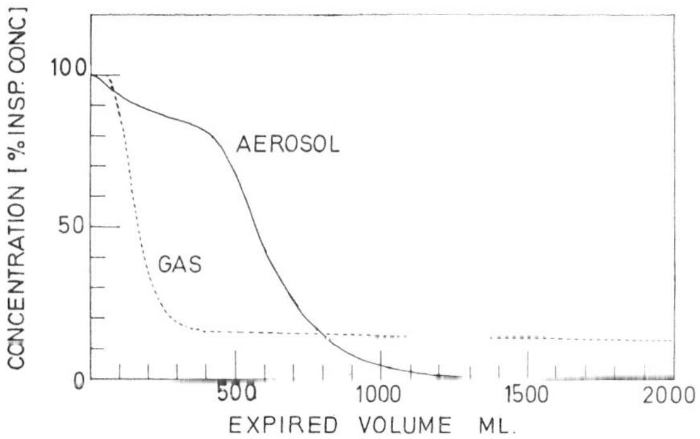

FIG. 4.

Dr Leopold. Some years ago, Drs Reid and Simon realised that the clinical and post-mortem bronchogram provided clinicians and pathologists with the means of observing many of the detailed features of lung histopathology that have been mentioned at this conference. Leopold and Gough (1963) published some of the results from their use of lead dust as the radiopaque material with which to coat the surfaces of bronchi and bronchioles and obtain highly-detailed post-mortem bronchograms. An unpublished aspect of this work has an important connection with the study carried out by Reid and Simon (1958). One feature of their publication was that it drew attention to the branching interval as an index to level in the bronchiolar system : a change in branching interval from one of ½–1 cm. to one of 1–2 cm. marked the level of the terminal bronchioles. Compared with the semi-fluid barium sulphate injections used by Reid, lead dust has shown greater detail at this peripheral level in the bronchogram. I find that the first branches separated by intervals of millimetre magnitude are often respiratory bronchioles and not terminal bronchioles. In our hands Microtrast paste (barium sulphate) gives the appearance at the periphery of the post-mortem bronchogram shown in Figure 5. The finest branches, which are separated from their neighbours by intervals of approximately 2 mm., show no structural detail. Their outline does not differ from that of more proximal bronchioles. The lead bronchogram shows comparable branches but, in contrast, these show the protrusions and feathery outlines which we have established by histological control to be due to the presence of alveoli (Fig. 6). If, however, there is a difference of opinion between myself and Reid and Simon concerning the level of the first millimetre branches it is of little importance and, as she has found and I too confirm, the level is subject to variation. However, I most strongly disagree with her statement that in a ‘ well-filled normal ’ clinical bronchogram all orders of respiratory bronchioles, etc. are usually free from contrast medium, because it serves to obscure the fact that when branches in a bronchogram (clinical or post-mortem) arise at such short interval as a millimetre or so, much of the contrast medium has entered the field of respiratory tissue ; depicted are the structures which show abnormality when emphysema exists.

Centrilobular spaces of emphysema are revealed in clinical and post-mortem bronchograms (Leopold & Seal, 1961 ; Leopold & Gough, 1963). The latter conclusion is supported by Wyatt *et al.*, (1961), who blew crystalline Micro-opaque into the lung. My lead bronchograms also differentiate between normal respiratory tissue and that affected by panacinar emphysema (compare Figs. 6 and 7).

My final comment concerns the anatomical state of the main conductive airways in chronic bronchitis. Much has been said at this meeting of the gross disturbance in pulmonary function that can result from chronic bronchitis. Notable is a considerably increased resistance to airflow. In a comparison of the post-mortem bronchograms of lungs with chronic bronchitis with the bronchograms of non-bronchitic controls, the most consistent abnormality I have found has been widespread (if only of modest degree) tubular bronchial and bronchiolar dilatation, not stenosis or stricture. Of course, ‘ the broken bough ’ appearance is seen in the post-mortem,

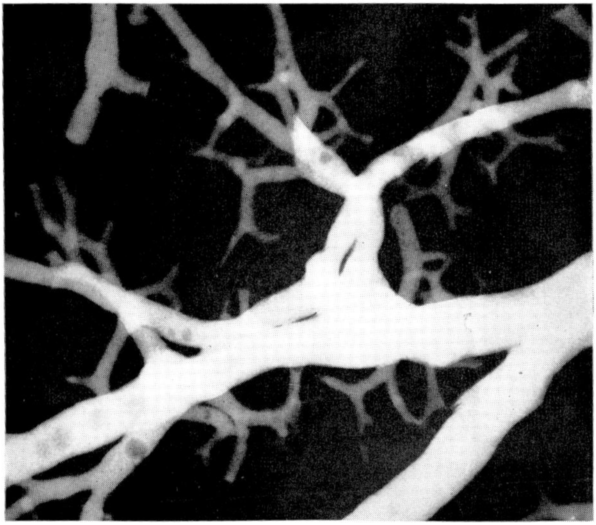

FIG. 5. Area of Microtrast bronchogram. Normal lung. The small branches with a short interval between divisions show no special morphological feature. Magn ×3.

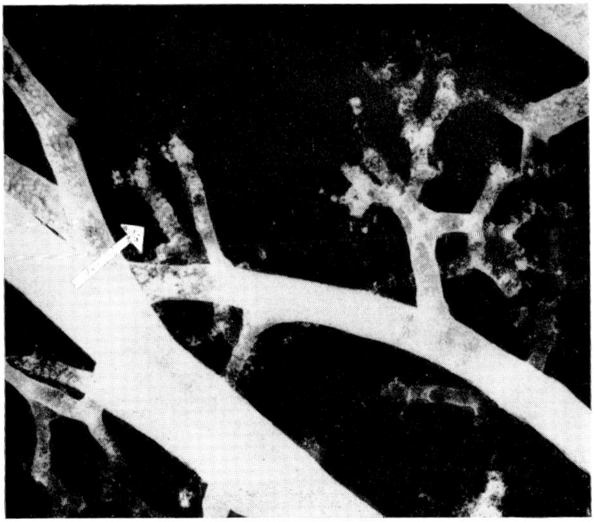

FIG. 6. Area of lead dust bronchogram. Normal lung. The branches separated by short intervals show alveoli, recognised as protrusions (see arrow) or as a feathery stippling of the bronchiole. Magn ×3.

[*To face page* 92

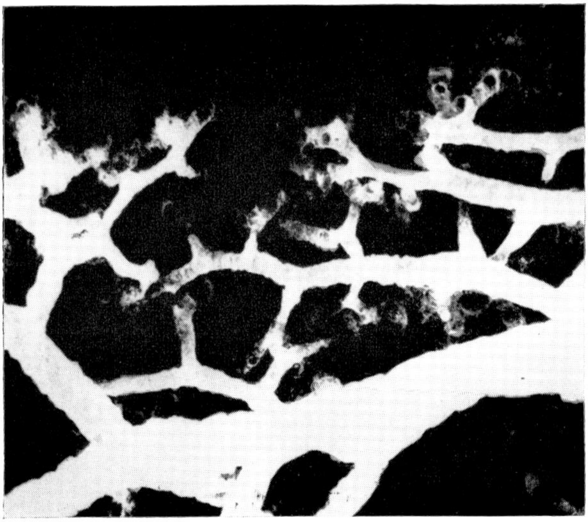

FIG. 7. Area of lead dust bronchogram. Dock labourer of 56 yr. with chronic bronchitis and slight panacinar emphysema. The respiratory bronchioles resemble a chain of soap bubbles. Magn ×3.

as in the clinical, bronchogram. It is interpreted as due to bronchial blockage by secretions : a state which we know in asthma can remain unrelieved for long periods (Sanerkin *et al.*, 1966).

Chairman. I have a question for Dr Cumming. Have you done any calculations assuming the area of the base of the model, the distance to the alveolar membrane, the time, the specific diffusibility of carbon dioxide and oxygen and the temperature—the relevant factors governing transfer—to find whether in fact the appropriate quantities of oxygen can get across ?

Dr Cumming. We are at the moment engaged in trying to find out whether gas transfer from the alveolar space into the blood is restricted at all, in rate and in quantity, by gaseous mixing within the airways. We're not in a position at the moment to make any comment about this but the indication is that, if the molecule of gas can get to the alveolar surface, the transfer function across the membrane is the same as in health, but the difficulty is in getting the molecules of gas to the alveolar surface.

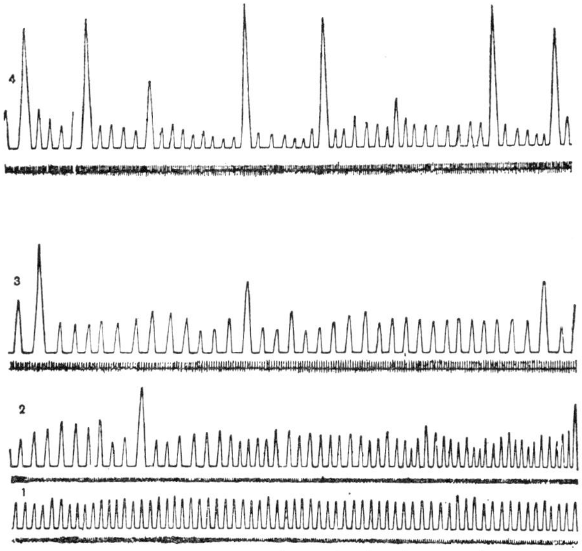

FIG. 8. Subject J.G.P. Concertina 'unlimited. Time marker = seconds. (1) Sitting. (2) Lying. (3) Sitting, with corsets. (4) Lying, with corsets.

Dr Filley. This whole question of series versus parallel (or in other words, stratified versus regional) is really a very old story. August Krogh's work in 1914 has been mentioned with regard to the idea that the lung has non-uniformity in series though Krogh did not draw the lung to illustrate this idea. Now Haldane (1919) didn't draw the lung, either. In contrast to modern physiologists who sketch the lung on the blackboard quite often and quite casually, it's very interesting that neither Krogh nor Haldane drew models. They thought about the lung (rather than drawing it) in terms of a series type of model which, at the present time, has tremendous clinical implications. To illustrate this point I present a reproduction (Fig. 8) of four spirometer tracings of the breathing pattern of J. S. Haldane's favourite ' guinea-pig,' Dr J. G. Priestley before and after his breathing was restricted by experimentally applied corsets. (These results were reported in Haldane's classic paper on ' The Effects of Shallow Breathing ', 1919). In tracing 1, the subject is seated and he spontaneously breathes at constant frequency and tidal volume. Lying down, a position known to be associated with an elevated position of the diaphragm at end expiration, is also associated with some irregularity of rate and an occasional sigh as in tracing 2. When corsets are applied to chest or abdomen (tracing 3), the breathing becomes either shallow or deep as the subject reacts to the restrictions imposed by the corsets. In tracing 4 the constriction

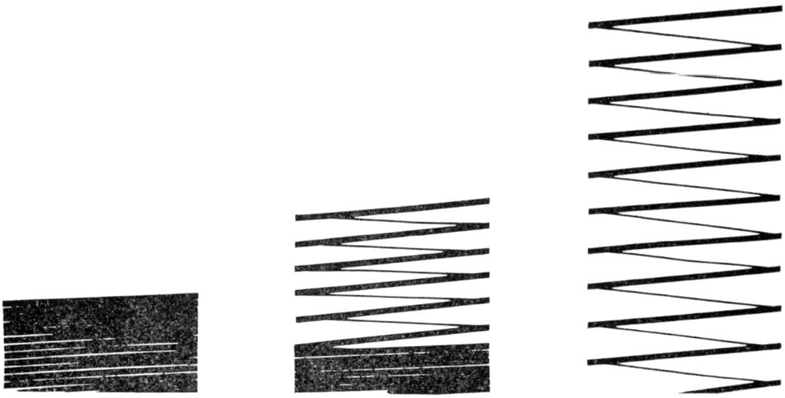

FIG. 9.

of corsets and recumbency produces a pattern of intermittent very deep breaths. Although Haldane did not use the phrase, it is clear from his paper that he visualised Priestley's need to ' open up the bases of the lungs ' as the cause of this breathing pattern.

It is only in the past few years that mechanical respirators designed for use in recumbent patients in respiratory failure have been programmed to administer a 'periodic deep breath' in order to prevent the alveolar collapse and $\dot{V}/\dot{Q}$ disturbances which were inferred by Haldane to result from shallow breathing. I think a case can be made for thinking about the lung as a transport organ which operates primarily with series non-uniformities rather than drawing it as a blackboard caricature with non-uniformities in parallel. The functional configuration of the lung seems to be more like a 'slinky spring' (Fig. 9) than like a bunch of grapes.

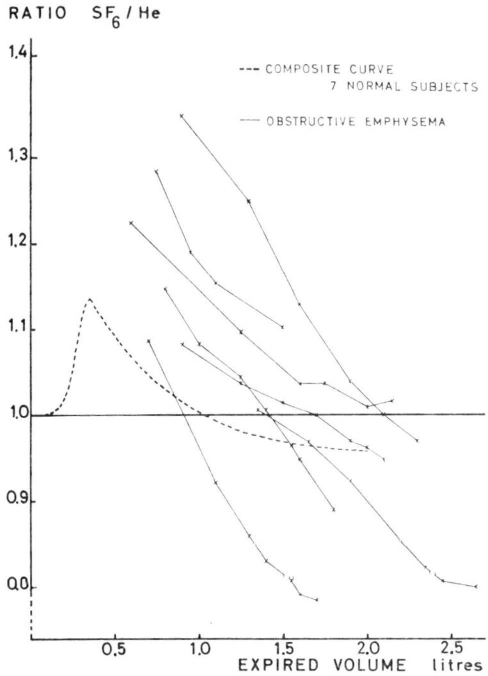

Fig. 10. The ratio SF_6/He in the expired air collected during a maximal expiration following a normal inspiration of a mixture containing the two gases. (Reprinted by permission from Clinical Science.)

Dr Georg. Some years ago we had the opportunity to carry out a series of experiments in many ways similar to the one described to you by Dr Cumming. We used He, Ne and SF_6 as inert tracers of widely different molecular weight and tried to demonstrate differences in their behaviour in the airways. Any such disparity must be caused by differences in diffusion velocity (Georg *et al.*, 1965).

The subjects were, at the end of a normal expiration, made to inhale about 500 ml. of a mixture of these three gases, and asked to exhale to residual volume immediately afterwards. Five to seven fractionated samples of the expired air were taken for analysis. In the normal subject it was always found that the first part of the expirate contained relatively more of the heaviest gas, whereas the last part contained more of the lightest gas. In emphysematous subjects the first part of the expirate contained the heavy gas in even higher proportions, and often it was not possible to obtain samples of expired air in which the lighter gas was predominating. The findings are depicted in Figure 10.

We took this to indicate that diffusion does occur in the airways proper in normal subjects, and that the diffusion space is likely to be greater in the emphysematous subjects, giving rise to a comparatively higher ratio of heavy to light gas in the first part of the expirate. Furthermore the experiment shows that some emphysematous subjects are not able to expire gas from the deeper parts of the lungs in which the lighter gas must have diffused out to a greater extent than the heavier gas.

As the volume of the larger bronchi is unlikely to be much different in normal and emphysematous subjects, the findings seem to be caused by a longitudinal diffusion in the bronchial tree rather than by a lateral diffusion in the major airways. The impossibility of obtaining representative samples of alveolar air in emphysematous subjects is also underlined by these findings. For this reason it has seemed to us unlikely that further approaches along the same lines would lead to new data, and we have tried instead to approach the problem from the alveolar side. The two inert gases krypton and hydrogen, employed as the isotopes ^{85}Kr and ^{3}H (tritium), have been used as indicators (Mellemgaard *et al.*, 1962).

When injected intravenously in saline these gases will to a large extent leave the blood in the alveoli on account of their very low solubility, only a small amount appearing in the arterial blood. Two factors contribute to this arterial recovery : right-to-left shunt and alveolar back pressure. The blood–gas partition coefficient of krypton is about 0·064 and that of tritium about 0·017. Thus if the same alveolar space is available to the two gases and all the gas injected comes into contact with the alveolar air, we shall expect the two gases to appear in the arterial blood in the proportion of $Kr/T_2 = \frac{0{\cdot}064}{0{\cdot}017} = 3{\cdot}8$ (or, with a small correction for loss with the blood, 3·7).

If the gases do not get into contact with alveolar air, *i.e.* are shunted from right to left, the proportion will be the one in which they are injected, by definition =1. The proportions of 1 and 3·7 are thus the two extremes between which we shall expect our recoveries to be placed. The nearer 3·7, the smaller the shunt; the nearer 1, the bigger the shunt. The simultaneous employment of these two gases enables us to get a reliable estimate of the true right-to-left shunt.

In Figure 11 are shown the average values for the recovery of krypton and tritium in the arterial blood (sampled for 5 to 30 seconds after intravenous injection) in nine normal and six emphysematous subjects. During normal respiration the recoveries are somewhat higher in the normal than in the emphysematous subjects. This may be explained by the difference in alveolar volume available to the gases in these two groups of subjects. The ratio between the recoveries of krypton and tritium are, however, nearly identical: 3·18 in the normal and 2·88 in the emphysematous subjects. Both groups thus have the same right-to-left shunt (about 0·3 per cent. of cardiac output).

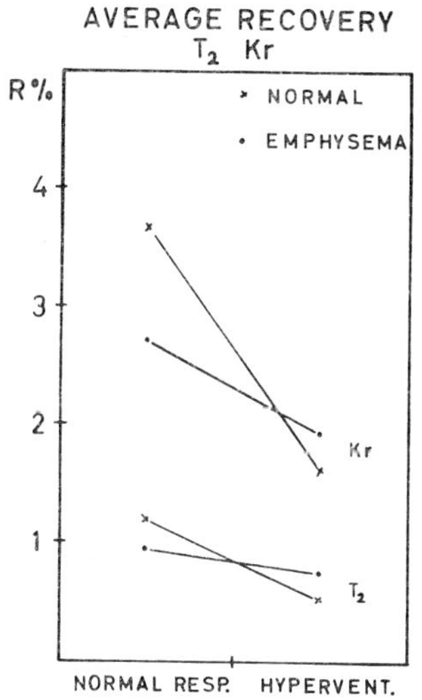

FIG. 11. The recovery of tritium and krypton in the arterial blood following an intravenous injection in normal and in emphysematous subjects.

The measurements were then repeated with the subjects hyperventilating during the procedure. This leads to a pronounced decrease in the recoveries in the normal subjects, but affected the emphysematous subjects to a much lesser degree. The ratio between the recoveries of krypton and tritium was virtually unchanged in the emphysematous subjects, whereas it increased in the normal subjects (*i.e.* indicating a decreased shunt).

We consider it unlikely that hyperventilation affects the true right-to-left shunt in normal subjects and not in emphysematous subjects. The findings are more reasonably explained by a change in the size of the alveolar space available to the two gases. In emphysema hyperventilation seems only to a very small degree to influence the alveolar space into which the two gases diffuse. In normal subjects hyperventilation leads to an increase in the available alveolar space, as evidenced by the decrease in the calculated right-to-left shunt. This decrease indicates a change in the assumptions underlying the calculation rather than any real change in the size of the shunt. Tritium, due to its more rapid diffusion, reaches regions where bulk transport begins, whereas the more slowly diffusing gas, krypton, distributes itself into a smaller space, less affected by the air flow in the conducting system. In the emphysematous subjects, however, hyperventilation has very little effect on the size of the space into which these two gases diffuse.

Thus we feel that these findings lend support to the hypothesis that a main factor in the pathophysiology of emphysema is an increase in the intrapulmonary diffusion space.

Dr Mead. Just a small point—it needs to be borne in mind that if you take two gases of different diffusivities and flow them through a tube in which there is a parabolic velocity profile across the tube, then the composition will change in the course of time because the gas of a lower density in the faster central region will tend to diffuse to the periphery and leave the central core enriched with the heavier gas. You've got to consider side-to-side differences in ventilation, as it were, before you can interpret the quick changes taking place during respiration.

Dr Cumming. This is absolutely true : if there is a parabolic velocity profile in the airways this is a very relevant objection. But the existence of a parabolic profile in the airways depends on two things : the rate at which the profile is moving forwards and the rate at which diffusion laterally is occurring to obliterate the velocity profile. The speed of linear movement in RBI is less than a millimetre per second and the speed of lateral diffusion and mixing is 40 times greater than this.

Chairman. Is the flow in the lung laminar or turbulent ?

Dr Horsfield. There's no doubt that the Reynold's number for the distal bronchi is very low and therefore the flow ought to be laminar. In a tube the fluid must traverse a length about ten times greater than the diameter in order to develop a significant velocity profile. Since most bronchi are shorter than this I am not at all sure that a fully developed parabolic profile ever occurs.

Dr West. Dr Hughes, in our laboratory, has been injecting radioactive xenon solution into a peripheral vein while the subject is breath-holding and then looking at the expired concentration of xenon as the lung is emptied. One might expect that the plateau would rise as expiration proceeded because if there were a diffusion concentration gradient in the airways, the gas exhaled last would have the highest concentration of tracer. But in fact Dr Hughes finds that the concentration of xenon falls in normal subjects during expiration after the anatomic dead space has been cleared. This suggests that if there is a diffusion gradient, it is being masked by regional differences in the rate of lung emptying under those conditions.

Dr Bates. I'd like to ask Dr Mead if one could infer from his discussion that the distribution of ventilation from the same lung volume would be independent of the velocity at which inspiration was made. Thus, in two experiments in which you began at either RV or FRC, does he think the velocity of inspiration to TLC would affect the distribution of ventilation ?

Dr Mead. In the normal lung, I would have thought that the time constants are so low that any deviation from the static distribution, even during a rapid inspiration, at the very low resistances that are developed in the airways at higher volumes would be very small. However, this would not be the case in diseased lungs where there might be a substantial increase in resistance in the smaller airways.

Dr Macklem. The interdependence versus the independence of units in parallel must, of course, have some size limitation. Two lungs will behave independently of one another and presumably two lobes will behave more or less independently of one another. When you get down to very small structures they are interdependent and I'm wondering if Dr Mead has any ideas, or any data, as to what size the structure has to be before it becomes relatively independent ?

Dr Mead. Lobes are independent. I can't really say at what sublobular level interdependence develops. In the goat and cow, however, it is certainly present at the lobular level.

Dr Permutt. In the model Dr Cumming has analysed—the sequential model—it occurs to me that it would be very easy to consider the abnormality in terms of dead space equivalent. In this model the greater the tidal volume the smaller the dead space. Perhaps Dr Cumming feels that some of the marked increase in the CO_2 dead space—the physiological dead space—that you see in the patient with chronic bronchitis or emphysema, might very well be due to the sequential aspect, as compared to the way that many others look at it, *i.e.* as very poorly perfused areas of the alveoli. Because, if that's so, there should be an experiment that could distinguish between these two : the sequential and the parallel. The parallel dead space caused by areas of very low perfusion certainly goes up as the tidal volume goes up. In the parallel model the ratio of the alveolar dead space to the total air going into the alveoli remains constant if a certain fraction of the lung is un-perfused with blood. I think it would be very interesting to see exactly what happens to the dead space in relation to tidal volume in the patient with a marked degree of emphysema. If it goes up, as I suspect it might, it would seem to me to suggest more of a parallel than a sequential type of dead space.

Dr Cumming. We have in fact done studies on this in a large series of bronchitics. We measured the decay curve and worked out, just as you've suggested, the equivalent dead space. I have now in mind a case who was grossly dyspnoeic and he had a tidal volume of 536, of which about 490 was dead space.

Dr Permutt. CO_2 dead space ?

Dr Cumming. This is the nitrogen–oxygen dead space, in fact. This was the thing we actually measured. When the man got a little better, the dead space diminished about 100 cc.

Dr Permutt. What I'm asking specifically is this : when you have these enormous ratios of dead space to tidal volume that I've seen, sometimes up to 65 or 70 per cent., if you now increase the tidal volume, does this dead space go up, or does it go down ? It's my impression that the CO_2 dead space increases with tidal volume so that at least a significant portion of the CO_2 dead space must be due to an actual parallel type of dead space.

Dr Cumming. I can't answer the question specifically—I've no figures on CO_2 dead space—but I would agree with you that the regional factors are important. If I may comment a little further, there seems to have grown up a belief that there is a conflict of opinion between the concepts of regional inhomogeneity and stratified. I believe there's no such conflict—certainly stratified inhomogeneity occurs and certainly regional does. There are two major defects of gas mixing : one is the type based on transit times, either due to the anatomical difference in transit pathway or to the distribution of intrapleural pressure up and down the lungs or, in other cases, it may be the distribution of elastic tissue. The second type is the poor mixing in a longitudinal direction. I think there's no conflict of opinion—the difficulty arises in ascribing quantitative figures to the part played by each one in a given region.

Dr Norman Jones. I have some data which may be of interest to Dr Permutt. We have studied CO_2 dead space in a large number of bronchitics and patients with emphysema during exercise. During exercise the tidal volume increases and, in the normal person, dead space increases roughly in relation to tidal volume. The slope of this relationship is certainly much steeper in patients with chronic airways obstruction. In other words, the dead space does increase to a greater degree with a given increase in tidal volume in these patients.

Dr Prime. In relation to this increase in resistance in the peripheral airways in chronic bronchitics it is really very uncommon to find abnormalities in blood gases in these patients until they are very severely disabled. You may have a quite considerable increase of airways resistance and a reduction in FEV of moderate degree, without abnormalities of blood gases. It seems to me, that if a rise of airways resistance were to be due mainly to obstruction to peripheral airways, one would expect abnormalities in blood gases to be much more common in the bronchitic than in fact they are. Have you any comment to make on this, Dr Mead ?

Dr Mead. There are certainly many other factors which determine gas exchange apart from obstruction in the peripheral airways—the ventilation/perfusion ratio, for one. You can get abnormal ventilation distribution without much in the way of abnormal gas exchange if perfusion is reduced in proportion to your ventilation. That might possibly be one explanation.

Chairman. Has anyone else anything to say as to whether there is any correlation between these physiological defects and the presence or absence of holes in the lung ?

Dr Thurlbeck. We have done lead bronchograms of the kind Drs Leopold and Gough (1963) described and we get very beautiful bronchograms this way. We see an enormous difference between the so-called normal lungs and our cases of bronchitis and emphysema.

The way I like to think of it is that there are two components to small airways disease : mucus in the tracheo-bronchial tree—the bronchioles in this case—which is a facet of chronic bronchitis; and bronchiolitis with inflammation around the bronchioles, bronchiolar narrowing and even bronchiolar obliteration in some instances. Whatever the exact mechanism of airways obstruction may be, a significant component is small airways disease. For instance, one patient died outside our hospital and didn't have the benefit of the usual tracheo-bronchial toilet, and this patient's whole bronchial tree was just stuffed up with inspissated mucus. He had by far the greatest airways resistance we have seen. Not that I am suggesting any close correlation here. We had another patient with a lot of mucus plugging and two others where it was relatively slight but the peripheral resistance was about the same in these three cases.

Dr Permutt. I'd like to make just one point, and perhaps speculate as to what the blood gas abnormalities actually are in these various types of disease. A number of people here today feel that the presence of cor pulmonale or abnormalities of blood gases is very frequent in patients with chronic bronchitis who do not have emphysema. Slides have been shown suggesting that the degree to which right ventricular hypertrophy and cor pulmonale occur, bears little relationship to the degree of emphysema. In my experience, in taking measurements of blood gases on abnormal patients, the impressive thing is that when they retain CO_2, they do so not because their total ventilations are down, but because they have enormous dead spaces. Very often the ventilations are perfectly normal in these people. Could it be that we are dealing here with a primary circulatory abnormality ?

Chairman. You think CO_2 retention is principally determined by gross $\dot{V}/\dot{Q}$ abnormalities ?

Dr Permutt. I am convinced that a patient who has a P_{CO_2} of 55 or 60 mm. of Hg will not have a marked abnormality in terms of total ventilation, unless, that is, he is in a deep coma—which he usually is not. His big problem is the fact that his ratio of dead space to tidal volume is 65 or 70 per cent. The cause of that may be circulatory—that he has areas of his lungs very poorly perfused with blood.

Dr Filley. May I comment on the statement that there's no relation between the right ventricular weight and the amount of emphysema, or the percentage of mucous glands—I think I'm quoting Dr Dunnill correctly. It should be pointed out that there is a difference between how much the right ventricle weighs after death and how much heart failure the patient had in life. Also a tremendous difference between what is thought to be cardiac enlargement on film and what is found at autopsy. In a long-term disease the temporal as well as the spatial, *i.e.* structural, considerations have to be taken into account. We can't say that just because something or other is found at autopsy, it is necessarily relevant to the pathogenesis of a process going on years before.

Professor Stuart-Harris. I'd like to continue along the lines on which Dr Permutt has been speculating. I agree with him, of course, that there's no question about the relationship between the tension of the carbon dioxide and the tendency to develop cor pulmonale and I'd like to refer briefly to some work done in Sheffield by Dr Penman, before he left for the United States. He was performing a three-compartment analysis, based on the ideas I think he acquired from Dr Riley in Baltimore. He was measuring the alveolar dead space in groups of normal subjects and in bronchitic subjects—those who had been in circulatory failure as well as those who had never shown cardiac complications. There was little doubt about the deadspace being increased, of course, in the bronchitics, but there was no real percentage difference in terms of the fraction of lung which was ventilated but not perfused between bronchitics who had not had cardiac complications and those who had. The third compartment—the compartment of the lung which is essentially unventilated but perfused, the blood-shunt compartment—was greatly increased in subjects who were either in cardiac failure or who had just come out of cardiac failure, compared with chronic bronchitics who did not actually have any cardiac complications. This tends to reinforce the suggestion that it is the circulation that determines whether or not there's going to be cor pulmonale and the actual amount of dead space doesn't seem to show any close correlation.

Dr Berglund. In this question of cor pulmonale the CO_2 retention has been mentioned but not the hypoxaemia, which I think is just as important. Dr Widimsky and I did a trial on a patient with bronchitis and CO_2 retention and hypoxaemia and the right ventricular failure was improved by giving oxygen without changing the CO_2. We shouldn't forget this fact.

Dr Campbell. A recent paper from Sydney by Pain and his colleagues (1965) examined the very difficult problem of the sudden increase of hypercapnia on being given oxygen, and threw some doubt on the conventional story that it is due to removal of the hypoxic drive. They came to the conclusion that perhaps a distortion of the pulmonary circulation may be important.

Dr Whitaker. I think it would be a great pity, having spent the afternoon living at academic levels, if we closed our eyes to the fact that is so obviously before us. I was startled that someone should ask if the disturbance in blood gas had anything to do with bronchitis. I think anyone who has ever seen cor pulmonale must know that the precipitating factor, whatever the underlying disease may be, is bronchitis. If you follow a group of 100 patients the usual thing that produces the acute disturbance in their oxygen saturation and CO_2 tension is an acute respiratory infection. I think one ought to say this quite clearly, in case anyone should go away from here thinking that cor pulmonale has nothing to do with bronchitis. However the primary underlying disease may eventually be defined, there's no doubt in my mind that the common precipitating factor is a respiratory infection.

Dr Macklem. I certainly think one can't deny the correlation between the presence of bronchitis and the presence of cor pulmonale in respiratory failure. I didn't mean in any way to attempt to deny this, but there's a big gap between the two and, to physiologists, when you say bronchitis, you imply a specific anatomical lesion. What I can't understand is how a lesion of the bronchi, purely of the bronchi, can produce abnormal blood gases—at least without causing such an incredible degree of airways obstruction that the patient would be virtually suffocating from that, before he got abnormal gas exchange.

Dr Whitaker. I'm really the wrong person to be speaking, because all my information comes from the work I saw in Professor Stuart-Harris's department, but the facts were there. These patients came in with respiratory infection. I think that in 53 per cent., or something like that, Professor Stuart-Harris cultured the pneumococcus, and if you treated these people with antibiotics they recovered from their respiratory infection and lost their heart failure and their blood gases returned to a level which we found in chronic bronchitics.

Dr Macklem. I would prefer to say, under those circumstances, that they got an exacerbation of chronic bronchiolitis, not bronchitis. I just think it may be wrong to take an anatomical diagnosis as the cause of development of the blood gas abnormality ; something else may be going on as well.

Chairman. I think we ought to accept that there is an inflammatory process and in the bronchi this must mean a narrowing, a reduction of the lumen, and the flow will vary according to the fourth-power relationship. The smaller the tube the greater will be the effect on flow. So an infection is bound to lead to narrowing of the tube which will result in greatly reduced flow or greatly increased pressure—one of the two.

Dr Macklem. I would quite agree with this because the resistance of the large airways is very much greater than the resistance of the small airways and in normal conditions normal people are very sensitive to narrowing of the large airways, which I take to be the bronchi. They are insensitive to narrowing of the peripheral airways. I have recently observed two or three patients who have had respiratory failure but their airway resistance is virtually normal. I cannot therefore attribute the hypercapnia in these cases to lesions in the large airways, the bronchi. Possibly in the bronchioles, yes, and possibly in the parenchyma but certainly not in the bronchi.

Chairman. The actual gas exchange area must have had a higher CO_2 tension if they had hypercapnia. Therefore it must have been poorly ventilated. There's no getting away from that.

Dr Bates. Some of our confusion is semantic and arises because we have got orientated to a definition of chronic bronchitis based essentially on epidemiological criteria. I think it's very important that we fully understand that there are several sub-divisions of chronic bronchitis and it seems to me that to lump gas exchange problems into epidemiologically defined chronic bronchitis is going to get us all into serious trouble. There's quite a lot of evidence to suggest that it's much too simple a way of looking at a disease process which goes all the way from mucous gland hypertrophy in big bronchi, reflected in infections probably at that site, to the kind of terminal airways obliteration which seems to us, to be perhaps, an earlier stage of the disease.

Dr Filley. This is the same problem we had with emphysema for a long time, until we clearly distinguished between morphological definitions and clinical ones. Chronic bronchitis, as we use the term, refers to a clinical state and mucous gland hyperplasia refers to a pathological state. They are obviously connected, but not necessarily directly.

Dr Fletcher. I must protest at the idea of 'epidemiological definition'; there's no such thing. Epidemiologists happened to be the first people to tackle the problem of definition by saying that they would call bronchitis a particular symptomatic syndrome. Since then three divisions have been proposed with a number of criteria and obviously what Dr Whitaker is talking about is mucopurulent bronchitis which, defined clinically, is someone who is producing pus in the sputum. Dr Macklem, on the other hand, is talking about bronchiolitis as seen on a slide. These may be totally different things.

Dr Campbell. When I went to Hammersmith I found Dr Fletcher describing patients who cough and spit and have low FEV/VC ratios, hypercapnia and hypoxaemia and in whom, when they died, the pathologists did not find emphysema. Travelling around the world I then got the impression from colleagues in the field elsewhere, that there was emphysema if only the people at Hammersmith knew where to look for it. Would it now be true to say that in such patients it's not a matter of finding emphysema if only one knew where to look for it, but that airways obstruction would be found if only one knew where to look for it?

Dr Thurlbeck. I think the situation would probably be this: we have come to the view that it is the small airways disease which is important in certain aspects of obstructive lung disease. In fact, one of the first descriptions of almost pure small airways disease comes from Hammersmith: it was Brian Heard (Easterly & Heard, 1965) who described multiple bronchiolar stenosis in a patient with irreversible airways obstruction, who had no, or very little emphysema and in addition had normal major bronchi. This was a non-bronchitic in terms of mucous gland hyperplasia and yet he had irreversible airways obstruction.

Dr Leopold. In considering airways obstruction from the pathologist's point of view, the only thing I can do is make a comparison between the person who is claimed to be a bronchitic and the person who's supposed to be normal. When this comparison is made, by and large, the major air pathways of the bronchitic are *wider* in calibre than the normal.

Dr Thurlbeck. But the small airways don't fill.

Dr Macklem. Just so. In attempting to define the site of obstruction by filling the airways with something, you've got the cards stacked against you, because you only fill the airways that are open, you don't fill the airways that are obstructed.

REFERENCES

ALTSHULER, B., PALMES, L., YARMUS, L., & NELSON, N. (1959). *J. appl. Physiol.* **14,** 321.

ANTHONISEN, N. R., BASS, H., PLACE, R. E. G. & BATES, D. V. *J. clin. Invest.* In press.

ANTHONISEN, N. R. & MILIC-EMILI, J. (1966). *J. appl. Physiol.* **21,** 760.

BALL, W. C., Jr., STEWART, P. B., NEWSHAM, L. G. S. & BATES, D. V. (1962). *J. clin. Invest.* **41,** 519.

BRYAN, A. C., BENTIVOGLIO, L. G., BEEREL, F., MACLEISH, H., ZIDULKA, A. & BATES, D. V. (1964). *J. appl. Physiol.* **19,** 395.

BRYAN, A. C., MILIC-EMILI, J. & PENGELLY, D. (1966). *J. appl. Physiol.* **21,** 778.

CUMMING, G. (1967). *Resp. Physiol., Neth.* **2,** 213.

CUMMING, G., CRANK, P., HORSFIELD, K. & PARKER, I. (1966). *Resp. Physiol., Neth.* **1,** 64.

CUMMING, G. HORSFIELD, K., JONES, J. G. & MUIR, D. C. F. (1967). *Resp. Physiol., Neth.* **2,** 386.

ESTERLY, J. R. & HEARD, B. E. (1965). *Thorax,* **20,** 309.

GEORG, J., LASSEN, N. A., MELLEMGAARD, K. & VINTHER, A. (1965). *Clin. Sci.* **29,** 525.

GLAZIER, J. B., HUGHES, J. M. B., MALONEY, J. E., PAIN, M. C. F. & WEST, J. B. (1966). *Lancet* **2,** 203.

HALDANE, J. S. (1919). *J. Physiol.* **52,** 433.

HOLLEY, H. S., MILIC-EMILI, J., BECKLAKE, M. R. & BATES, D. V. (1967). *J. clin. Invest.* **46,** 475.

HORSFIELD, K. & CUMMING, G. (1967). *J. appl. Physiol.* In press.

HORSFIELD, K., CUMMING, G. & HICKEN, P. (1966). *Am. Rev. resp. Dis.* **93,** 900.

HYATT, R. E. & FLATH, R. E. (1966). *J. appl. Physiol.* **21,** 1448.

KANEKO, K., MILIC-EMILI, J., DOLOVICH, M. B., DAWSON, A. & BATES, D. V. Regional distribution of ventilation and perfusion as a function of body position. *J. appl. Physiol.* **21,** 767 (1966).

KROGH, A. & LINDHARD, J. (1917). *J. Physiol.* **51,** 59.

KREUGER, J. J., BAIN, T. & PATTERSON, J. L., Jr. (1961). *J. appl. Physiol.* **16,** 465.

LEOPOLD, J. G. & GOUGH, J. (1963). *Thorax,* **18,** 172.

LEOPOLD, J. G. & SEAL, R. M. E. (1961). *Thorax,* **16,** 70.

MCLEAN, K. H. (1958). *Am. J. Med.* **25,** 62.

MACKLEM, P. T. & MEAD, J. (1967). *J. appl. Physiol.* **22,** 395.

MEAD, J. & WHITTENBERGER, J. L. (1953). *J. appl. Physiol.* **5**, 779.
MELLEMGAARD, K., LASSEN, N. A. & GEORG, J. (1962). *J. appl. Physiol.* **17**, 778.
MILIC-EMILI, J., HENDERSON, J. A. M., DOLOVICH, D. V., TROP, D. & KANEKO, K. (1966). *J. appl. Physiol.* **21**, 749.
MILIC-EMILI, J., MEAD, J. & TURNER, J. M. (1964). *J. appl. Physiol.* **19**, 212.
MUIR, D. C. F. (1967). *J. appl. Physiol.* **23**, 210.
OTIS, A. C., MCKERROW, C. B., BARTLETT, R. A., MEAD, J., MCELROY, M. B., SILVERSTONE, N. J. & RADFORD, E. P., Jr. (1956). *J. appl. Physiol.* **88**, 427.
PAIN, M. C. F., READ, D. J. C. & READ, J. (1965). *Australas. Ann. Med.* **14**, 195.
RADFORD, E. P., Jr. (1964 *a*). In *Aging of the Lung*, p. 152, ed. CANDER, L. New York : Grune & Stratton,
RADFORD, E. P., Jr. (1964 *b*). In *Handbook of Physiology*, Sec. 3, vol. I, p. 429. ed. FENN, W. O. & RAHN, H. Washington D.C. : American Physiological Society.
RAUWERDA, P. E. (1946). Thesis Groningen University.
REID, L. & SIMON, G. (1958). *Thorax*, **13**, 103.
ROBERTSON, J. S., SIRI, W. E. & JONES, H. B. (1950). *J. clin. Invest.* **29**, 577.
SANERKIN, N. G., SEAL, R. M. E. & LEOPOLD, J. G. (1966). *Ann. Allergy*, **24**, 586.
TENNEY, S. M. & MILLER, R. M. (1956). *J. appl. Physiol.* **9**, 321.
TURNER, J. M. (1962). *Physiologist* (*Wash.*), **5**, 223.
WEST, J. B. (1965). In *Ventilation/Blood Flow and Gas Exchange*. p. 31. Oxford : Blackwell Scientific Publications,
WEST, J. B. & DOLLERY, C. T. (1960). *J. appl. Physiol.* **15**, 405.
WOOD, E. H., NOLAN, A. C., DONALD, D. E. & CRONIN, L. (1963). *Fedn. Proc. Fedn. Am. Socs. exp. Biol.* **22**, 1024.
WYATT, J. P., FISHER, V. W. & SWEET, H. (1961). *Lab. Invest.* **10**, 159.
YOUNG, A. C. & MARTIN, C. J. (1966). *Resp. Physiol.* **1**, 372.

SESSION THREE

THE FACTORS DETERMINING BLOOD FLOW IN THE PULMONARY CIRCULATION

Chairman : Alfred P. Fishman

RECENT WORK ON THE DISTRIBUTION OF PULMONARY BLOOD FLOW AND TOPOGRAPHICAL DIFFERENCES IN ALVEOLAR SIZE[1]

J. B. WEST, J. B. GLAZIER, J. M. B. HUGHES and J. E. MALONEY

IN this presentation, I shall first summarise some older material on the distribution of pulmonary blood flow and ventilation, and then discuss some recent findings.

DISTRIBUTION OF BLOOD FLOW AT MODERATELY HIGH LUNG VOLUMES

Figure 1 shows the distribution of blood flow in the normal

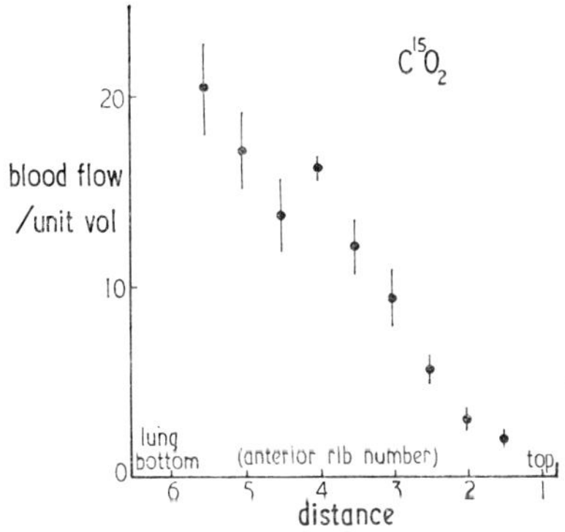

FIG. 1. Normal distribution of blood flow in the upright human lung at a moderately high lung volume as measured with radioactive carbon dioxide in 16 normal volunteers. Means and standard errors. Note the steady decrease from the bottom to the top of the lung; flow is almost nil at the apex. (Modified from the *Journal of Applied Physiology*.)

upright lung at a moderately high lung volume as measured in a series of healthy volunteers. It can be seen that blood flow decreases fairly steadily from the bottom to the top there being virtually no flow at the apex. These results were obtained with radioactive carbon dioxide (West & Dollery, 1960), and the general pattern has been confirmed with xenon (Bryan *et al.*, 1964). This normal

[1] Supported by the Medical Research Council.

distribution is affected by change of posture and exercise. It has been shown that when the subject lies supine, apical blood flow increases until it is approximately the same as basal flow. On mild exercise, apical blood flow increases more than the basal flow so that the distribution becomes more uniform. Pathology also affects the normal distribution of blood flow. Left-to-right intracardiac shunts which increase the pulmonary blood flow produce the same pattern as exercise. Pulmonary hypertension not associated with an increased pulmonary blood flow results in a more even distribution than in the normal lung. Diseases in which the pulmonary venous pressure is moderately raised cause an even distribution while higher venous pressures may be associated with an inversion of the normal pattern of flow so that apical blood flow exceeds basal flow.

CAUSE OF THE NORMAL DISTRIBUTION OF BLOOD FLOW

This has been studied using an isolated lung preparation (West *et al.*, 1964) and a scheme which satisfactorily accounts for the findings is shown in Figure 3. The lung is divided into three zones by the relative magnitude of the pulmonary arterial, venous and alveolar pressures.

In *zone* 1, pulmonary arterial pressure is less than alveolar pressure and there is no flow. Here we are taking into account the hydrostatic gradient in the pulmonary arteries whereby the perfusing pressure falls by 1 cm. H_2O/cm. distance up the lung. The cause of the absence of blood flow is that the delicate pulmonary capillaries are directly exposed to alveolar pressure and therefore collapse when this exceeds the perfusing pressure. Thus any fall in arterial pressure or rise in alveolar pressure will enlarge this zone. If lung in this zone is rapidly frozen by inundating the surface of the lung with liquid freon cooled to $-150°$ C while the lung is being perfused, the alveolar walls are seen to be very thin and contain very few red blood cells (Fig. 2 A). Actually we now know that these collapsible vessels are protected from alveolar pressure to the extent of a few centimetres of water by a pressure developed by the surface tension of the alveolar lining layer and that, as a result, the pericapillary pressure depends to some extent on the volume history of the lung (Pain & West, 1966).

In zone 2, arterial pressure exceeds alveolar pressure which in turn exceeds venous pressure. Here the vessels behave as Starling resistors (Permutt *et al.*, 1962), that is, collapsible tubes surrounded by a pressure chamber, and flow is determined by arterial pressure minus

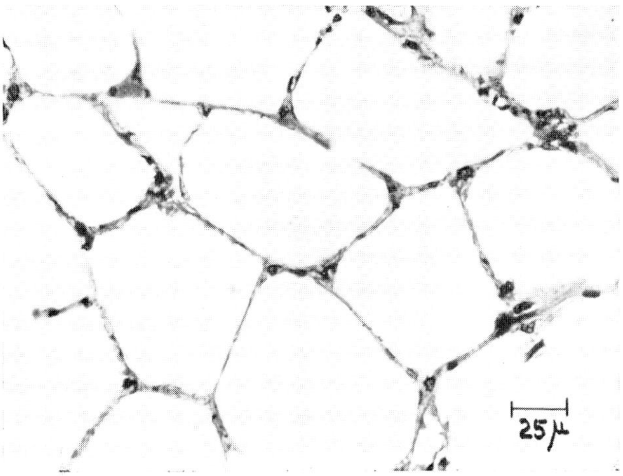

(A)

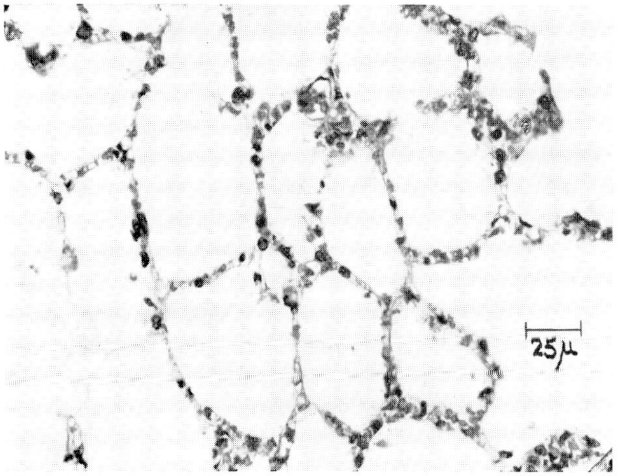

(B)

FIG. 2A. Section of an isolated lung rapidly frozen 7 cm. above the junction between zones 1 and 2. There was no blood flow in this region of the lung because the pulmonary arterial pressure was less than alveolar pressure. Note the thin alveolar septa containing few red blood cells.
FIG. 2B. Section rapidly frozen from same lung 10 cm. below the junction of zones 1 and 2. There was blood flow in this region and many red blood cells can be seen in the alveolar septa.

[*To face page* 112

alveolar, not arterial pressure minus venous pressure. In rubber tube models, the tube develops a constriction in its downstream end until the pressure inside the tube is equal to chamber pressure. Thus

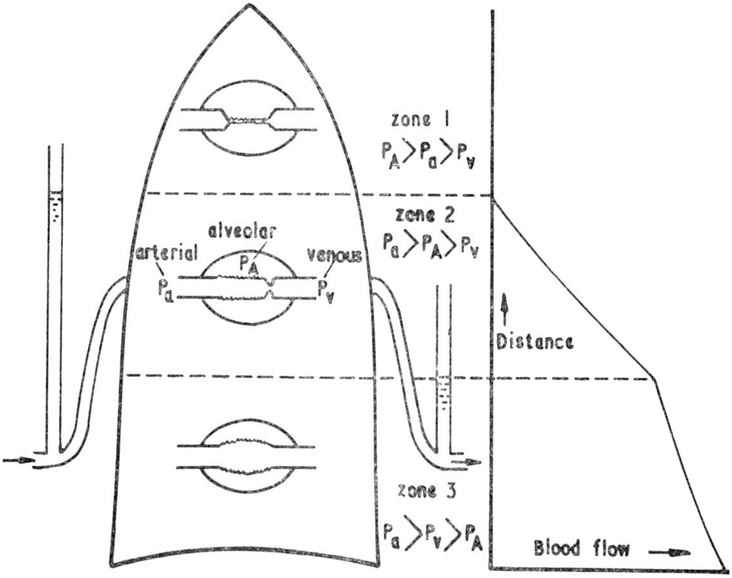

FIG. 3. Diagram to explain the topographical distribution of blood flow in the lung. The lung is divided into 3 zones by the relative magnitude of the pulmonary arterial, venous and alveolar pressure. In zone 1, arterial pressure is less than alveolar and there is no flow presumably because collapsible vessels are directly exposed to alveolar pressure. In zone 2, arterial pressure exceeds alveolar, but alveolar exceeds venous pressure. Here the vessels behave like Starling resistors and flow is determined by the difference between arterial pressure (which is increasing down the lung) and alveolar pressure (which is constant). In zone 3, venous pressure exceeds alveolar and flow is determined by the arterial-venous difference. Flow increases down this zone because the transmural pressure of the vessels increases so that the vessels have a larger calibre and also perhaps because new vessels open up. (From the *Journal of Applied Physiology*.)

the pressure gradient responsible for flow is the perfusing pressure minus chamber pressure. Since arterial pressure increases steadily down the zone while alveolar pressure is constant throughout the lung, blood flow increases down this zone. The rate of increase is slow at first and then faster, presumably because of the opening of more and more vascular units, and the distention of those already open. Figure 2 B shows that rapidly frozen lung from zone 2 has strings of red blood cells in the alveolar septa.

In the bottom zone, *zone* 3, venous pressure exceeds alveolar pressure and flow is determined by the usual arterial-venous pressure difference. The increase in blood flow observed down this zone is apparently caused by distension of the vessels as a result of the rising transmural pressure, and by the opening up of more vessels. In the isolated dog lung, the rate of increase of blood flow down zone 3 is almost as rapid as down zone 2 and it is consistent with the pressure-flow relations of whole lobes (Fowler *et al.*, 1966). The vessels which show a fall in resistance down zone 3 are exposed to alveolar pressure (West & Dollery, 1965).

Application of this scheme to man is complicated by the pulsatile nature of the pulmonary arterial pressure. Does the junction between zones 1 and 2 move up and down with the pulmonary arterial pressure so that the apical capillaries wink open and shut with each heart beat, or is the distribution of blood flow determined by the mean pressure? Recently Bergel, Maloney and their colleagues in our laboratory have studied the propagation of the pulsatility through the blood vessels of an isolated lung and shown that the system is very highly damped. At physiological frequencies, only 15 per cent of the flow pulsations in the pulmonary artery appeared in the veins, and only 30 per cent. of the pressure pulsation was transmitted from the pulmonary artery to the small collapsible vessels. Thus it appears that the level to which blood rises is determined chiefly by the mean pulmonary arterial pressure.

DISTRIBUTION OF BLOOD FLOW AT LOW LUNG VOLUMES

Recently Dr Hughes and his collaborators have studied the effects of changing lung volume on the distribution of blood flow. The method of Anthonisen and Milic-Emili (1966) was used in order to obtain blood flow per alveolus. The radioactive xenon was injected into normal volunteers at a given lung volume and after it had all reached the lung, the subject inhaled to total lung capacity and the lung was scanned. Figure 4 shows some of the results obtained.

It can be seen that although at total lung capacity blood flow increased more or less steadily from the base to the apex, at lower lung volumes there was a region of reduced blood flow or increased vascular resistance in the most dependent zones. Thus at functional residual capacity, blood flow per alveolus began to decrease 8 cm.

above the bottom of the lung and a further reduction of the proportion of pulmonary blood flow to the base was seen at residual volume where apical flow exceeded basal flow.

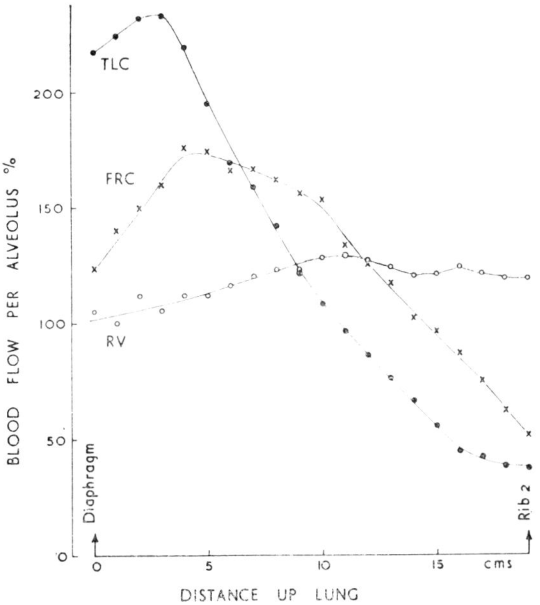

FIG. 4. Distribution of blood flow in an upright normal subject at total lung capacity (TLC), functional residual capacity (FRC), and residual volume (RV). Blood flow per alveolus plotted against lung distance as a percentage of that expected had all alveoli been perfused equally. Note the reduction of basal blood flow particularly at lower lung volumes. (From *The Lancet.*)

These patterns cannot be explained on the basis of the 3 zone model depicted in Figure 3 which is concerned with the pressure-flow relations of the small vessels exposed to alveolar pressure and we believe that the vascular resistance of the larger extra-alveolar vessels must be considered. Before doing this however, some recent data on regional differences of alveolar size in the lung will be reviewed.

VERTICAL GRADIENT OF ALVEOLAR SIZE

There have been several reports that the intra-pleural pressure is less negative at the base of the upright lung than at the apex (Krueger *et al.*, 1961 ; Daly & Bondurant, 1963 ; Wood *et al.*, 1963). Regional differences in intra-pleural pressure mean that the apex and base of the lung are exposed to different expanding pressures so that they imply differences of alveolar size down the lung. There have been frequent histological studies of the lung since the original report of Stephen Hales in 1731 that the alveoli of a calf's lung were about 1/100 in. in diameter. No study has revealed any systematic regional differences in alveolar size. In most cases however, the lung has been re-inflated outside the chest before fixation, with the result that any differences in intra-pleural pressure were abolished, and in no instance can it be said with certainty that the measurements reflected the state of the lung *in situ*.

It is clear that in order to demonstrate any histological differences in alveolar size it is essential to fix the lungs inside the chest. Dr Glazier and his co-workers (1966) have accomplished this by freezing anaesthetised dogs by surrounding them with solid carbon dioxide at −78° C. Under these circumstances, the architecture of the alveoli is well preserved but, because the central parts of the lung take 4 to 6 hours to freeze, there is some destruction of tissue at the cellular level because of ice crystal formation.

Figure 10 A shows the appearance of alveoli taken from the apex of the lung of a greyhound dog frozen in the vertical (head up) position. Compare this with a section taken 20 cm. below this level in the same animal (Fig. 10 B). The smaller size of the alveoli is apparent.

In order to compare the volume of the alveoli at different levels, statistical morphometric techniques as described by Weibel (1963) were used. A grid consisting of 21 test lines was placed on various fields chosen by stratified random sampling, and from the number of intersections of the test lines with alveolar walls, the volume-to-surface ratio of the alveoli was obtained. From this, the average volume of the alveoli at different levels could be compared.

Figure 5 shows the pooled results obtained in five greyhound dogs frozen in the vertical (head up) position. It can be seen that the alveoli at the apex of the lung were some four times larger than those at the base, the major change in volume being in the uppermost 10 cm. When dogs were frozen in the horizontal position, the dependent alveoli were always smaller than the uppermost ones though the apical and basal alveoli were the same size (Fig. 6). Thus, in a supine dog, the dorsal alveoli were the smallest while in a dog frozen in the prone position, the dependent ventral alveoli were the smallest. Three dogs frozen in the right lateral position had smaller alveoli in the dependent right lung than in the left. Distention of the lung by

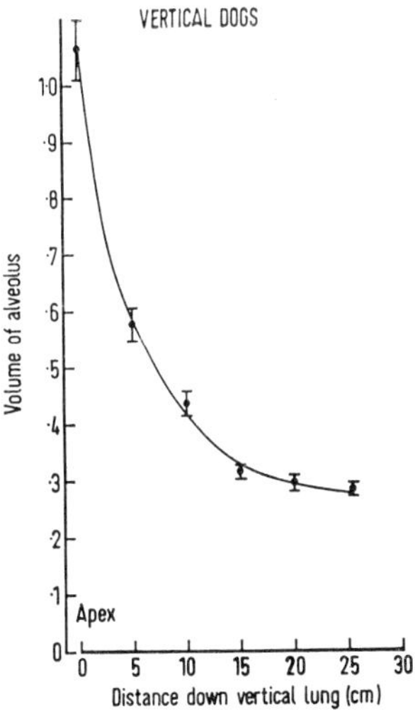

FIG. 5. Volume of alveoli at 5 cm. intervals from apex to base measured in five frozen vertical (head up) greyhound dogs. Means and standard errors. The apical alveoli are about four times larger than the basal alveoli. (From the *Journal of Applied Physiology*.)

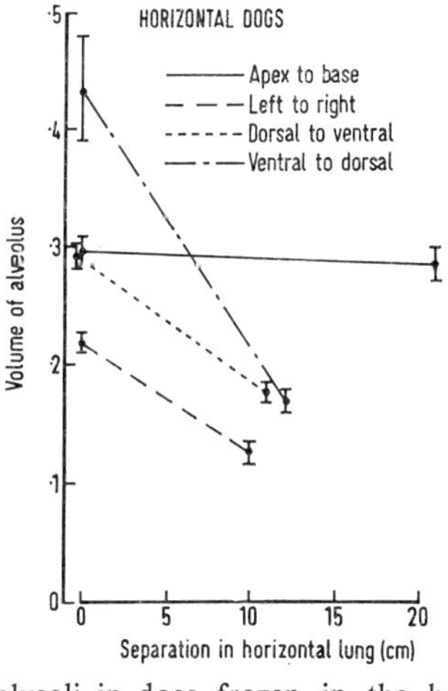

FIG. 6. Volume of alveoli in dogs frozen in the horizontal position. Note that the apical and basal alveoli were the same size but that in dogs frozen in the supine, prone and right lateral positions, the dependent alveoli were always smaller than the uppermost alveoli. (From the *Journal of Applied Physiology*.)

positive pressure inflation during freezing reduced the regional differences in alveolar size, while exposing the animal to increased G on a centrifuge exaggerated the differences (Fig. 7). Surprisingly, the alveoli of dogs frozen in the inverted position were uniform in

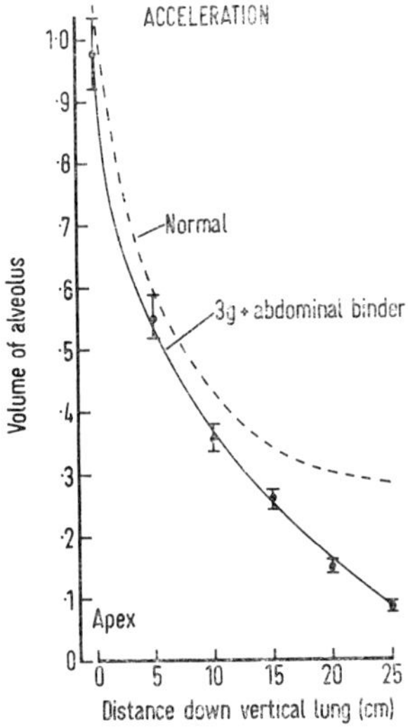

FIG. 7. Volume of alveoli in a dog exposed to a headward acceleration of 3G on a centrifuge while freezing. An abdominal binder (G suit) was applied to prevent descent of the diaphragm. Note that there was no significant change in size of the apical alveoli but that the basal alveoli became much smaller, the vertical gradient of volume now being 11 to 1. (From the *Journal of Applied Physiology*.)

size (Fig. 8). No systematic differences were found between hilar and peripheral regions at any given level of the lung in the vertical dogs ; the volume of alveolar ducts and alveoli changed to the same extent down the lung.

In an attempt to explain these results, we have considered the way in which the lung is supported inside the chest. Suppose that the lung below a given level is supported by the many fibres acting across the cross sectional area of the thoracic cavity at that level (Fig. 9) : then the total force acting across this plane is the weight of the lung, and the distending pressure will be given by the weight divided by the cross sectional area. It is clear that on this hypothesis, the distending pressure will be high at the apex where the weight of the lung below is great but the cross sectional area is small. Dr Glazier

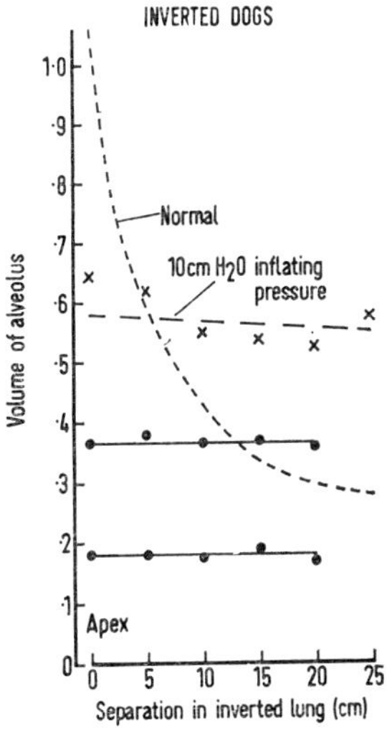

FIG. 8. Alveolar volume in 3 dogs in the inverted (head down) position. 10 cm. H_2O positive inflating pressure was applied to the trachea of one of the dogs during freezing. Note that, surprisingly, there were no differences in alveolar size down the lung. (From the *Journal of Applied Physiology.*)

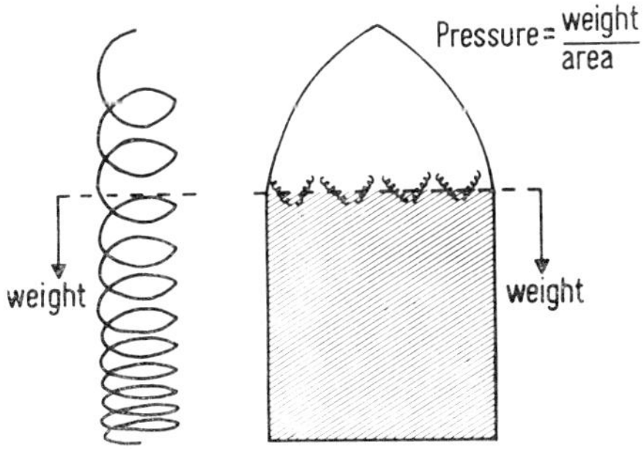

FIG. 9. Model to account for the vertical differences in alveolar size. In a spring supported at the top, the distending force is determined by the weight of the spring below any point. By analogy, the weight of the lung below any horizontal plane is supposed to be taken by the parenchymal fibres in the plane so that the distending pressure is the dependent weight divided by the cross sectional area. This simple hypothesis fits the observed differences in alveolar size in both the vertical and inverted dogs.

has calculated the differences in alveolar size which would be expected according to this hypothesis and has shown that both the large gradient of alveolar size in the upright lung and the uniform pattern in the inverted lung can be explained in this way. The latter result is due to the fact that while the weight increases up the inverted lung, the measured cross sectional area increases at approximately the same rate.

ALVEOLAR AND EXTRA-ALVEOLAR VESSELS

We have seen that the parenchyma at the bottom of the upright lung is less well expanded than that at the top. How can this explain the zone of reduced blood flow in the dependent regions of the lung at less than maximal volume (Fig. 4) ? We believe that the answer to this question lies in the important distinction between pulmonary blood vessels exposed to alveolar pressure and those outside the influence of alveolar pressure : the ' extra-alveolar ' vessels (Mead and Whittenberger, 1964).

Figure 11 shows a section of dog lung in which the alveolar walls with their capillaries can be clearly seen. There is good reason to believe that these small vessels are exposed to alveolar pressure (or very nearly so) because when alveolar pressure exceeds arterial pressure, these vessels collapse (Fig. 2 A). In fact, close examination of a series of similar sections showed that no vessels with diameters less than 30 microns were open under these conditions (Fowler *et al.*, 1966). Since vessels up to approximately 100 microns have extremely thin walls with small amounts of elastic tissue and little if any muscle, we concluded from these measurements that the vessels up to about 30 microns or so were directly exposed to alveolar pressure (modified by surface forces).

Figure 11 also shows a larger pulmonary vessel with its surrounding interstitial tissue which includes the potential perivascular space. This sheath is a prolongation of the mediastinum into the peripheral parts of the lung and contains many lymphatics (von Hayek, 1960). There is good evidence that vessels such as these (say larger than 100 microns in diameter) are exposed to a pressure which may be considerably lower than either alveolar or pleural pressures, and we would say that these extra-alveolar vessels are exposed to interstitial pressure. Macklin showed that inflation of the lung increased the capacity of the pulmonary arteries and veins. Howell *et al.*, (1961) suggested that as the lung parenchyma expanded, a low pressure was generated around these extra-alveolar vessels. Recently Mead (1968) has argued that the effective distending

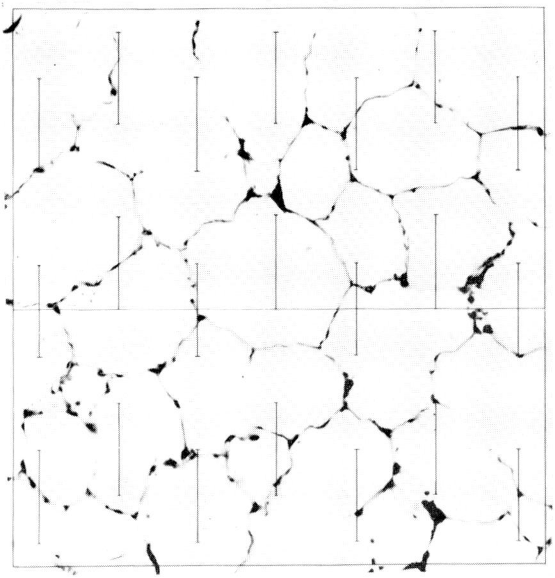

(A)

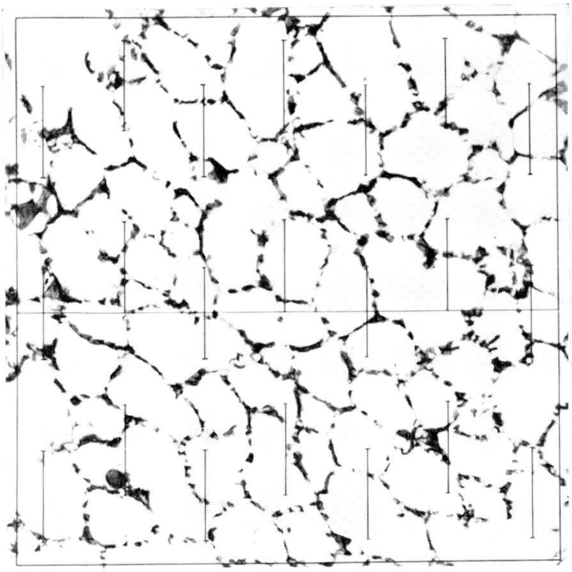

(B)

FIG. 10. Sections of lung from (A) apex and (B) 20 cm. lower down the lung of an anaesthetized greyhound dog frozen in the vertical (head up) position. The grid used for determining alveolar size is superimposed on the fields. Each of the test lines is equivalent to 100 microns. (From the *Journal of Applied Physiology*.)

[*To face page* 120

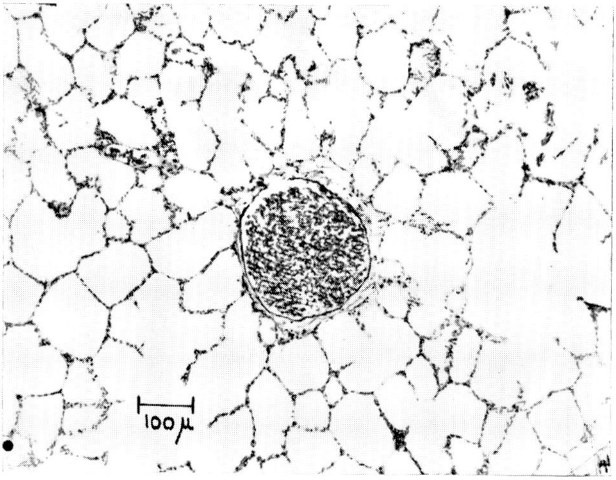

FIG. 11. Photomicrograph of dog lung showing alveolar walls containing 'alveolar' vessels and a larger 'extra-alveolar' vessel with its surrounding interstitial tissue and potential perivascular space.

pressure on the larger vessels is related to the departure of the area of the unit from the area which it would achieve if it distended identically with its surroundings. This implies that these relatively poorly distensible vessels may be exposed to expanding pressures considerably greater than transpulmonary pressure.

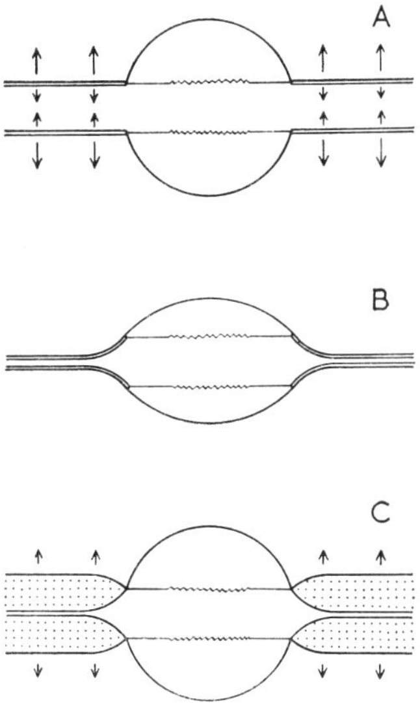

FIG. 12. A shows the subdivision of the pulmonary blood vessels into 'alveolar' and 'extra-alveolar'. The alveolar vessels (contained within the circle) are exposed to alveolar pressure. The extra-alveolar vessels are surrounded by a low interstitial pressure developed by the expansion of the lung parenchyma. B shows that in the collapsed lung, the extra-alveolar vessels close because of the inherent tension in their walls. C shows that in the presence of oedema fluid in the perivascular space, the vessels are isolated from the normal expanding pull and close. (From *Circulation Research*.)

Figure 12 A is a schematic representation of a pulmonary blood vessel showing the central part exposed to alveolar pressure while on either side of this are the extra-alveolar portions. The pressures acting on the alveolar part of the vessel have been considered in Figure 3 ; these pressures are responsible for the increase in blood flow from the top to the bottom of the upright lung. There is accumulating evidence that the calibre of the extra-alveolar vessels is determined by a balance between several forces. The tension of the elastic tissue in their walls and the inherent tone of the wall muscle tends to close them, while they tend to be held open by the outward pull developed by the expansion of the lung parenchyma. Thus the vascular resistance of collapsed lung is high (Fig. 12 B) because the extra-alveolar vessels are not pulled open and they collapse due to the inherent tension in their walls.

Since the parenchyma at the base of the vertical lung is less well expanded than that at the apex (Fig. 5), the resistance of the extra-alveolar vessels at the base will be higher. We believe that this is the explanation of the zone of increased vascular resistance seen in the dependent zone of the normal upright lung at medium and low lung volumes (Fig. 4). However at high lung volumes the expanding pull on the extra-alveolar vessels is much increased, and in any case, all the alveoli have nearly the same volume. The result is that the region of increased vascular resistance at the base of the lung is abolished.

A further cause of increased vascular resistance of these lower zone vessels is fluid in the interstitial perivascular space. It has been known for many years that these extra-alveolar vessels, particularly on the arterial side, are surrounded by a potential perivascular space which is a prolongation of the mediastinal space into the lung (for example, von Hayek, 1960). This space contains many of the lymphatics which transport lymph from the capillaries to the hilum and any increase in lymph drainage is accompanied by an increase in the amount of fluid in this space. Dr Hughes has shown that when dextran solution is infused into intact vertical dogs, there is a rise in pulmonary venous and arterial pressures, and the perivascular resistance in the dependent zone of the lung can be demonstrated with radioactive xenon. This observation complements an earlier one that isolated lungs which develop interstitial oedema may show a gross reduction of lower zone blood flow in the presence of a raised venous pressure (West *et al.*, 1965).

We believe that the explanation of this rise in regional vascular resistance is that the perivascular oedema isolates the vessel from the normal expanding action of the lung parenchyma, with the result that it closes by virtue of the inherent tension in its wall (Fig. 12). The phenomenon is of clinical interest because it is known that a reduction in blood flow in the lower zone of the lung is frequently seen in severe mitral stenosis (Fig. 13) (Dollery & West, 1960) and acute left ventricular failure (Ueda *et al.*, 1964) where an increase in size of the perivascular space is often found (Heath & Hicken 1960). Characteristic changes in the pulmonary vasculature can be seen on radiographs in these conditions, particularly in the lower zones. It seems likely that an increase in pulmonary interstitial pressure with its resultant effects on the extra-alveolar vessels is the initiating factor in these vascular changes.

An interesting observation is that in the isolated dog lung an area of increased vascular resistance is regularly seen at the lung base even in the absence of histological perivascular oedema. This area of high resistance can be exaggerated by vasoconstrictor drugs, reduced by vasodilator drugs, and abolished by inflation to high lung volumes.

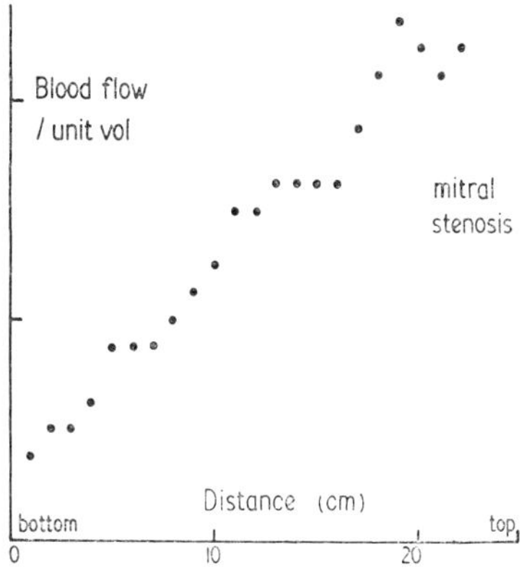

FIG. 13. Distribution of pulmonary blood flow in a housewife, aged 43, with severe mitral stenosis. The measurement was made at a moderately high lung volume. Note the inversion of the normal pattern of distribution (compare Fig. 1). It is likely that a raised interstitial pressure with its resultant effects on the extra-alveolar vessels is the initiating factor in these vascular changes. (Modified from *The Lancet.*)

These features strongly implicate the extra-alveolar vessels in spite of the fact that alveolar size is uniform in this preparation. An attractive explanation is that the perivascular pressure is inherently higher at the bottom of the lung because the lymphatics form a continuous system in which there is presumably a hydrostatic gradient of pressure.

Figure 14 shows how the three-zone diagram of Figure 3 can be modified to take account of the reduction of blood flow of the most dependent zone of the lung as a result of a raised interstitial pressure (Hughes *et al.*, 1968). At the top is shown the zone of capillary collapse where the pressure outside the vessels (alveolar, or nearly so) exceeds the pressure inside. Next comes the waterfall zone where flow is determined by the difference between pulmonary arterial and alveolar pressures and there is a rapid increase in flow with distance down the lung. In the zone labelled ' distension ', blood flow is determined by the difference between arterial and venous pressures and the increase in flow down the zone is caused by distension of the vessels and an increase in the number which are perfused. In these three zones, it is the relations between arterial, alveolar and venous pressures on the *alveolar* vessels which determine the differences in

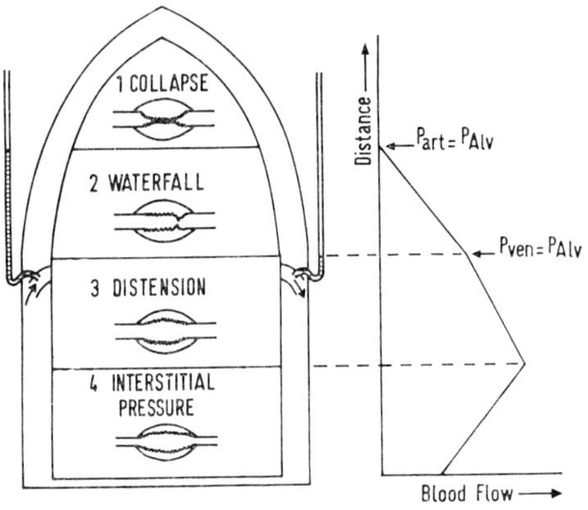

FIG. 14. Modification of the 3 zone model shown in Figure 3 to take account of the reduction in blood flow in the most dependent regions of the normal lung. This reduction is thought to be caused by the effects of raised interstitial pressure on the extra-alveolar vessels. In the normal lung at less than maximal volumes, the interstitial pressure at the base is raised because the lung parenchyma is less well expanded than at the apex (compare Fig. 5). Under pathological conditions, interstitial oedema may further raise the interstitial pressure (Fig. 12) thus further reducing basal blood flow. (From *Respiration Physiology*.)

blood flow. Finally, there may be a zone where the vascular resistance of the *extra-alveolar* vessels becomes significant because of a rise in interstitial pressure. As we have seen, this occurs in the normal lung at volumes below total lung capacity because of the relatively poor expansion of the lung parenchyma in the dependent zones. Furthermore a pathological rise of interstitial pressure caused, for example, by interstitial oedema can exaggerate this zone of reduced blood flow.

RECENT OBSERVATIONS ON THE MEASUREMENT OF REGIONAL $\dot{V}/\dot{Q}$ RATIOS IN CHRONIC LUNG DISEASE

D. V. BATES, N. R. ANTHONISEN, H. BASS,
T. HECKSCHER and A. ORIOL

INTRODUCTION

IT has been recognised for many years that the principal effect of many types of chronic lung disease is to produce an imbalance within the lung ventilation and perfusion distribution. Measurements of uneven gas distribution have existed in various forms for the past 100 years, and the period since 1945 has seen a progressive development of new techniques designed to measure the consequences of ventilation/perfusion differences in patients (Bates & Christie, 1964). These methods have been based on recent development of understanding of the consequences of ventilation/perfusion imbalance ; they have included measurements of differences of gas tensions between alveolar gas and arterial blood (Klocke & Rahn, 1961) as well as ingenious analyses of lung performance described in terms of theoretical compartments each having its own volume, ventilation, and perfusion distribution (Ruch & Patton, 1965).

The introduction of radioactive gases in the study of lung function added a new tool to these existing methods, and permitted measurements of regional ventilation distribution and perfusion distribution to be accomplished without difficulty in the normal or the diseased lung (Knipping *et al.*, 1961 ; Dollery & Hugh-Jones, 1963 ; Ball *et al.*, 1962). Up till the present time, however, such methods have involved the quantitation of ventilation by analysis of distribution of inspired gas, and of perfusion distribution by delivery of radioactive xenon dissolved in saline into alveolar gas via the pulmonary artery (Bentivoglio *et al.*, 1963). There was no assurance that the resulting data actually represented the performance of any particular part of the lung in its overall ventilation/perfusion relationship. The results of studies of the distribution of ventilation and perfusion measured in patients with emphysema by these two techniques have been presented elsewhere (Bentivoglio *et al.*, 1963) and in that paper we drew attention to the observation that discrepancies between the washout curves of inhaled and injected xenon had been observed in one subject with emphysema. We have recently published details of a new method of steady-state measurement of regional ventilation/perfusion ratios (Anthonisen *et al.*, 1966), and we now wish to report some recent data using this technique in the study of patients with lung disease.

MATERIALS AND METHODS

Radioactive gas technique

The full details of this method as applied to normal man have been described elsewhere (Anthonisen *et al.*, 1966), but some details will be amplified in clarification of the method. The theory of the method is the following : if a solution of ^{133}Xe is infused intravenously at a constant rate, it will evolve into the lung gas and, provided neither tidal volume nor perfusion change, will attain a steady alveolar concentration. This will be detected by an external scintillation counter, which will, therefore, reach a stable plateau after a period of 2 or 3 minutes. It can be appreciated intuititively that the count rate so observed will be dependent on lung geometry, chest wall radioactivity (if any), and—most importantly—by the ratio that exists within that counter zone between delivery of xenon (perfusion) and clearance of xenon (alveolar ventilation). We have explored elsewhere the complex problem of handling the deadspace distribution within the lung, and this will not be discussed further in this paper.

The actual study is accomplished by the alignment of 10 or 12 scintillation counters with 17 cm. tubular collimators over various regions of both lungs in the subject who is lying supine. The respiratory circuitry is so arranged that the subject can either breathe through open circuit, in which case the mixed expired xenon is analysed by a scintillation counter with a 2 in. diameter crystal placed after a mixing chamber and recording into a digital rate meter, or he can breathe to equilibrium with a closed spirometer circuit which also contains a scintillation counter. When the minute volume of the subject appeared to be steady, a solution of ^{133}Xe in saline contained in a syringe driven by a Harvard Pump, was infused for 5 minutes at a rate of approximately 2 mc. per minute into a previously prepared left antecubital vein. The subject was unaware when the xenon infusion began. The output from the scintillation counters positioned over the chest was monitored, and the infusion was continued until these became steady, but in any event, for no longer than 10 minutes in order to restrict the dose of radioactivity which the subject would receive. At the end of this time the infusion pump was turned off, and the subject continued to breathe at a normal tidal volume clearing ^{133}Xenon from his lungs. The rate of clearance was recorded by all chest counters and from the mixed expired line. At some time during this procedure, the cardiac output was measured by a dye dilution technique with injection into the right heart, and collection either using an arterial cuvette, or an ear oximeter.

The second part of the experiment consisted in equilibrating the subject with a spirometer circuit containing trace amounts of xenon until both the spirometer count rates and the regional count rates over the lung were stable, oxygen being added at a rate sufficient to keep the spirometer volume constant. After steady regional count rates had been attained, the subject was turned out of the closed circuit and again allowed to breathe room air. Once again the rate of clearance of xenon from the lung was observed by chest counters and the scintillation detector over the expired gas line. Correction for chest wall count rate was performed as previously described.

The data from these experiments were analysed in terms of $\dot{V}/\dot{Q}$ ratio existing in each counter zone, the T1/2 for clearance of xenon from each counter zone being calculated firstly after perfusion delivery of xenon at the end of the continuous injection study ; and secondly, after switchout following equilibrium with xenon in the spirometer circuit. The clearance of xenon in expired gas was analysed as described in the same two experiments.

PATIENT SELECTION

Studies have been conducted of the performance of different lung zones in 10 patients under the age of 35 known to be suffering from bronchial asthma, 20 patients of average age 54 who, on standard pulmonary function tests and radiological criteria as well as on clinical evidence, were believed to have some degree of pulmonary emphysema, and 10 patients of average age 48, who have been subjects in a department of Veterans Affairs study on chronic bronchitis (Bates *et al.*, 1966). The average lung radiation dose from a total study was 200 millirads ; the object and purposes of the study were carefully explained to each patient in advance. The physicians taking part in the project acted as a normal group in this experimental pattern.

RESULTS

Pulmonary emphysema

In a previous study (Bentivoglio *et al.*, 1963) we noted that discrepancy was observed between the pattern of xenon zonal clearance in the ventilation and perfusion experiments (Bates & Christie, 1964: Fig. 4.1). The conclusions from the present studies performed of 10 zones in 20 patients with emphysema may be summarised as follows: (1) By this technique, the $\dot{V}/\dot{Q}$ ratios measured over most lung zones in emphysema are low. High $\dot{V}/\dot{Q}$ regions are not observed although, in patients who have suffered from pulmonary emboli, high $\dot{V}/\dot{Q}$ regions can be detected using the same technique (Bass *et al.*, in the press). (2) In approximately half of the zones a clear discrepancy can be demonstrated between the rate of xenon clearance after perfusion delivery and after equilibration. (3) In every instance, the rate of clearance from perfusion delivered xenon is slower, than clearance after the lungs have been equilibrated with the spirometer.

Spasmodic asthma

(1) Although regional impairment of ventilation was found in a number of zones in patients with spasmodic asthma, there was little or no discrepancy between the rate of clearance of xenon delivered by the two routes, even in zones to which total ventilation was much reduced. (2) Little regional impairment of ventilation could be demonstrated unless the maximal ventilatory capacity had been reduced below 50 per cent. of that predicted.

Chronic bronchitis

(1) The 10 patients with chronic bronchitis had the least reduction of total pulmonary function of any of these groups, since in many of them the ventilation was well preserved and the maximal ventilatory ability was nearly normal. (2) In 8 of the 10 patients, however, a discrepancy was found in at least one counter zone between clearance of xenon from perfusion delivery and from ventilation. The results of one such study are shown in Figure 1. It will be seen from this figure that the patient, aged 48, was capable of a maximal ventilation of 94 litres per minutes and had a normal uptake of carbon monoxide indicating the probable integrity of his lung parenchyma. There was, however, chronic overinflation of the lung shown both radiologically and by elevation of the ratio of residual volume to total lung capacity. Detailed study of pulmonary mechanics on this man revealed that he had a normal elastic recoil, and no significant increase in measurable airway resistance as studied in a volume plethysmograph. In spite of these relatively normal findings in a man who was fully at work and not in any sense incapacitated, a clear divergence between the xenon clearance rates

was observed in a number of counters. Figure 1 shows the discrepancy observed by counter R4 (the fourth counter from the apex of the lung on the right side) and counter L2 positioned over the left lung. The reciprocal of the half time of clearance from the perfusion study was 12 and from the ventilation study was 35 for counter zone

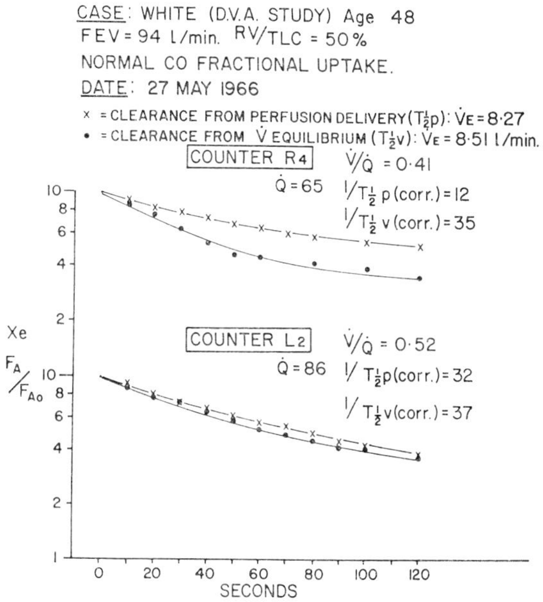

Fig. 1. Comparison of the clearance of Xenon[133] from two counter-fields (R_4 and L_2) in a patient with clinical chronic bronchitis, but with preservation of good ventilatory function and little disability. Note that in counter R_4 the clearance from perfusion delivery is delayed compared to clearance from ventilation equilibrium, whereas, during the same experiment there is no time discrepancy in the field of counter L_2.
FEV = forced expiratory volume corrected to maximal ventilatory volume.
RV/TLC = residual volume/total lung capacity.
$\dot{V}_E$ = minute volume during each experiment.

R4, and the overall $\dot{V}/\dot{Q}$ of the zone was 0·41. The $\dot{V}/\dot{Q}$ of zone L2 was higher, and there was no measurable divergence in this zone between the rate of clearance of radioactive xenon in the two experiments.

Figure 2 shows the significance of this observation of regional discrepancies of clearance in terms of xenon removal as a whole in the same patient, whose results appear in Figure 1. The expired gas xenon declined much more rapidly after the lung had been

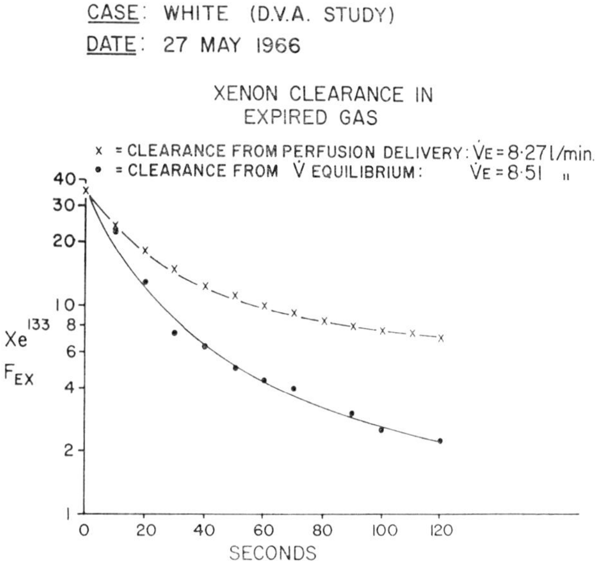

FIG. 2. Xenon analysis in expired gas during the same two experiments plotted in Figure 1. Note that the cumulative effect of a number of zones in which clearance after perfusion delivery is retarded compared to that after equilibrium, results in a considerable discrepancy between xenon in expired gas recorded at the mouth during open circuit breathing.

equilibrated with xenon in the gas phase than after the perfusion delivery experiment. This indicates that the functional discrepancy observed in discrete counter zones over the chest is detectable by comparison of clearance rates at the mouth in the two experiments.

Figure 3 shows the results from a second patient with chronic bronchitis with more impairment of ventilatory capability since the FEV value was only 30 litres per minute. In this patient one of the counterfields (R3) showed no discrepancy whatever between perfusion and ventilation clearance, whereas in another counter to which flow was greater (L3) and in which the total $\dot{V}/\dot{Q}$ was similar to R3, there was a measurable discrepancy between the xenon clearances. It has been our experience of studying 10 patients with chronic bronchitis that this kind of discrepancy is frequently observed in such patients, many of whom have very little impairment of total ventilatory function.

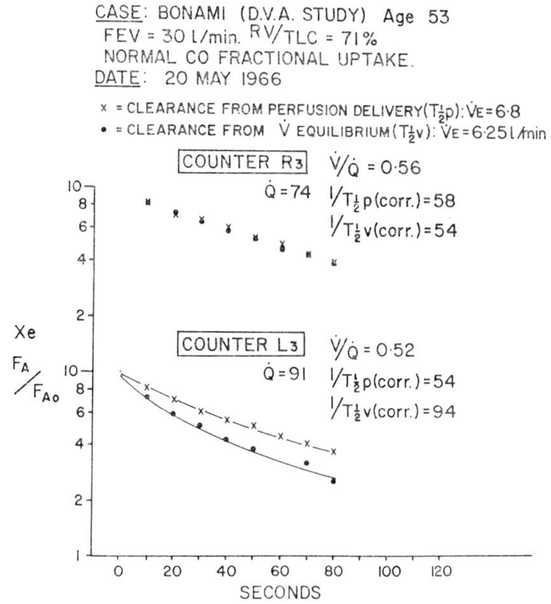

FIG. 3. Data and abbreviations as in Figure 1. In a second patient with more ventilatory defect (FEV = 30 litres per minute), counter L_3 shows discrepancy whereas another counter (R_3 on the right) shows no discrepancy of clearance between xenon after perfusion delivery and after $\dot{V}$ equilibrium.

DISCUSSION

In 1963, we observed discrepant clearance in a patient with pulmonary emphysema. The autopsy on this patient 2 years later revealed that the counters in which this phenomenon had been observed must have been positioned over lung whose architecture had been severely destroyed by pulmonary emphysema. When we observed that the discrepant clearance of xenon was not found in patients with spasmodic asthma, even with considerable ventilatory disability, it was naturally tempting to assume that the observation of discrepant clearance would indicate that lung architecture had been seriously deranged. However, such a conclusion is contradicted by the present data which has revealed significant clearance discrepancy in patients with chronic bronchitis, whose lung parenchyma is most probably intact. It seems to us likely that the patients with chronic bronchitis are suffering from considerable obstruction and disease in small bronchioles leading to regions of poor ventilation within each counter field, and it is the presence of these zones which is causing the discrepancies between xenon delivered by perfusion and from equilibration. It is quite clear that much further work lies ahead of us in clarifying the exact meaning of this phenomenon, but it seems to us to represent a useful addition to existing methods to quantitate ventilation/perfusion abnormalities.

It cannot be maintained that the methods of study which we have described are simple to perform. Care must be taken that the patient is quite comfortable ; it is essential that the tidal volume should not vary greatly between the two studies, and total minute volume should be comparable (as indicated in Figs. 1 and 3). Furthermore, it is necessary to make a measurement of cardiac output during the procedure since otherwise the mixed venous concentration of xenon cannot be precisely calculated. However, the present method probably gives a more reliable indication of the total behaviour of each counter zone than has been possible with previous techniques using radioactive xenon or $C^{15}O_2$. It is essential to realise, however, that each counter zone is composed of units which must be behaving very differently, and the zone cannot be regarded as a uniform field. It is important that conclusions derived from these regional $\dot{V}/\dot{Q}$ measurements should be tempered by the realisation of the comparatively large parts of the lung which are being surveyed, though it is not to be supposed that different results would necessarily be obtained by using smaller detectors in larger numbers. It is known from previously described techniques that low $\dot{V}/\dot{Q}$ regions are common in emphysema (Hilton, 1959) and, to that extent, the present data in regard to the patients with emphysema conform to expectation. However, it is obvious that high $\dot{V}/\dot{Q}$ regions must exist either within each counter field, or conceivably in zones not covered by the present counters. It is our view that the most likely explanation of our inability to demonstrate high $\dot{V}/\dot{Q}$ regions in any of the patients with emphysema studied (though high $\dot{V}/\dot{Q}$ alveoli must certainly exist in these lungs) is probably to be explained by the fact that their volume representation is small. Indeed, it might be postulated that the high $\dot{V}/\dot{Q}$ regions of the lung in emphysema are essentially zones through which air is passing on its way to low $\dot{V}/\dot{Q}$ regions. One might visualise high $\dot{V}/\dot{Q}$ alveoli as being alveoli positioned off the walls of terminal bronchioles which have maintained a reasonable perfusion and which perforce have good ventilation. If gross alveolar destruction is present beyond the terminal bronchiole, it is possible to suggest that the high $\dot{V}/\dot{Q}$ regions must consist of alveoli positioned adjacent to or opening into bronchioles fairly close to divisions from major bronchi. However this may be, it is clear that the volume representation of high $\dot{V}/\dot{Q}$ regions must be small, since low $\dot{V}/\dot{Q}$ regions dominate the total $\dot{V}/\dot{Q}$ pattern in every counter field that we have so studied in emphysema.

It is of course unfortunate that such an elaborate technique is required to demonstrate significant changes of function in patients whose total function is minimally disturbed, but it is the inevitable task of newly developed methods to push back the frontiers of diagnosis. It seems likely that the demonstration of marked regional abnormalities of function in men with minimal clinical chronic bronchitis, may represent an important contribution to our understanding of the earliest stages of this disease. It is inevitable that one cannot immediately confirm the view that the lung in these subjects is involved with terminal airway disease, nor prove that some degree of pulmonary emphysema does not exist, but the evidence would certainly suggest that no gross disorganisation of the lung architecture can have occurred in these subjects.

These data have been presented to illustrate new methods of studying regional pulmonary function in patients with different types of chronic lung disease.

SUMMARY

1. The results of a study of 20 patients with pulmonary emphysema, 10 patients with spasmodic asthma and 10 patients with chronic bronchitis by a steady-state xenon technique are described.

2. It was found that the regional lung function of patients with pulmonary emphysema showed a low $\dot{V}/\dot{Q}$ ratio in most counter zones. Zones of high $\dot{V}/\dot{Q}$ ratio could not be demonstrated. In more than half of the two hundred zones studied, significant discrepancy was observed between the clearance of xenon delivered via perfusion of the lung and clearance of xenon after equilibration of the lung with a spirometer.

3. In patients with spasmodic asthma, considerable regional impairment of ventilation exists, but discrepancy between clearance of xenon from the two experiments was only rarely observed.

4. In patients with chronic bronchitis, even with preservation of normal total pulmonary function as judged by routine tests, regional zonal abnormalities could be demonstrated in 8 out of the 10 patients

studied. These commonly consisted of discrepancy between the rate of clearance of xenon from the lung after perfusion delivery compared to xenon clearance from the same lung zone after the lungs had been equilibrated with a spirometer containing xenon. This discrepancy is thought to indicate that significant small airway obstruction (or disease) must exist in patients with minimal clinical bronchitis, leading to collateral ventilation of significant regions of the lung as a result of small airway obstruction. The possibility that the discrepancy of xenon clearances is attributable to a mild degree of centrilobular emphysema in these patients cannot be completely excluded.

5. These data are presented to illustrate the use of a new radioactive isotope technique in studying differences between different types of chronic respiratory disease, and to emphasise the probable future usefulness of steady state techniques using radioactive xenon in the early detection of significant function abnormality in patients with clinically minimal chronic bronchitis.

THE ORIGINS OF PULMONARY HYPERTENSION IN PATIENTS WITH CHRONIC BRONCHITIS AND EMPHYSEMA

J. M. Bishop

Pulmonary hypertension is frequently, but by no means invariably, present in patients with chronic bronchitis and emphysema. The purpose of this paper is to review what is known of the causes of the pulmonary hypertension, to suggest which of these factors are of major importance and to raise some questions concerning the relationship of some of these to alterations in the structure of the lung.

In Figure 1 are presented some data about the extent and frequency of pulmonary hypertension, at rest, in a group of 50 patients with chronic bronchitis. The patients have been studied in considerable detail but are unselected except that all are moderately or severely disabled. The range of pulmonary arterial pressure is from levels which are almost normal to very high values. The

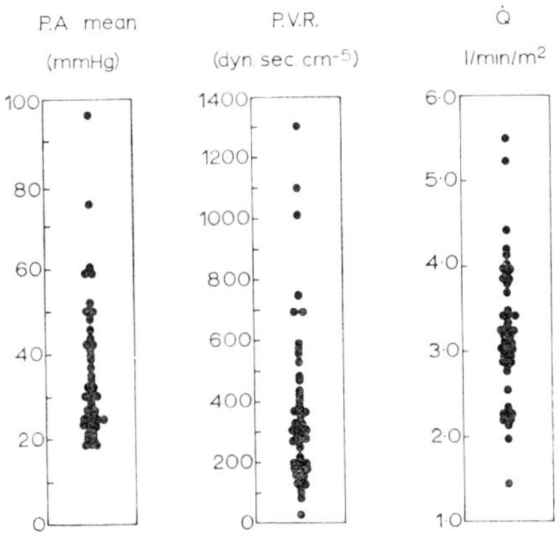

FIG. 1. Pulmonary arterial mean pressure, pulmonary vascular resistance and cardiac output at rest in fifty patients with chronic bronchitis.

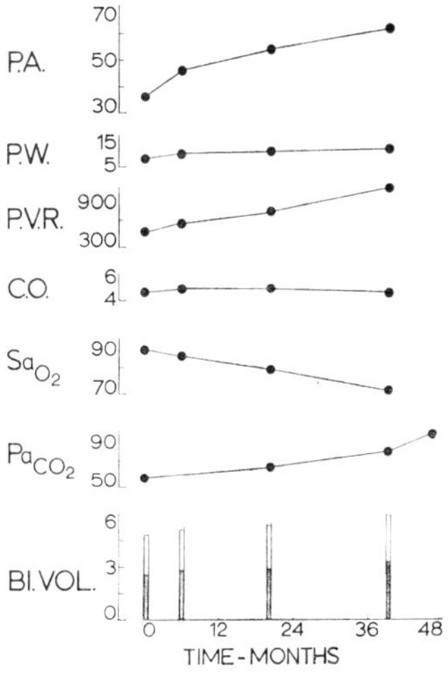

Fig. 2. Serial measurements in one patient with chronic bronchitis during a period of 4 years. Values are shown for pulmonary arterial mean (P.A.) and pulmonary wedge (P.W.) pressure, pulmonary vascular resistance (P.V.R.), cardiac output (C.O.), arterial oxygen saturation (Sa_{O_2}) and partial pressure of carbon dioxide (Pa_{CO_2}), and blood volume (Bl. vol.) with plasma volume hatched.

pulmonary vascular resistance is also shown and follows the pattern of distribution of pulmonary arterial pressure. The cardiac output, on the other hand, was within the normal range for our laboratory except in a few instances.

These differences in pulmonary arterial pressure do not result simply from the observations having been made at various stages of the disease. Serial measurements have been made and they indicate that the pulmonary arterial pressure may or may not show progressive changes in an individual patient with the passing years. The results illustrated in Figure 2 relate to a patient with marked hypoxaemia, polycythaemia and pulmonary hypertension. Pulmonary arterial pressure rose progressively over a period of nearly four years while arterial oxygen content decreased. By contrast, in two equally disabled patients (Fig. 3) pulmonary arterial pressure

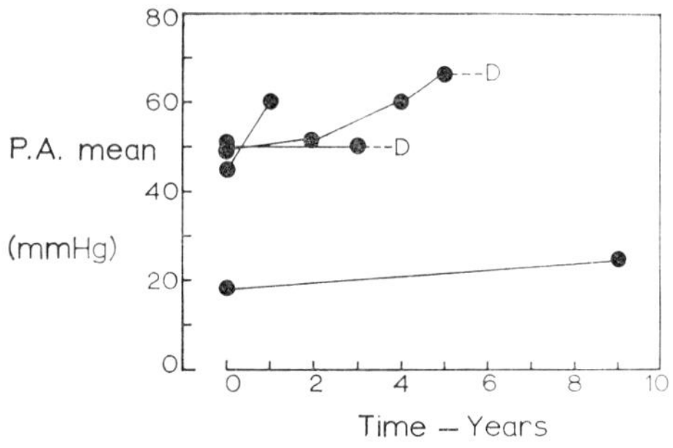

FIG. 3. Serial measurements of pulmonary arterial mean pressure in four patients with chronic bronchitis, two of whom subsequently died as indicated (D).

did not increase during periods of 3 to 9 years. More observations of this kind are needed but the time course of the pulmonary hypertension is clearly variable.

Further alterations in pulmonary arterial pressure are seen in individual patients over a short period of time when they develop congestive failure. Figure 4 shows the results of measurements of pulmonary arterial pressure in our own patients and in the patients described by Harvey *et al.* (1951) and Whitaker (1954). The fall in pressure with recovery is evident and consistent.

In considering some of the factors which may affect pulmonary arterial pressure in these various circumstances, mention must first be made of the structural changes in pulmonary blood vessels. These are considered in full in the following paper and the characteristic changes, present in all patients with pulmonary hypertension, are described. These cannot, of course, explain the variable element in pulmonary arterial pressure and the factors which may be important here will now be discussed.

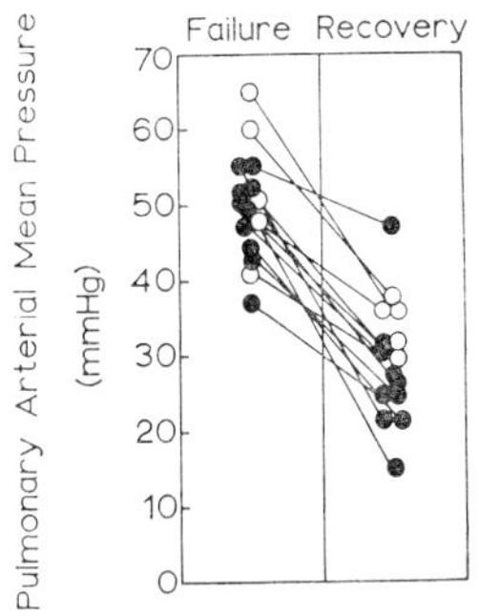

FIG. 4. Pulmonary arterial mean pressure measured when in congestive failure and after recovery in 15 patients with chronic bronchitis. Data from Harvey *et al.*, 1951 (closed circles) and Whitaker, 1954 (open circles).

As already noted, the cardiac output is not consistently raised in the steady state but pulmonary vascular resistance is increased. Even in the acute stages of congestive failure we have not found any increase in cardiac output. Earlier workers reported such an increase, however, and there is some evidence that it was formerly a more frequent feature (Harvey *et al.*, 1965) of such acute episodes.

The effects of hypoxia upon the pulmonary circulation are now well established and the vasoconstrictive action is demonstrable in patients with chronic bronchitis and emphysema as in normal subjects. The vasoconstriction appears to be due to a local effect of hypoxia upon the wall of the blood vessel, and not to a nervous reflex. It has long appeared tempting to relate the pulmonary hypertension to the known hypoxaemia in these patients. Like many other workers we have found a negative correlation between pulmonary arterial mean pressure and arterial oxygen saturation or oxygen tension, and we found similar correlations for pulmonary vascular resistance. This does not necessarily imply any causal relationship, although such is possible. The relationship could simply mean that both hypoxaemia and pulmonary hypertension were features of a particular kind of disease or structural disorder. An observation which has been invoked to suggest that hypoxia is not a major factor in the pulmonary hypertension, is that the administration of oxygen to such patients causes at most a small reduction in pulmonary arterial pressure. This is certainly true for patients in the steady state, but evidence presented below suggests that the effect of oxygen may be greater in patients with congestive failure.

We have also found a direct correlation between the arterial carbon dioxide tension and pulmonary arterial pressure, but again the meaning is uncertain. By contrast with hypoxia, however, the administration of carbon dioxide mixtures has not been shown consistently to cause pulmonary vasoconstriction in man, either healthy or when suffering from chronic bronchitis and emphysema (Fishman *et al.*, 1960).

Liljestrand (1958) suggested that the effects of both hypoxia and hypercapnia upon the pulmonary circulation were mediated by changes in hydrogen ion concentration. Once again there is a positive correlation between pulmonary arterial pressure and hydrogen ion concentration. Enson and his colleagues showed that infusions of either sodium bicarbonate or THAM led to a fall in pulmonary arterial pressure in some but no change in other patients. Since this was always associated with a rise in cardiac output, the infusions appeared to have caused pulmonary vasodilatation. However in the course of studies for another purpose, during which THAM infusions were given over a much longer period of time (Aber *et al.*, 1963), no change in either pulmonary arterial pressure or cardiac output was observed. Enson *et al.* also describe one patient in whom an infusion of hydrochloric acid caused changes suggesting pulmonary vasoconstriction. We have been unable to confirm this observation and, as illustrated in Figure 5, found a small but significant fall of pulmonary vascular resistance during such an infusion in a group of six patients with chronic bronchitis (E. Housley, unpublished observations). More information is clearly needed but, to say the least, the effects of isolated alterations in hydrogen ion concentration are doubtful, although the effects may be greater at higher concentrations of hydrogen ion.

Some of these patients have an increased blood volume and a correlation was found between total blood volume and pulmonary arterial pressure (Segel & Bishop, 1966), while all pulmonary vascular pressures rose following an infusion of human serum albumen. These results were obtained during the course of an investigation into the effects of increased blood viscosity, another factor which may influence the pulmonary arterial pressure. Markedly increased viscosity is associated with polycythaemia which is itself comparatively rare in chronic bronchitis. In a group of such patients we reduced viscosity to normal by repeated venesection during 7–10

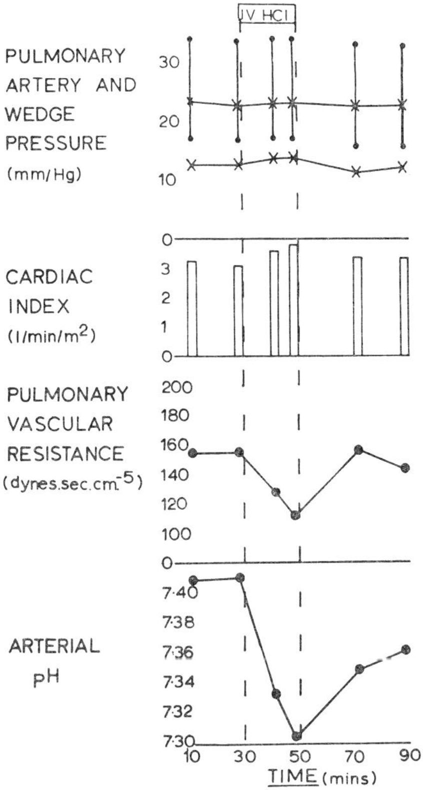

FIG. 5 Effect of an intravenous infusion of hydrochloric acid upon pulmonary arterial and wedge pressure, cardiac output, pulmonary vascular resistance and arterial pH. Mean values for six patients with chronic bronchitis.

days and found that pulmonary arterial pressure fell in some but not in others. Examining the results it was evident that the size of this fall depended upon the extent of the reduction in blood volume

(Fig. 6). It appeared therefore that increased blood viscosity played a relatively minor role, but that increased blood volume was of greater importance.

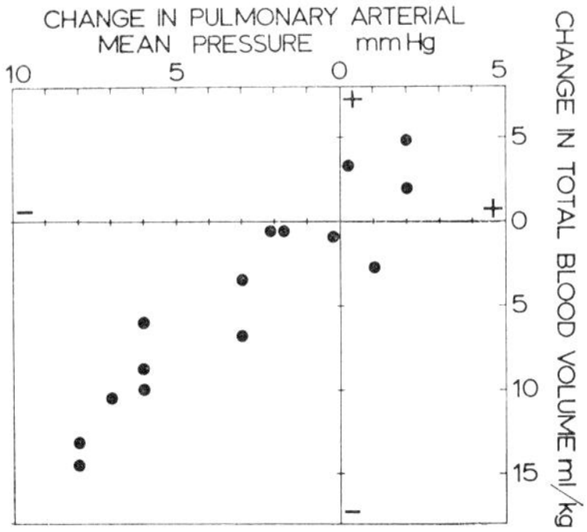

FIG. 6. Relationship between change in pulmonary arterial mean pressure and change in total blood volume in patients with chronic bronchitis and secondary polycythaemia. Measurements were made before and after repeated venesection over a period of 1 week.

Consideration of the effects which alterations in the mechanical properties of the lung may have upon the pulmonary arterial pressure reveals two quite separate mechanisms which may play a part. The first of these is concerned with the effect of the raised mean alveolar pressure which is a feature of airway obstruction. Rodbard (1953) was one of the first to suggest that if alveolar pressure rises sufficiently then compression of parts of the pulmonary vascular bed results, with increased pulmonary vascular resistance. One is obliged to be rather vague in describing the site of this compression since it is uncertain which kinds of the pulmonary blood vessels are situated in such a position that they would be subject to compression. This hypothesis, however, fails to explain why many patients with undoubted severe airway obstruction have normal, or near normal, pulmonary arterial pressures while other patients with a similar degree of airway obstruction have severe pulmonary hypertension.

The raised alveolar pressure seems likely, on the other hand, to account for the raised pulmonary wedge pressure seen in a proportion of patients, as shown in Figure 7. During exercise an even larger proportion of patients have an abnormally high wedge pressure (Horsfield *et al.*, 1967). It appears probable that under these conditions alveolar pressure has exceeded the pulmonary venous pressure and the vessels containing the static column of blood have been occluded. The pressure so recorded as pulmonary wedge now reflects alveolar pressure rather than pulmonary venous or left atrial pressure.

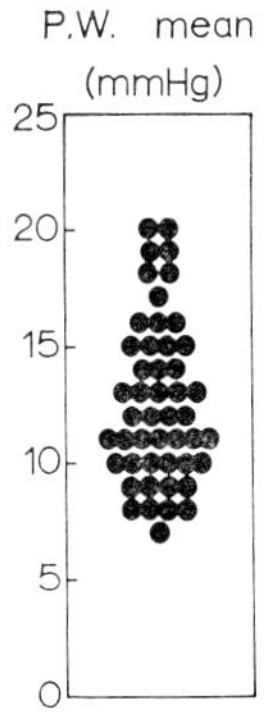

FIG. 7. Pulmonary wedge pressure at rest in 50 patients with chronic bronchitis.

The second mechanism which might influence the pulmonary blood vessels is the interstitial pressure surrounding the pulmonary resistance vessels. Permutt (1965) has suggested that those vessels which lie outside the alveolar territory are subjected to a surrounding pressure which is more negative than intrapleural pressure and which is opposed to the force of the muscle tone in the wall of the vessel. If this state of affairs does exist then emphysema is one of several conditions in which this surrounding interstitial pressure will be higher than normal, with the possible consequence that a stimulus to contraction in the arterial wall may lead to a greater degree of narrowing of the lumen than normal. For example one might expect, in these circumstances, an exaggerated response to hypoxia. This is an interesting concept, but its practical importance depends upon morphological considerations. Where are those vessels situated which contain circular smooth muscle and which constitute the site of the variable pulmonary vascular resistance? Are they situated outside the 'alveolar territory', as the hypothesis requires? What, in any case, constitutes the 'alveolar territory' and what are its boundaries? Answers to these questions are required before it is possible to evaluate the importance of the proposed mechanism.

Since patients with respiratory and congestive failure show, as already noted, a marked element of reversibility in their pulmonary hypertension, it seemed possible that study of such patients might be profitable. We have made serial observations during the first 5 days as the patient improves under the influence of treatment, and have compared the results with those obtained 2 or 3 weeks later after full recovery from the acute episode (A. S. Abraham, unpublished observations). Three findings from these investigations are worthy of mention.

In the first place we observed that the fall in pulmonary arterial pressure always preceded a decrease in blood volume, which was initially well above the normal level. Blood volume did not seem to be of major importance at this stage of the disease.

Secondly, although the number of studies is as yet small, it appears that the administration of a mixture containing 28 per cent. oxygen caused a definite fall in pulmonary arterial pressure during the acute stage of the illness, and that the extent of this reduction diminished progressively as the patient recovered and the pulmonary hypertension declined (Fig. 8).

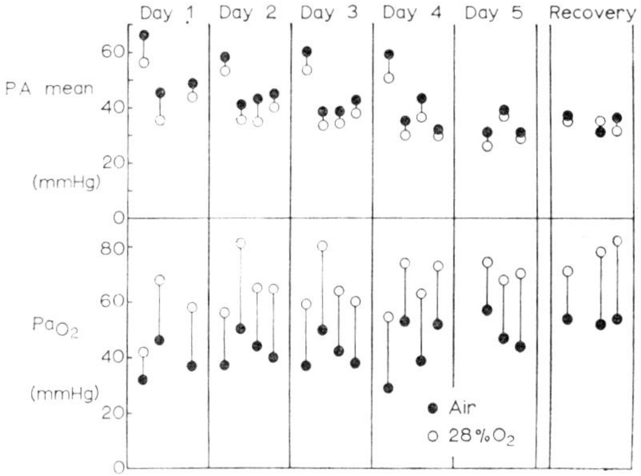

FIG. 8. Serial measurements of pulmonary arterial mean pressure and arterial oxygen tension in four patients with chronic bronchitis and congestive failure. Measurements were made on five successive days and again after full recovery from congestive failure. Values are shown when breathing air (closed circles) and 28 per cent. oxygen (open circles). Each patient occupies the same position in the chart for each day.

The third observation was that acetylcholine infused into the pulmonary artery reduced pulmonary arterial pressure (Fig. 9), and in one patient the fall was to the level at which pressure finally stabilised after recovery. The rise in pulmonary arterial pressure accompanying the acute illness in this patient was therefore due almost entirely to active pulmonary vasoconstriction. Mechanical factors, increased blood volume and increased blood viscosity cannot have played any important part. These results differ from those of Chidsey *et al.* (1960) who gave acetylcholine to patients with emphysema in a stable state and observed little or no change in pulmonary arterial pressure.

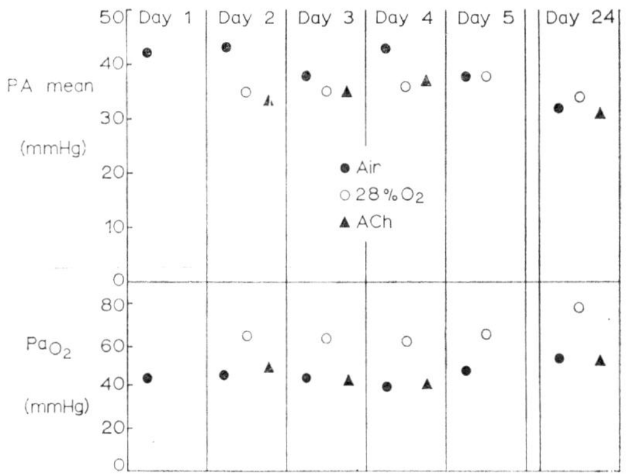

FIG. 9. Serial measurements of pulmonary arterial mean pressure and arterial oxygen tension in one patient with chronic bronchitis and congestive failure during a period of 5 days and again after recovery from congestive failure. Values are shown when breathing air (closed circle), breathing 28 per cent. oxygen (open circle) and when breathing air with an infusion of acetylcholine into the right atrium (triangle).

Further study of the factors responsible for the reversible part of the pulmonary hypertension of acute respiratory and congestive failure should be informative. It could well be that these same factors also initiated the changes which led to the persistent structural changes in pulmonary blood vessels through long continued and oft-repeated functional vasoconstriction.

It is evident from this review that the number of factors possibly contributing to the pulmonary hypertension is considerable and no single one is obviously the unique cause. The pulmonary vasoconstriction may have a multifactorial causation and if this is so it is possible that these factors interact rather than that they are simply additive. A few studies of such possible interactions have recently been reported. Rudolph and Yuan (1966) showed an interaction between the effects of hydrogen ion concentration and hypoxia in the newborn calf. Pulmonary vasoconstriction was greater in the presence of acidaemia, and the threshold for hypoxic vasoconstriction was also raised. One hypothesis which would be consistent with the data presented by Enson *et al.* (1964) is that such an interaction also occurs in patients with emphysema. On the other hand we could find no potentiation of the effect of hypoxia by acutely induced acidaemia in a series of patients with chronic bronchitis (E. Housley, unpublished observations).

We have also looked for any interaction between expansion of the blood volume and hypoxia (Abraham *et al.*, 1967). Again we found no evidence of potentiation, and the level of pulmonary arterial pressure reached with hypoxia after expansion of blood volume was the same as with hypoxia alone (Fig. 10). There are

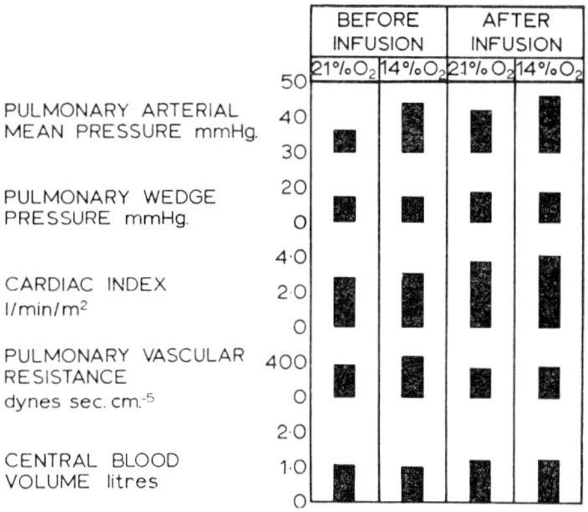

FIG. 10. Effect of acute hypoxia before and after expansion of blood volume in a group of 12 patients with chronic bronchitis. Measurements were made of pulmonary arterial mean and pulmonary wedge pressures, cardiac output, pulmonary vascular resistance and central blood volume when breathing air and 14 per cent. oxygen before and after the infusion of one litre of a solution of human serum albumen.

several other interactions which require study although the experiments will be complex.

From this account there emerges the suggestion that the most important factor leading to the variable pulmonary hypertension is hypoxia, possibly potentiated by acidaemia. The altered interstitial pressure surrounding the pulmonary resistance vessels may play some part, but this is not as yet established. An essential piece of information in the evaluation of these possibilities is a knowledge of the structural and spatial relationships between the relevant blood vessels and the air spaces. Active vasoconstriction implies the presence of smooth muscle in the wall of the vessels concerned. The pulmonary arteriole normally contains little or no muscle, although in emphysema with pulmonary hypertension a layer of circular muscle is seen. These vessels are normally surrounded by alveoli and are presumably affected by variations in their immediate gaseous environment. The observations of Staub (1961) and Jameson (1963) indicate the likelihood that considerably larger vessels, perhaps small and medium sized muscular pulmonary arteries, are also situated so close to air spaces as to be capable of gas exchange across their walls. We know little of the detailed relationships of these vessels to the bronchioles and alveoli in the normal lung and knowledge of how these vessels are related to the abnormal air spaces, alveolar and bronchiolar, in emphysema is even less. It seems reasonable to suggest that the vasoconstriction of acute episodes of respiratory and congestive failure occurs in vessels whose local environment has been rendered hypoxic, and also that the walls of arterioles which show hypertrophy in their circular muscle coat are similarly hypoxic. Is it possible then, to explain the wide variations in the structural changes in the arterioles in terms of different spatial relationships between these vessels and the air spaces, or in terms of different structural changes in the air spaces themselves leading to lower oxygen tensions in the distal spaces in some patients than in others ?

Similarly, if the place of mechanical factors is to be evaluated we need to know which of the vessels we have discussed are likely to be subject to variations in alveolar pressure and which, if any, lie outside the zone of alveolar pressure and might be surrounded by a low interstitial pressure. If there are such vessels, are they the ones which are the seat of the variable pulmonary vascular resistance, or are they, perhaps, larger and unlikely to be capable of vasomotor activity ?

In conclusion it is suggested that although further physiological investigations are clearly necessary, their interpretation is likely to remain incomplete until we have a better understanding of the detailed structural relationships in the normal and diseased lung in quantitative terms.

DISCUSSION OF SESSION THREE

Dr Mead. What do you mean, Dr West, by 'isolation' of vessels by a cuff of oedema ?

Dr West. In the presence of perivascular oedema these vessels could show an increase in vascular resistance for two reasons : on the one hand, you could argue that the perivascular cuffs simply compress the vessels. We are not particularly happy about this because if you look at a distensible organ like the lung, it is difficult to see how interstitial pressure could compress the vessels within it. It has been demonstrated that interstitial pressure in a solid organ with a capsule like the kidney could do this (Hinshaw *et al.*, 1959) but in the lung it's more difficult to conceive it happening. On the other hand, if you allow that the vessels have an inherent tendency to close—and this is demonstrated by the fact that when the lung is allowed to collapse the vascular resistance goes up—then we can argue that the interstitial oedema isolates these vessels from the normal distending force. Thus it allows them to pull away from the normal force which is expanding them and they close by virtue of the inherent tension in their walls.

Professor Wade. Does the space the fluid occupies have to be perivascular ? Suppose there was fluid in the pleural cavity at the base of the lung ?

Dr West. One would expect that an accumulation of fluid in the pleural space would reduce the state of lung expansion at the bottom of the lung and in that way would increase the vascular resistance of the extra-alveolar vessels.

Professor Wade. Well, from that, does it follow that what you're looking at is just a space-occupying lesion ? It doesn't really matter where the lesion is ?

Dr West. I would imagine that for a given amount of space occupied, the effect on vascular resistance would be much greater in this critical region—the perivascular space—than outside the lung.

Dr Permutt. One of the first slides that Dr West showed gives the impression that the alveolar vessels are chiefly limited to the small vessels within the septa of the alveoli and presumably then, would be capillaries. Our work indicates, however, that the vessels which are exposed to alveolar pressure are probably the chief volume-containing vessels of the lung. If this is so, the alveolar vessels certainly consist of much more than capillaries and they probably include venules and perhaps certain parts of the arterial system.

Dr West. The reason why we say alveolar pressure is limited to the vessels below 50μ or so in diameter, is that vessels above that size remain open when alveolar pressure exceeds arterial pressure. If you look at their walls they are exceedingly delicate and thin ; they contain virtually no muscle and exceedingly little elastic tissue. Thus, if they remain open, it seems likely that they are not exposed to alveolar pressure.

Dr Heath. These extra-alveolar vessels are presumably arterioles. Now of course, the structure of arterioles in mitral stenosis varies throughout the lung. As you suggest, these extra-alveolar vessels at the apex and in the upper lobes will be thin-walled vessels consisting of a single elastic lamina but in the lower zones they will consist of thick muscular tubes composed both of circularly and longitudinally orientated smooth muscle fibres, and I'm wondering whether in fact you've taken sufficient cognisance of this complete difference in structure ?

Dr West. I'm very glad you raised that because I don't want to leave the impression that we attribute the reduction in blood flow at the bottom of the lung in established mitral stenosis to interstitial oedema. We certainly don't do that because there's a wealth of morbid anatomical evidence that the structure of vessels changes over the years and the vessels at the bottom of the lung suffer more changes than those at the top and this must be important. But what we are suggesting here is that in a condition like left ventricular failure, where the vessels previously may well have been quite normal, this is the likely initiating factor.

Dr Macklem. I was very interested in the analogy you drew between the interstitial space and the pleural space and it strikes me that there's an additional degree of similarity and this is that in both the interstitial space and the pleura, the pulmonary and the systemic circulations are in very close contact with one another. Theoretically therefore, you could get interstitial oedema from disorders of either circulation. Presumably, in mitral stenosis, it results from the pulmonary circulation but do you know of any evidence that you can get interstitial oedema in right ventricular failure as well ? You can presumably get a hydrothorax from right ventricular failure ?

Dr West. I do not have evidence on this point. Interstitial oedema is a difficult thing to study. I'm very disappointed, for instance, in the amount of interstitial oedema one generally sees at post-mortem ; whereas if you take bits of lung at biopsy you often see it.

Professor Stuart-Harris. Do you make any distinction between arterioles and venules in this regard ? This is a very vital point, because the muscular pulmonary arteries and arterioles follow the line of the respiratory bronchioles and the alveolar ducts, whereas the venules move away immediately from the alveoli to the septa. Presumably therefore, the sort of mechanical stress to which the venules are subjected, is going to be rather different from that to which the arterioles are going to be subjected. One would imagine that the arterioles are more liable to be affected by alveolar pressure than the venules, which lie further away in the septa.

Dr West. We are quite interested in the differences between the arterial and the venous side ; it's our impression that you get interstitial oedema earlier on the arterial side and a little bit later around the bronchi and the veins. There is potential perivascular space along the veins, as well as the arteries—occasionally people have denied this but it's certainly been seen by us. It is quite true of course that the position of the arteries and the veins in the lungs is different.

Professor Stuart-Harris. What is the reason for reduction in blood flow if the airway to a lobe, for instance, is blocked ? As soon as collapse appears, the blood flow immediately drops off. Is this due to an absence of retracting forces ?

Dr West. It would fit in quite well with the sort of model I presented, that if the airways are closed and that part of the lung collapses, the parenchyma is under less stress and therefore the pull on the extra-alveolar vessels is less. Therefore they close, because of the inherent tone of their walls, and the vascular resistance rises.

Chairman. If acute atelectasis is produced by obstructing an airway in the open-chest dog, the amount of reduction of blood flow through the collapsed lung is of the order of 10 to 20 per cent. It is not a very dramatic fall. Only with time, as the lung stays collapsed, does the reduction reach levels of 40 to 50 per cent. So, even through acute collapse of a lung does curtail pulmonary blood flow, the effect is not a very dramatic one.

Dr West. That's not the experience we have had with isolated lungs. There is an enormous rise in vascular resistance when the lung collapses and trans-pulmonary pressure goes down to nil. Probably most of the airways are still open and the alveoli certainly contain some gas, yet there is a great rise in pulmonary vascular resistance.

Chairman. I should like to make one other point with respect to Dr West's presentation. Morkin, Skalak, Szidon and Ingram, working in my laboratory, have shown that blood flow throughout the lung, including the veins, is exceedingly pulsatile. In our studies, pulsatility in the pulmonary venous flow pattern was much more marked than in the observations which Dr West has shown on the isolated lung. Perhaps the difference is attributable to the preparations which we used. We used the intact, unanaesthetised dog with an electro-magnetic flow probe on the artery and on the vein. By using these flow probes in conjunction with body plethysmography, we could follow the transformation of the pressure and the flow pulse from the artery to the capillaries and to the veins. Remarkably, there may be only a 50 per cent. decrease in the amplitude and little change in the contour of the pulmonary venous flow pulse even though the pressure pulse is considerably damped in travelling from the arterial to the venous side. I should also note that pulmonary venous flow pulsatility does not arise from the left atrium since it persists in the perfused lung in situ, even though a reservoir is substituted for the left atrium. Finally, as Szidon and Ingram have recently shown, pulmonary oedema decreases markedly the amplitude of the pulmonary venous pulsations in flow.

Dr West. We do see pulsations on the venous side—it's just that they are much less than the pulsations on the arterial side. There's no question about pulsatile flow but when we find it we measure it to be much less.

Dr Heath. Everybody's been talking this morning about this nebulous entity, the extra-alveolar vessel and I think it really ought to be defined much more closely. For instance, you said that when the lung collapsed the vessels constricted due to their inherent tone. So far as I know, the major extra-alveolar vessels are arterioles which don't have any muscle in them. The first class of vessels that have muscle are the small muscular pulmonary arteries which, as Professor Harris has shown, will be in justaposition to relatively indistensible things like small bronchi or bronchioles.

Dr West. I think it's well defined, if I may say so—operationally defined. By extra-alveolar vessels we mean the vessels not exposed to alveolar pressure. Now that's a very tight definition. We don't know precisely what these vessels are but we've got them defined operationally quite accurately. We do feel though, that this probably includes most of the larger vessels. The very small vessels, for example the capillaries, are excluded, as are the main pulmonary arteries as they enter the lung, and the main pulmonary veins just as they come out. The last two are exposed to pulmonary pressure.

Dr Permutt. If you could show, under a variety of circumstances, that some of the blood vessels of the lung act as though they were exposed to alveolar pressure, whatever they are and wherever they are, then by definition those are alveolar vessels, the others extra-alveolar. The difficulty arises when we come to apply the operational definition to a particular blood-vessel !

Turning now to Dr Bates's paper, one of the criticisms of determining the $\dot{V}/\dot{Q}$ ratio by the xenon technique is that the counter covers a very large area. Within the area covered by the counter, if there's not homogeneity, this method gives an average $\dot{V}/\dot{Q}$ ratio of the whole area ; it does not indicate the discrepancies within that area. The clinical evidence and the crude pulmonary function tests that have been used in the past suggest the presence of areas of very high $\dot{V}/\dot{Q}$ ratios. The counter shows essentially no such areas but our work shows they must be there. Would you agree that in an area in which you have measured a low $\dot{V}/\dot{Q}$ ratio, there might be countless areas that have exceedingly high $\dot{V}/\dot{Q}$ ratios ?

Dr Bates. There must be but their volume representation must be small.

Dr West. I feel very strongly about this. We're seeing quite large proportions of the lung under these counters and the results are the means from large areas of lung. It can be misleading to argue from the $\dot{V}/\dot{Q}$ ratios obtained in this way.

Chairman. If one had holes in the lung with little blood supply left, one would be very apt to see alveoli hyperventilated with respect to perfusion. Whereas in bronchitis, where the disease is largely obstructive, one might be less apt to do so. You must have in your own mind, Dr Bates, some idea of what the anatomy looks like in these people who have mild chronic bronchitis.

Dr Bates. I find this very hard to answer. I would have to say that there must be, in the cigarette-smoking population, significant abnormalities and they could be, of course, just plugs, temporary obstructions of some kind. There must be significant abnormalities out in the distal airways which have not been noticed, and probably such a lung would be passed as normal at autopsy. There would be some mucous gland hyperplasia but not tremendous. The trouble is that people don't come to autopsy at this stage of the disease.

Dr Dunnill. If you do a post-mortem on an asthmatic who's symptom-free—and I've been fortunate enough to do post mortems on four people killed in motor-car accidents who were known asthmatics—you see mucous plugs, particularly in the lower lobes. There's some evidence that these mucous plugs stay in the bronchi for weeks, months, even years, without altering, and you can see the decayed cells of necrotic material in the centre of them. I think that may be important.

Dr Reid. Dr Gregg, a general practitioner, has done some extremely interesting work just using straight peak flows on patients in a general practice who were smokers but have given it up. He finds (Gregg, 1966) that there are patients who may have impaired F.E.V.$_{1}$ and regular sputum production. In some of those, when they stop smoking their sputum disappears and their F.E.V.$_{1}$ goes back to normal. In others, the sputum disappears but the F.E.V.$_1$ does *not* go back to normal. This is simply some evidence that one can pick up an early group of mildly affected cases in which the changes are already irreversible.

Dr Thurlbeck. We've actually been exercising ourselves trying to guess at what may be the structural abnormality in the lungs in these people. From a random series of necropsies, in the age group 45–54, we find that a chronic bronchitic male has a 90 per cent. chance of having emphysema (Thurlbeck, 1966). However, this still leaves open the question whether this structural parenchymal change is sufficient to account for the disturbance of function. Now the question I have for Dr Reid is this : what are the lesions in the small airways in a smoking male bronchitic between 45 and 54 who doesn't have parenchymal disease, by which I mean loss of alveolar walls ?

Dr Reid. I can't answer strictly within the terms of the question in that I can't say I've looked at men of the age group you mentioned who have smoked but have not died of chronic bronchitis. But if you take a group of bronchitics who have died for other reasons or whose lungs were obtained at surgery one does find that the goblet cells extend in a most striking way right the way down the bronchial tree, where there are hardly any goblet cells under ordinary circumstances. One also finds patchily distributed signs of chronic inflammation and an increase in the fibrous tissue and this is usually irregularly disposed through the walls, so that there are multiple incomplete stenoses, and of course this will produce irregularity of the epithelium. What has particularly struck us, looking at the bronchograms of some of these smoking early bronchitics with perhaps even more normal function than the ones Dr Bates has mentioned, is the surprising degree to which you can pick out the lesions of bronchiolectasis. You see pools of radio-opaque material a few millimetres across and smooth and still within the bronchial tree. They are at terminal, or pre-terminal bronchiolar level. So that there are signs of bronchiolar damage, irregularly distributed, even in early cases.

Chairman. You are referring to the group just described, to the type of patient Dr Bates has been talking about ?

Dr Reid. Yes. Or a smoker whose functions do not go back to normal when he stops smoking.

Dr Cumming. Dr Bates, I was fascinated to see the two curves of different rates of clearance with the injected xenon and the re-breathed xenon. It occurred to me that these areas of high $\dot{V}/\dot{Q}$ which you might expect to see, might in fact be in the respiratory bronchiolar area. It's a small step from there to say the high $\dot{V}/\dot{Q}$ area is a pathological change in the airways around this area. What would be the possible functional consequences of such a high $\dot{V}/\dot{Q}$? If you re-breathe the xenon, and gas mixing is not complete, the rate of clearance would be high. If you put the xenon into the alveolus from the capillaries, diffusion from the alveolus into the dilated respiratory bronchiole must occur before clearance can start and the rate of this would be very much slower than it would be from the re-breathing technique. So I think you've shown very elegantly that the physical functional disability in these people is that of stratified inhomogeneity.

Dr Whitaker. In considering the mechanical factors that could be playing a part in this reversible pulmonary hypertension in acute illness, Professor Bishop mentioned that airways obstruction could be a factor. I wonder if he has any observations correlating measurements of airways obstruction with changes in the pulmonary artery blood pressures in and out of failure?

Professor Bishop. No, we don't have any information on that yet.

Professor Stuart-Harris. In some recent work that we've been doing in Sheffield with the body plethysmograph we found in anoxic patients that breathing 30 per cent. oxygen caused a reduction in the increased airways resistance of such patients. There is no similar effect in normal subjects. The effect in patients is inversely correlated with the lowering in oxygen tension of the arterial blood and not only is there a change in airways resistance but, as one would anticipate, there is a reduction in the work of breathing. This effect on the airways must be taken into account though exactly how it can bear on changes in the pulmonary artery pressure, one can only speculate.

Dr Whitaker. This really is terribly interesting. It suggests that when you give oxygen to patients who have pulmonary hypertension with congestive heart failure, the fall in pulmonary artery blood pressure that is observed may be due to the change in airways obstruction and not to a change in vascular resistance produced by the alteration in the blood oxygen tension as had previously been believed.

Dr Cotes. In reply to Professor Stuart-Harris, Dr Pisa and I have some information on the effect of oxygen on the pulmonary artery pressure and cardiac output in patients with chronic respiratory failure. We found on average a 10 per cent. drop in pulmonary artery pressure associated with a 7 per cent. drop in cardiac output. Thus most of the change in pulmonary artery pressure could superficially be explained in terms of the change in cardiac output and the point of my remark is that this change in cardiac output was almost entirely due to a drop in cardiac frequency.

Dr Permutt. I have attempted to put these factors together over the years. I won't go into all my reasons at this time—I will simply state my view that I would really completely dismiss alveolar pressure as being a significant factor causing pulmonary hypertension in the patients with chronic lung disease. Alveolar pressure goes up during expiration but you can look at it rather like pleural pressure. The patients I have studied with pulmonary hypertension and chronic lung disease have high pulmonary artery pressures relative to pleural pressure, so the expiratory phase does not account for the rise in pulmonary arterial pressure.

Much of the real significance of hypoxia is overlooked because of the lack of consideration of the proper time scale. A good model to think about under these circumstances is what happens to cows when they are taken up to high altitudes. If you make a cow hypoxic by making it breathe a hypoxic mixture, the rise in pulmonary artery pressure will be rather trivial. If you now take the cow up to 11,000 feet, it gets a progressive rise in pulmonary artery pressure taking place over a period of weeks. If you then give it oxygen to breathe, it gets an acute fall in pulmonary artery pressure, but the pulmonary artery pressure doesn't go anywhere near back to its normal level. Finally, if you now bring the cow down to a normal altitude, its pulmonary artery pressures come back to a normal level over a period of 6–8 weeks. This response to hypoxia must be thought of in terms of a prolonged time-scale. It is always accompanied by structural changes in the pulmonary artery, increased smooth muscle, etc., and it's also typical of the people who live at high altitudes.

Chairman. I can support this. In a group of patients with cystic fibrosis of the pancreas, who suffered from obstructive lung disease, pure oxygen decreased pulmonary arterial pressure with little effect on airway resistance. The cardiac output did not change appreciably.

Professor Bishop. Would Dr Permutt agree with the suggestion that these high pulmonary wedge pressures that we've been recording could well be reflecting alveolar pressure ?

Dr Permutt. They very well could be. We have evidence in the dog that we can produce wedge pressures considerably higher than left atrial pressures by elevating alveolar pressure. Even a normal subject can have a high wedge pressure if the tip of the catheter is high relative to the left atrium because of collapse of vessels between the tip of the catheter and the left atrium. If you adhere to the criteria of Dexter—in other words if you are always able to draw oxygenated blood and if you are always able to see left atrial pulsation—then you will probably be recording the left atrial pressure. But many times people stick a catheter in, they wedge it, they are unable to draw blood back, they don't get left atrial pulsations and so the tip of the catheter might very well be in a place that has absolutely no communication at all with the left atrium.

Dr West. Some years ago when we were working with the isolated lung and a cardiac catheter, two or three times we wedged a catheter and were able to show that as you lowered the venous reservoir, you saw a falling wedge pressure. Then, once venous pressure fell below alveolar pressure, the pressure seen by the wedge catheter did not change, exactly as you would predict from the Starling resistor model. Thus when venous pressure was below alveolar pressure, you saw alveolar pressure with the catheter.

Dr Whitaker. I think we ought to put on record that we don't believe that the wedge pressure measures the left atrial pressure at all.

Chairman. Bell and his group have shown that, despite conventional criteria for adequate wedging, it is possible to be measuring something entirely unrelated to left atrial pressure. For example, the catheter may impinge on the vascular wall instead of facing the lumen and record beautiful but meaningless wiggles. This type of artefact is most apt to occur in normal lungs and is least likely when the vascular tree is congested. Thus, when venous pressure is high, it is difficult to convince yourself that you're not measuring left atrial pressure. Indeed, if you record the wedge pressure and left atrial pressure simultaneously during pulmonary venous congestion, the two tracings bear a remarkable resemblance to each other.

Dr Whitaker. You're really saying, sir, that if it measures what you think it ought to measure, then you accept it !

Chairman. Then we have tremendous confidence in it !

Professor Harris. I would like to take issue over alveolar pressure. I think it is a very important determinant. If you increase the mouth pressure in normal persons, you will increase their pulmonary wedge pressure, their pulmonary arterial pressure and their pulmonary vascular resistance. The increase in the wedge pressure under those circumstances is not itself a reflection of alveolar pressure because if you do it in somebody with a small atrial septal defect you find that the wedge pressure goes up at the same time as the left atrial pressure and to the same extent. The fact that you can increase the pulmonary vascular resistance by increasing the mouth pressure to my mind means that you must be able to compress some vessels which are under the influence of the pressure in the alveolus. To take the opposite extreme, as Professor Bishop has just shown us, if you infuse albumen or in some other way increase the static pressure inside these vessels and finally distend them, you find they are relatively indistensible. The pulmonary vascular resistance does not change. So if you have wide phasic variations in alveolar pressure, then during inspiration you wouldn't expect the vessels which are in contact with the alveoli to widen very much, but in expiration you could expect them to narrow. That is to say, the overall mean effect during the cycle of inspiration/expiration, would be that the vessels would narrow and their resistance would be raised. You can demonstrate this very easily in patients with chronic bronchitis. If you make them hyperventilate, the pulmonary arterial pressure goes up and their pulmonary vascular resistance also increases, whereas of course this doesn't occur in a normal person.

Dr West. Following that, it's very difficult for me to see how the pulmonary arterial pressure could go up more than alveolar pressure. I don't know how far the alveolar pressure goes up on expiration, but I think it could only account for a small rise in arterial pressure.

Dr Reid. To facilitate comparison between normal and diseased lungs of the size of the medial coat of the pulmonary artery and its branches, an attempt was made to relate the size of a given artery to that of its accompanying airway. This did not prove useful, but it was found possible, if the vessels were injected under standard conditions, to predict to a surprisingly high degree the structure and size of an artery according to its external diameter.

The pulmonary artery and its branches were injected at a pressure of 100 cm. H_2O with a micropaque and gelatine mixture which allowed routine microscopical examination. The wall thickness (W.T.) was expressed as a percentage of the external diameter (E.D.) according to the formula $\frac{2 \times \text{W.T.}}{\text{E.D.}} \times 100$.

For arteries above 150 μ in external diameter, the structure and wall thickness can be closely predicted to within 1 per cent. (Elliott, 1964, Elliott & Reid, 1965, Reid, 1967). Arteries below 2,000 μ in external diameter are muscular ; above this figure they are elastic or transitional.

In the elastic arteries the wall thickness is between 3 per cent. and 5 per cent. of external diameter ; it falls gradually until at the beginning of the muscular region the percentage is between 1·5 and 2·5, and in vessels of 1,000 μ it is 1 per cent. Distal to this the ratio assumes an upward trend, giving arteries below 200 μ in diameter relatively the thickest wall. This peripheral increase is not the result of failure to distend the smaller vessels as in the smaller vessels the medial area also shows an increase proportional to the size of external diameter (Fig. 1).

Along any arterial pathway a point is reached where the complete muscle coat (' completely muscular ') gives way to a spiral (' partially muscular ') of muscle, before it disappears (' non-muscular ') (Fig. 2). The arterial size at which these changes occur is not constant

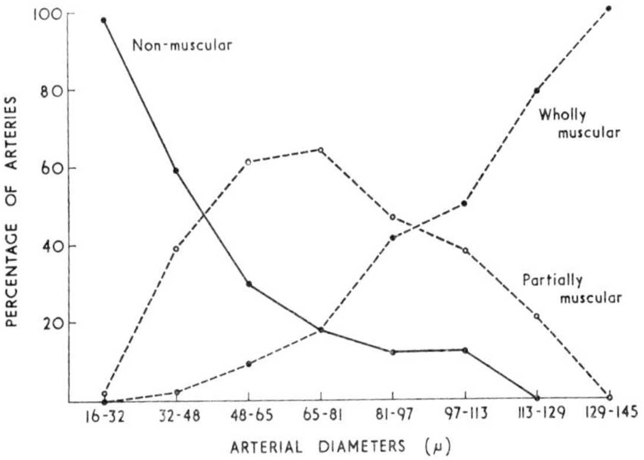

FIG. 1. Distribution of arterial types in vessels below 145 μ. Completely muscular arteries are gradually replaced by partially and non-muscular arteries.

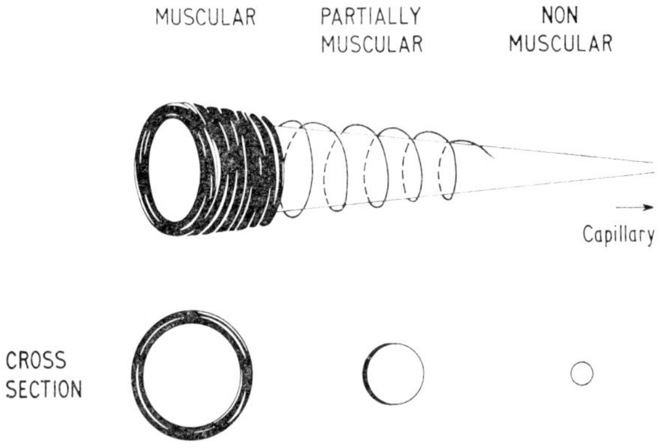

FIG. 2. Along any artery, the completely muscular coat gives way to a spiral of muscle before being lost. The lower row of circles shows that in the partially muscular arteries only a crescent of muscle is seen.

so that at any diameter below 150 μ the arterial population is mixed. (Fig. 3). For the completely muscular arteries below 150 μ the wall thickness can be predicted from external diameter.

To study arteries in this size range it is necessary to estimate, for a given diameter, the proportion of vessels which fall into each category as well as the wall thickness of the muscular vessels. The ‘ partially muscular ’ artery has virtually a capillary wall, making gas

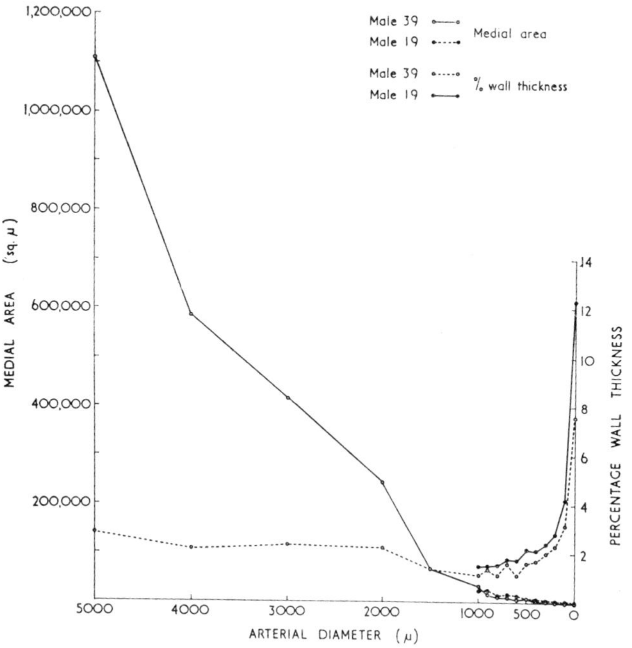

FIG. 3. Medial area and wall thickness showing relative increase in wall thickness in smaller arteries. Medial area falls with size of artery but at point where wall thickness is increasing the medial area falls less sharply, suggesting that the wall thickness increase is not the result of incomplete distension.

exchange possible, as well as a spiral of muscle, capable of contraction. This spiral is in direct continuity with the small muscular vessels which are relatively the most muscular in the lung, and presumably contract actively. Against a given pressure, tone is more easily maintained in narrower than in wider vessels (cf. Poiseuille’s Law) so that the smaller the vessel, the less the muscle needed for this purpose. The work of physiologists, in particular the experiments of von Euler and Liljestrand (1946) have shown that hypoxia increases pulmonary resistance by direct action at the level of the alveoli. Hilton (1959 : 1963) has shown in systemic vessels that variations in tone arise from impulses conducted directly from muscle fibre to muscle fibre without intermediate nervous reflexes or circulatory humoral mediation. If this work can be transferred to the pulmonary system a stimulus to constriction arising in the partially muscular vessels can quickly produce constriction in the small completely muscular vessels—this region is structurally a veritable ' stopcock ' (Elliott 1964).

REFERENCES

Aber, G. M., Bayley, T. J. & Bishop, J. M. (1963). *Clin. Sci.* **25,** 171.

Abraham, A. S., Hedworth-Whitty, R. B. & Bishop, J. M. (1967). *Clin. Sci.* **33,** 371.

Anthonisen, N. R., Dolovich, M. B. & Bates, D. V. (1966). *J. clin. Invest.* **45,** 1349.

Anthonisen, N. R., Milic-Emili, J. (1966). *J. appl. Physiol.* **21,** 760.

Ball, W. C., Jr., Stewart, P. B., Newsham, L. G. S. & Bates, D. V. (1962). *J. clin. Invest.* **41,** 519.

Bass, H., Heckscher, T. & Anthonisen, N. R. A. In press.

Bates, D. V. & Christie, R. V. (1964). *Respiratory Function in Disease.* Philadelphia : Saunders.

Bates, D. V., Gordon, C. A., Place, R. E. G., Snidal, D. P. & Woolf, C. R. (1966). *Med. Ser. J. Can.* **22,** 5.

Bentivoglio, L. G., Beerel, F., Stewart, P. B., Bryan, A. C., Ball, W. C., Jr. Bates, D. V. (1963). *Am. Rev. resp. Dis.* **88,** 315.

Bergel, D. H., Glazier, J. B., Hughes, J. M. B., Maloney, J. E. & West, J. B. (1966). *J. Physiol., Lond.,* **189,** 28.

Bryan, A. C., Bentivoglio, L. G., Beerel, F., MacLeish, H., Zidulka, A. & Bates, D. V. (1964). *J. appl. Physiol.* **19,** 395.

Chidsey, C. A., Fritts, H. W., Zocche, G. P., Himmelstein, A. & Courand, A. (1960). *Malatt. cardiovasc.* **1,** 15.

Daly, W. J. & Bondurant, S. (1963). *J. appl. Physiol.* **18,** 513.

Dollery, C. T. & Hugh-Jones, P. (1963). *Br. med. Bull.* **19,** 59.

Dollery, C. T. & West, J. B. (1960). *Circulation Res.* **8,** 765.

Elliott, F. M. (1964). Ph.D. Thesis, University of London.

Elliott, F. M. & Reid, L. (1965). *Clin. Radiol.* **16,** 193.

Enson, Y., Guintini, C., Lewis, M. L., Morris, T. Q., Ferrer, M. I. & Harvey, R. M. (1964). *J. clin. Invest.* **43,** 1146.

Euler, V. S. von & Liljestrand, G. (1946). *Acta physiol. scand.* **12,** 301.

Fishman, A. P., Fritts, H. W. & Cournand, A. (1960). *Circulation,* **22,** 220.

Fowler, K. T., Pain, M. C. F., West, J. B. (1966). *J. Physiol. Lond.,* **185,** 44P.

Fowler, K. T., West, J. B., & Pain, M. C. F. (1966). *Resp. Physiol., Neth.* **1,** 88.

Glazier, J. B., Hughes, J. M. B., Maloney, J. E., Pain, M. C. F. & West, J. B. (1966). *Lancet* **2,** 203.

Gregg, I. (1966). *J. Coll. gen. Practnrs.* **11,** Suppl. 2, 36.

Hales, S. (1731). *Vegetable Staticks.* p. 241. London.

Harvey, R. M., Enson, Y., Cournand, A. &. Ferrer, M. I. (1965). *Arch. Kreislaufforsch.* **46,** 7.

Harvey, R. M., Ferrer, M. I., Richards, D. W. & Cournand, A. (1951). *Am. J. Med.* **10,** 719.

Hayek, H. von (1960). *The Human Lung.* New York : Haffner Publishing Co.

Heath, D. & Hicken, P. (1960). *Thorax,* **15,** 54.

Hilton, S. M. (1959). *J. Physiol., Lond.,* **149,** 93.

Hilton, S. M. (1962). *Physiol. Rev.* **42,** Suppl. No. 5, p. 265.

HINSHAW, L. B., DAY, S. B. & CARLSON, C. H. (1959). *Am. J. Physiol.* **197,** 309.
HORSFIELD, K., SEGEL, N. & BISHOP, J. M. (1967). *Clin. Sci.* **34.** In press.
HOWELL, J. B. L., PERMUTT, S., PROCTOR, D. F. & RILEY, R. L. (1961). *J. appl. Physiol.* **16,** 71.
HUGHES, J. M. B., GLAZIER, J. B., MALONEY, J. E. & WEST, J. B. (1968). *Res. Physiol., Neth.* In press.
JAMESON, A. G. (1963). *Science, N.Y.* **139,** 826.
KLOCKE, F. J. & RAHN, H. (1961). *J. clin. Invest.* **40,** 286.
KNIPPING, H. W., BOLT, W., VALENTIN, H., VENRATH, H., & ENDLER, P. (1961). *Z. Tuberk.* **117,** 51.
KRUEGER, J. J., BAIN, T. & PATTERSON, J. L. (1961). *J. appl. Physiol.* **16,** 465.
LILJESTRAND, G. (1958). *Acta. physiol. scand.* **44,** 216.
MEAD, J. & WHITTENBERGER, J. L. (1964). In *Handbook of Physiology*, Sec. 3, Vol. I. p. 477. ed. Fenn, & Rahn, H., Washington D.C. : *American Physiological Society*,
PAIN, M. C. F. & WEST, J. B. (1966). *J. appl. Physiol.* **21,** 1545.
PERMUTT, S. (1965). *Med. Thorac.* **22,** 118–131.
PERMUTT, S., BROMBERGER-BARNEA, B., & BANE, H. N. (1962). *Med. Thorac.* **19,** 239.
REID, L. (1966). Structural and functional reappraisal of the pulmonary artery circulation. *Basic Science of Medicine Lecture, Series* **1966–1967,** London : Athlone Press.
REID, L. (1967). In *The Pathology of Emphysema*, London : Lloyd-Luke.
RODBARD, S. (1953). *Am. J. Med.* **15,** 356.
RUCH, T. C. & PATTON, H. D. (1965). *Physiology and Biophysics.* Philadelphia : Saunders.
RUDOLPH, A. M. & YUAN, S. (1966). *J. clin. Invest.* **45,** 399.
SEGEL, N. & BISHOP, J. M. (1966). *J. clin. Invest.* **35,** 1555.
STAUB, N. C. (1961). *Fend. Proc. Fedn. Am. Socs. exp. Biol.* **20,** 107.
THURLBECK, W. H. (1966). In *Emphysema in Industry*, p. 1 ed. de Treville, R. T. P. Pittsburg : Industrial Hygiene Foundation of America.
UEDA, H., IIO, M. & KAIHARA, S. (1964). *Jap. Heart J.* **5,** 431.
WEIBEL, E. R. (1963). *Morphometry of the Human Lung.* p. 9. Berlin : Springer.
WEST, J. B. & DOLLERY, C. T. (1960). *J. appl. Phsyiol.* **15,** 405.
WEST, J. B. & DOLLERY, C. T. (1965). *J. appl. Physiol.* **20,** 175.
WEST, J. B., DOLLERY, C. T. & HEARD, B. E. (1965). *Circulation Res.* **17,** 191.
WEST, J. B., DOLLERY, C. T. & NAIMARK, A. (1964). *J. appl. Physiol.* **19,** 713.
WHITAKER, W. (1954). *Q. Jl Med.* **23,** 57.
WOOD, E. H., NOLAN, A. C., DONALD, D. E. & CRONIN, L. (1963). *Fedn. Proc. Fedn. Am Socs. exp. Biol.* **22,** 1024.

SESSION FOUR

THE DEVELOPMENT OF PULMONARY HYPERTENSION AND ITS RELATION TO STRUCTURAL CHANGES

Chairman: ALFRED P. FISHMAN

HYPERTENSIVE PULMONARY VASCULAR DISEASE IN EMPHYSEMA AND STATES OF CHRONIC HYPOXIA

DONALD HEATH

MY task this afternoon is to describe the structural changes that occur in the pulmonary blood vessels in emphysema, with special reference to those associated with the development of cor pulmonale in this condition. At Birmingham we have carried out studies of the pulmonary vascular disease associated both with emphysema (Hicken *et al.*, 1965) and with other conditions associated with chronic hypoxia such as the Pickwickian syndrome (Hasleton *et al.*, 1967).

In our first study, namely that confined to emphysema, we studied both lungs from 19 cases of emphysema. We found it difficult to detect the presence of emphysema and to determine its type using untreated necropsy material. This was particularly so in bronchiolar emphysema since the small abnormal air spaces were hidden by blood and fluid and by the partial collapse of the lung. Hence in all instances the lungs were inflated and fixed by the formalin steam method of Weibel and Vidone (1961). Examination of sagittal slices cut from lungs fixed in this manner enabled us to distinguish the type of emphysema present with some confidence. Our series consisted of 11 cases of alveolar (*i.e.* alveolar duct and pan acinar emphysema), 6 cases of bronchiolar (*i.e.* centrilobular emphysema) and 2 cases of bullous emphysema. We excluded from this study cases of simple overdistension of lung, such as occurs in status asthmaticus, and cases with pronounced interstitial fibrosis of lung. We also excluded cases of emphysema in which there was associated mitral stenosis, or some other form of chronic rheumatic heart disease, or an abnormally hypertrophied and dilated left ventricle, since all these conditions may themselves give rise to pulmonary vascular disease which is brought about by altered haemodynamics and unrelated to emphysema.

In all cases we weighed the free wall of the right ventricle according to the method of Fulton *et al.*, (1952) and we accepted the figure of 65 G. as the upper limit of normal. We accepted right ventricular hypertrophy, that is a right ventricle exceeding 65 G. in weight, as an indication of chronic pulmonary arterial hypertension.

Blocks of tissue were examined from the upper and lower lobes of both lungs in each case. We studied muscular pulmonary arteries and pulmonary arterioles. A muscular pulmonary artery, according to the criteria of Brenner (1935) is between 100 and 1,000 μ in diameter (Fig. 1). It has a thin media of circular muscle which normally lies in the range of 2·8 to 6·8 per cent. of the external diameter of the vessel (Heath & Best 1958). They normally have no longitudinal muscle in the media or intima. A pulmonary arteriole is less than 100 μ and usually less than 80 μ in diameter. Its wall consists of a single elastic lamina (Fig. 2). In each instance the thickness of the media of circular muscle in the muscular pulmonary arteries and muscularised pulmonary arterioles was expressed as a percentage of the external diameter of the vessel. The thickness of a layer of longitudinal muscle found in the intima was also expressed as a percentage of the external diameter.

Clearly the questions we have to ask ourselves from such an investigation are as follows :

1. Do pulmonary vascular lesions exist in emphysema ?
2. If so, are any of them associated with emphysema *per se* ?
3. Are any of them associated with pulmonary hypertension and the development of cor pulmonale ?
4. Are the pulmonary vascular lesions identical in alveolar and bronchiolar forms of emphysema ?

From the results of our investigation we suggest that in describing the pulmonary vascular disease of emphysema, one must consider the following :

1. The development of longitudinal muscle in the intima of muscular pulmonary arteries and pulmonary arterioles.
2. The state of the original media of circular muscle in the muscular pulmonary arteries.
3. The muscularisation of pulmonary arterioles.
4. Intimal fibres in the pulmonary arteries and arterioles.

I should like to consider each of these features briefly.

1. *The development of longitudinal muscle in the intima.* In 16 of the 19 cases longitudinal muscle was found in the intima of muscular pulmonary arteries and pulmonary arterioles, the range of diameter of affected vessels being 800 to 45 μ. There appears to be a cycle of events in the intima beginning with the development of a few longitudinal muscle fibres in the intima (Fig. 3). This layer of intimal longitudinal muscle becomes thicker (Fig. 4). Elastic fibrils appear between individual muscle fibres (Fig. 5). Some of these may be accounted for by the development of new elastic fibrils ; some may be due to splitting of the internal elastic lamina. Collagen fibres appear to develop subsequently and eventually the

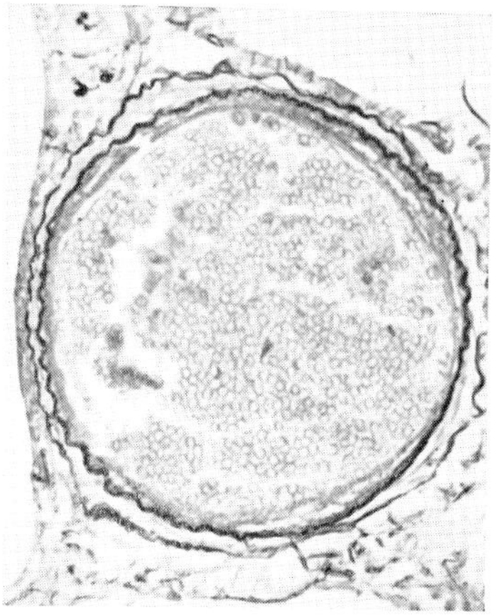

FIG. 1. Normal 'muscular pulmonary artery' with a thin media composed of circularly orientated smooth muscle fibres. The media is sandwiched between inner and outer elastic laminae. In this and the remaining photomicrographs in this paper the section was stained by the Lawson modification of the Weigert-Sheridan method for elastic tissue and counterstained with Van Gieson's stain. (×187).

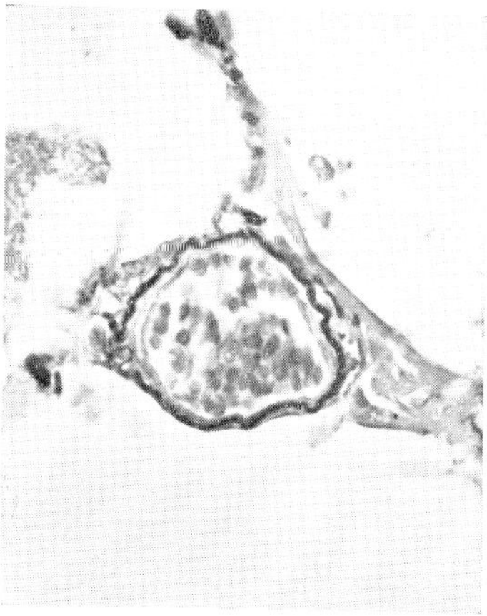

FIG. 2. Normal pulmonary arteriole with a wall composed of a single elastic lamina. From a case of alveolar emphysema with a normal right ventricle. (×337).

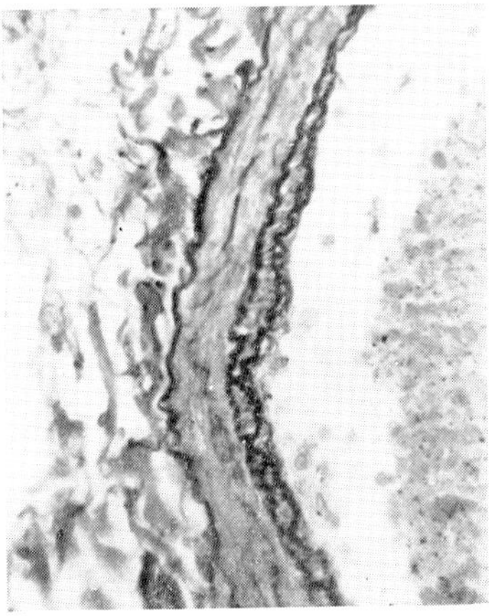

FIGS 3; 4; and 5. Pulmonary arterial vessels from a case of bronchiolar emphysema with right ventricular hypertrophy illustrating the development of longitudinal muscle and subsequent elastosis in the intima. Fig. 3. Muscular pulmonary artery showing early development of intimal longitudinal muscle with a covering elastic lamina. (× 337).

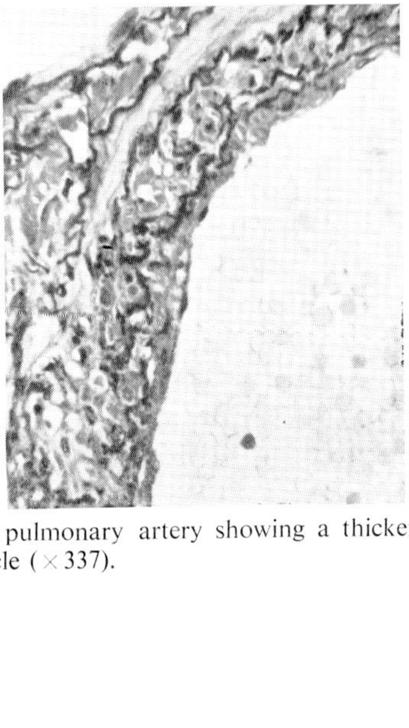

Fig. 4. Muscular pulmonary artery showing a thicker layer of intimal longitudinal muscle (× 337).

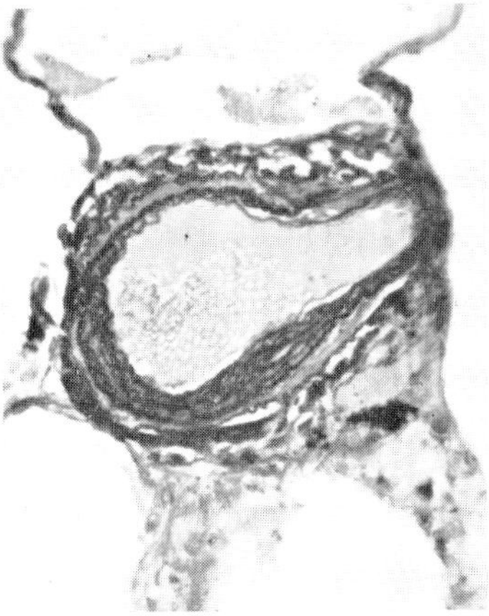

Fig. 5. Pulmonary arteriole showing the subsequent elastosis arouud longitudinal muscle in the intima. (×187).

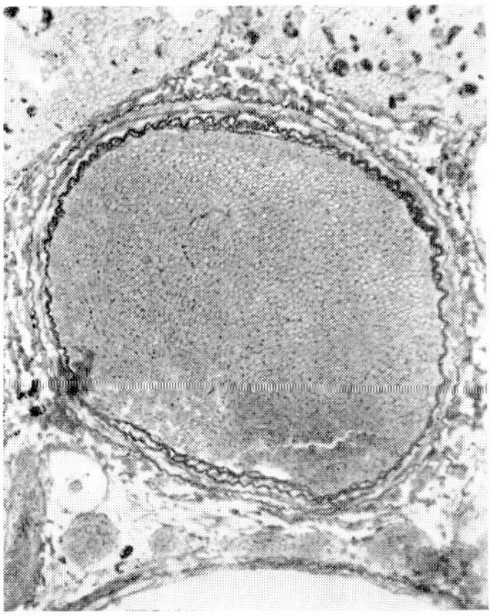

Figs. 6 and 7. 'Muscular pulmonary arteries' from cases of alveolar emphysema. Both show a normal thin media. In neither is there any form of intimal proliferation. (Both ×112).
Fig. 6. From a case with a normal right ventricle.

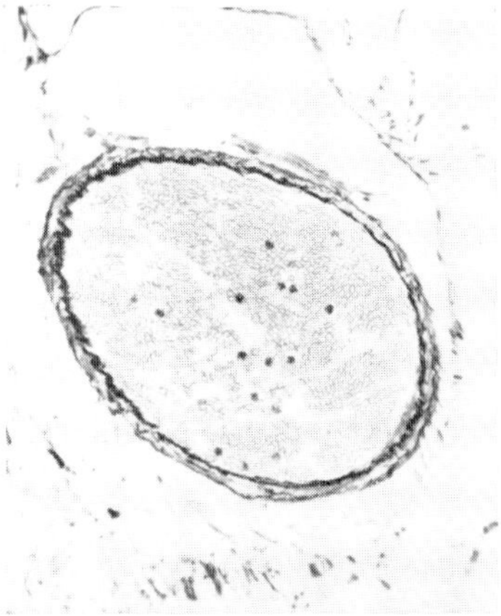

Fig. 7. From a case with right ventricular hypertrophy.

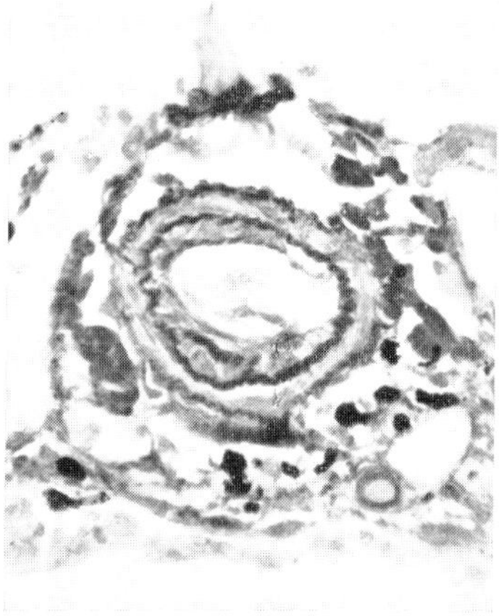

FIG. 8. Pulmonary arteriole showing a distinct media of circular muscle sandwiched between internal and external elastic laminae. There is also longitudinal muscle in the intima. From a case of bronchiolar emphysema with right ventricular hypertrophy. (× 337).

appearances are those of a thick layer of intimal fibrosis. If one is not aware that this fibrous layer represents the end result of a cycle of changes, one may misinterpret it as ‘ non-specific intimal fibrosis ’ or ‘ intimal sclerosis ’ as was done by McLean (1958). The thickness of the layer of longitudinal muscle may reach as much as 12 per cent. of the diameter of the affected vessel . In our series intimal longitudinal muscle was found with equal frequency in alveolar and bronchiolar emphysema. Muscle so orientated occurs equally commonly in those cases with right ventricular hypertrophy and in those without.

Previous studies (Heath 1963) have suggested that the development of longitudinal muscle in pulmonary arteries is a reaction to the combined stimulus of repeated stretching and increased intravascular pressure. The present study indicates that in emphysema the former factor is the more important since we have found that the development of longitudinal muscle is not related to right ventricular hypertrophy and pulmonary hypertension. Dunnill (1961) has suggested that muscular pulmonary arteries in bronchiolar emphysema may be distorted by the abnormal air sacs in the centres of secondary lung lobules. This stretching associated sometimes with pulmonary arterial hypertension may be the basis for the development of longitudinal muscle in the pulmonary arteries in this type of emphysema. Liebow (1964) states that he has seen longitudinal muscle in pulmonary arteries stretched around emphysematous bullae ; the results of this study confirm this observation.

The presence of longitudinal muscle in emphysema and other states characterised by chronic hypoxia is often striking and it is surprising that this anatomical feature was not mentioned at the fifth annual conference on research in emphysema at Aspen, Colorado. The reason for its development in the intima and its function are both obscure. Longitudinal muscle develops in the pulmonary arteries in a wide variety of congenital and acquired lesions of the heart but it usually forms external to the outer elastic lamina. However, the characteristic of the longitudinal muscle in hypoxic states is its distribution in the intima and at the moment we can offer no explanation for its predilection for this site.

2. *The thickness of the original media of circular muscle in the small pulmonary arteries.* In all cases there was no increase in thickness of the original media of circular muscle of the ‘ muscular pulmonary arteries ’ (Figs. 6 and 7). The range of medial thickness of the circular muscle media was 2·3 to 6·7 per cent., which is normal.

One would expect to find a media of normal thickness in the small pulmonary arteries in the 10 cases of emphysema with a right ventricle of normal weight (Fig. 6). It is, however, surprising that there was no evidence of medial hypertrophy in the muscular pulmonary arteries in the nine cases with right ventricular hypertrophy and hence presumably chronic pulmonary hypertension (Fig. 7). The early stages of most forms of hypertensive pulmonary vascular disease complicating mitral stenosis or congenital cardiac shunts show increased thickness of the circular muscle of muscular pulmonary arteries. How is this to be explained ? It may be due to the fact that in the majority of cases of emphysema the degree of pulmonary hypertension is less severe than in mitral stenosis or congenital heart disease. Furthermore the pulmonary hypertension of emphysema tends to be periodic rather than sustained, occurring during bouts of respiratory infection with congestive cardiac failure.

3. *Muscularised pulmonary arterioles.* Abnormal pulmonary arterioles with a distinct media of circular muscle between inner and outer elastic laminae were seen in nine cases (Fig. 8). In eight of these there was right ventricular hypertrophy, and even in the ninth case the right ventricular weight was at the upper limit of normal. In three cases the right ventricular weight was 200 G. or over and there were numerous muscularised arterioles of this type. All but one of the 10 cases with normal pulmonary arterioles had a right ventricle of normal weight.

These results suggest a close relationship between muscularisation of pulmonary arterioles and right ventricular hypertrophy in emphysema. Probably such abnormal arterioles form the organic basis for increased pulmonary vascular resistance in emphysema just as in other forms of hypertensive pulmonary vascular disease. The predominance of these muscularised arterioles in the bronchiolar types of emphysema suggests that this form of the disease is prominent in predisposing to pulmonary hypertension. This supports the observation of Leopold and Gough (1957) who found that 41 of their 75 cases of bronchiolar emphysema had right ventricular hypertrophy whereas only 9 of their 65 cases of alveolar emphysema had enlargement of this chamber.

The development of longitudinal muscle in these abnormal muscularised arterioles (Fig. 8) indicates that new muscle is formed and that the increase in their medial thickness is not to be accounted for solely on the basis of constriction of pre-existing circular muscle. The effects of constriction of such longitudinally orientated muscle would certainly be complex, and not at all like the simple vascular closure envisaged by many physiologists and clinicians.

4. *The development of intimal fibrosis.* In the absence of longitudinal muscle only sparse intimal fibrosis was present. In 16 of the 19 cases the mean percentage thickness of intimal fibrosis with regard to the inner diameter of the vessel was less than 10. The fibrous tissue was acellular and quite unlike the coarse fibro-elastosis seen in the pulmonary arteries in congenital heart disease.

Slight intimal fibrosis of this type is probably of little or no significance in bringing about increased pulmonary vascular resistance in emphysema. It produces no appreciable occlusion of the vascular lumen, and the presence of such a thin rim of intimal fibrosis can hardly render the pulmonary arteries resistant to normal distension since this degree of intimal fibrosis is present in the normal pulmonary artery as an ageing change (Brenner, 1935).

Hence the small pulmonary arterial vessels present a characteristic triad of histological features in emphysema with right ventricular hypertrophy. The triad consists of the formation of longitudinal muscle in the intima of muscular pulmonary arteries and pulmonary arterioles, the muscularisation of pulmonary arterioles by the development of a distinct media of circular muscle and the lack of hypertrophy of the media of circular muscle of the 'muscular pulmonary arteries' of Brenner (1935) (*i.e.* vessels between 100 and 1,000 μ in diameter). The full development of this triad occurs in both main types of emphysema but appears to be commoner in the bronchiolar form.

HYPOXIC HYPERTENSIVE PULMONARY VASCULAR DISEASE

Hasleton and his associates at Birmingham (1967) have demonstrated that this triad of microanatomical lesions is not peculiar to emphysema but has also been found in patients with right ventricular hypertrophy in several other conditions characterised by chronic hypoxia. Thus this complex of vascular changes has been found in (1) healthy subjects, free of cardiopulmonary disease, living at high altitudes, (2) Monge's disease ('chronic mountain sickness'), (3) the Pickwickian syndrome and (4) kyphoscoliosis.

This being so it appears that this triad may be considered as a form of hypertensive pulmonary vascular disease characteristic of states of chronic hypoxia. Hanley *et al.* (1958) reported that the small pulmonary arteries from cases of kyphoscoliotic heart disease with right ventricular hypertrophy did not show the features of severe hypertensive pulmonary vascular disease. Arias-Stella and Saldaña (1963) reported muscularised pulmonary arterioles in

Peruvian Indians indigenous to high altitudes. Naeye reported similar muscularisation of pulmonary arterioles in subjects living at high altitude (1961 *a*), in the Pickwickian syndrome (1961 *a*) and in kyphoscoliosis (1961 *b*).

Similar muscularisation of small pulmonary arterial vessels occurs in cats (Figs. 9 and 10), dogs (Figs. 11 and 12), and cows living at high altitude where they suffer from the effects of chronic hypoxia (Fig. 13). In contrast, there does not appear to be any muscularisation of similar vessels in the llama (Fig. 14), indicating a species difference and an adaptation to life at high altitude. Naeye and Bickerman (1957) reported similar findings in rats kept in room air at low barometric pressure and in hypoxic air at normal barometric pressure.

HYPOXIA AND PULMONARY HYPERTENSION

There is good clinical and experimental evidence of a close relationship between hypoxia and pulmonary hypertension. Such a relationship has been shown in normal subjects breathing a mixture of air low in oxygen (Fishman *et al.*, 1960), in patients with emphysema or bronchiectasis (Whitaker 1954), and in cats exposed to hypoxia (von Euler & Liljestrand, 1946, Duke, 1954). There is some controversy as to the precise stimulus causing an elevation of pulmonary arterial pressure in the clinical groups with chronic hypoxia listed above because in most of them there is associated carbon dioxide retention. Thus in these patients hypercarbia rather than hypoxia might be the more important factor in leading to pulmonary hypertension. It is, however, important to remember that healthy subjects indigenous to high altitude present chronic hypocarbia in association with chronic hypoxia and these people also show the characteristic triad of pulmonary vascular lesions described above. It would appear that the common factor in the causation of this form of pulmonary vascular disease is chronic hypoxia.

The mode of action of the hypoxia is obscure. Von Euler and Liljestrand (1946) found that the elevation of pulmonary arterial pressure produced by breathing 10 per cent. oxygen in nitrogen was unrelieved by vagotomy or removal of the stellate ganglion. This suggested that there was a direct effect of hypoxia on the small pulmonary arterial vessels. The results of recent histological studies at Birmingham by Hasleton and associates (1967) are certainly consistent with this view. Our studies have shown that the segments

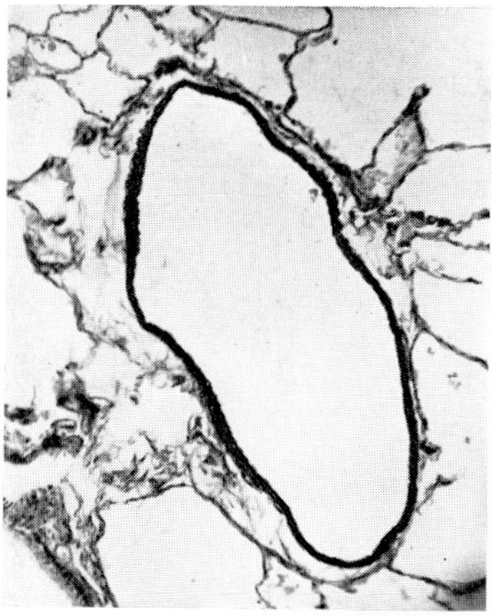

FIG. 9. Muscular pulmonary artery of a cat living at low altitude (Birmingham, England). The media is thin. (×112).

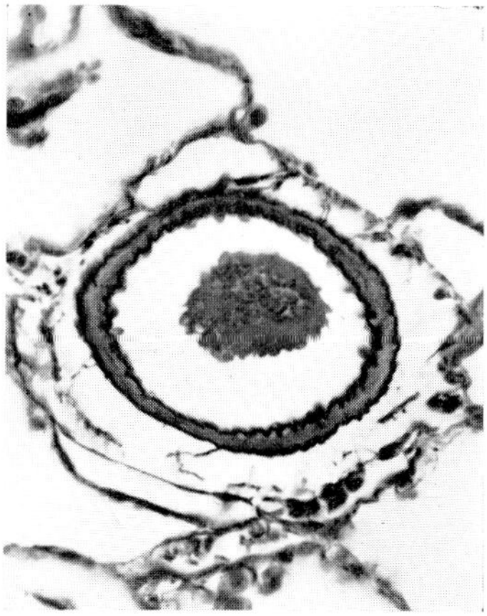

FIG. 10. Small muscular pulmonary artery of a cat living at high altitude (Cerro de Pasco in the Peruvian Andes, 14,250 feet above sea level). The media is thick. (×337).

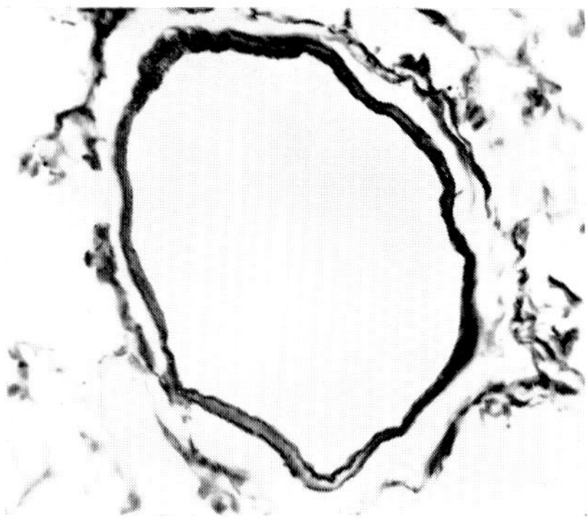

FIG. 11. Muscular pulmonary artery of a dog living at low altitude. The media is thin. (×337).

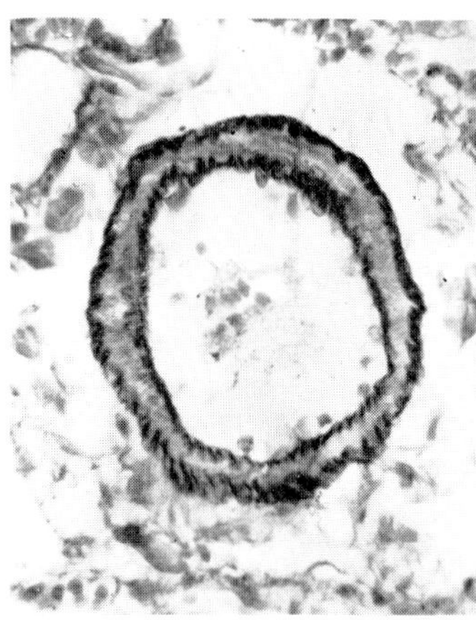

FIG. 12. Muscular pulmonary artery of a dog living at high altitude (Cerro de Pasco). (×337). The media is thick.

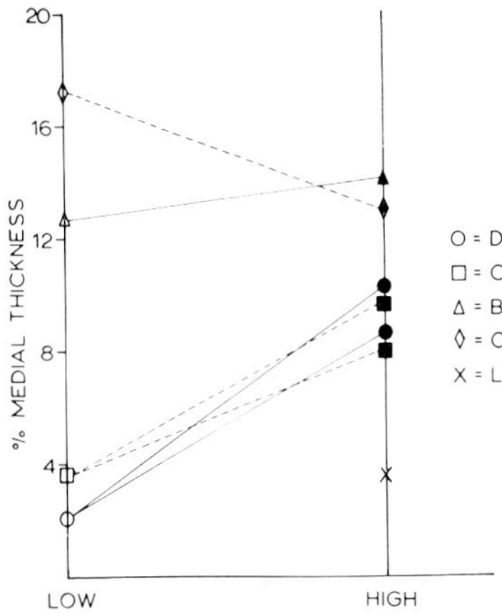

FIG. 13. Mean percentage medial thickness of muscular pulmonary arteries from various species at low (Birmingham, England) and high altitudes (Cerro de Pasco, Peruvian Andes, 14,250 feet above sea level).

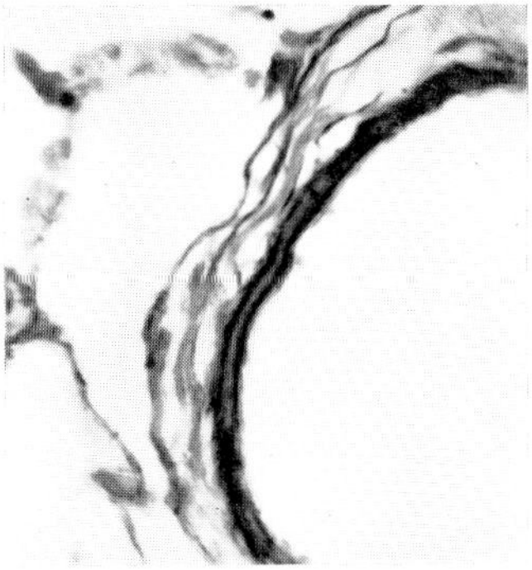

FIG. 14. Part of a muscular pulmonary artery from a llama living at high altitude in Peru showing the very thin media. (×450).

of the pulmonary vasculature which undergo such muscularisation lie in contact with alveolar ducts and spaces where they may come directly into contact with hypoxic alveolar air. This conclusion is also apparent from the diagrams published by Arias-Stella and Saldaña (1963). There is certainly much evidence to suggest that the form of hypertensive pulmonary vascular disease described here is the result of constriction secondary to chronic hypoxia.

REVERSIBILITY

Whatever the precise mechanism, and site, of action of hypoxia on the pulmonary vasculature the present histological studies suggest that the hypertensive pulmonary vascular disease of chronic hypoxia is reversible. The apparent organic basis for increased pulmonary vascular resistance is the muscularised arterioles. There is no intimal fibrosis or vascular occlusion so that when the alveolar oxygen tension is increased to normal levels, the arterioles relax and the pulmonary arterial pressure falls. Heath *et al.*, (1958) showed a similar effect of inhalation of oxygen in the early stages of hypertensive pulmonary vascular disease associated with cardiac shunts.

There is also much clinical and experimental evidence to suggest that hypoxic hypertensive pulmonary vascular disease is to a large extent reversible. Lack of time prevents me from giving more than two examples of this.

1. Peñaloza *et al.* (1963) showed that administration of 35 per cent. oxygen at high altitudes to subjects indigenous to such conditions produced a normal Po_2 and reduced their pulmonary arterial pressure. Pulmonary hypertension was reduced even further by acetyl choline. People living all their lives in the Andes had a normal pulmonary arterial pressure after 2 years residence at sea level.

2. Vogel *et al.* (1966) have recently shown that ligation of the left pulmonary artery of a newborn calf at 5,000 ft. above sea level produces an elevation of pulmonary arterial pressure but at sea level it does not. Acetyl choline diminishes the pulmonary hypertension at high altitude and oxygen inhalation reduces it even further. When acetyl choline and oxygen are given together for 12 days the pulmonary arterial pressure falls almost to normal levels. When the calf was brought down to sea level the pulmonary arterial pressure was normal within 16 hours.

CONCLUSION

Hence we may conclude that in cases of emphysema, be they alveolar or bronchiolar in type, the small pulmonary blood vessels show a characteristic triad of changes. This consists of the development of longitudinal muscle in the intima of pulmonary arterioles and muscular pulmonary arteries, a lack of hypertrophy of the original media of circular muscle in the muscular pulmonary arteries and muscularisation of the pulmonary arterioles. The latter change occurs in those cases of emphysema with right ventricular hypertrophy and appears to be the basis for increased pulmonary vascular resistance.

Similar changes in the pulmonary vasculature occur in normal subjects living at high altitude, in patients with Monge's disease and in patients with cor pulmonale due to kyphoscoliosis or the Pickwickian syndrome. Hence it would appear that the vascular changes in the lung in emphysema are really a form of hypertensive pulmonary vascular disease common to all states of chronic hypoxia.

Its histological features are consistent with the clinical and experimental observations that the pulmonary hypertension of chronic hypoxia is reversible. Affected arterial vessels have been shown to be related to those segments of the bronchial tree where they could come into immediate contact with alveolar air, suggesting that the hypoxia acts directly on the affected pulmonary blood vessels.

ON THE INDEPENDENCE OF PULMONARY HYPERTENSION AND ANATOMIC EMPHYSEMA[1]

JOHN P. WYATT and SADAMU ISHIKAWA

INTRODUCTION

IT has been generally accepted that two major factors influence the production of pulmonary hypertension, namely, organic and functional changes of the pulmonary circulation. Organic changes were the major impress in producing pulmonary hypertension in the experimental cor pulmonale studies of Ando (1965) and Naeye (1967). The important cause of pulmonary hypertension in cases of fibrosing pneumoconiosis is serious reduction of the lung vascular bed by organic disease (Lavenne, 1951 ; Harvey & Ferrer, 1960 ; Evans *et al.*, 1963).

The evidence for the role of the functional factor in pulmonary hypertension was experimentally demonstrated by Von Euler and Liljestrand (1946) as due to anoxia producing reactive arteriolar

[1] Supported in part by Medical Research Council of Canada Grant No. 01–365–47.

spasm. This experimental evidence found confirmation in man through the studies of Motley and Tomashefski (1950). That pulmonary hypertension might be labile and reversible, as in the experimental form, is suggested by the studies of Reeve *et al.* (1966) in patients with high pulmonary artery wedge pressure relieved by cardiac surgery.

Support for the importance of functional factors in the production of pulmonary hypertension has been added from our recent morphometric studies into the cardio-pulmonary alterations in cystic fibrosis. In this disease, disruptive emphysema was eliminated by stereoscopic assessment and the air blood interface was found to be intact. It was our conclusion from that investigation that the prominence of right ventricular hypertrophy was probably initiated by chronic hypoxia in the early phases of the disease (Bowden *et al.*, 1965).

In emphysema the common finding of a heart, normal in size, in the presence of extensive destruction of the lung tissue has left an unresolved, discursive and highly speculative clinico-pathological dilemma (Wyatt *et al.*, 1964). The problems involved in unravelling the factors concerned in emphysema-heart disease might be better expressed by this parody utilizing Edward Lear's limerick style.

> 'There was an old man with blocked air
> Whose heart was remarkably square
> Speculation was rife
> On the cause of the strife
> And the pathology gave only despair.'

This manuscript is an analysis of the complex morphological and physiological aspects concerned in emphysema-heart disease with the correlations between heart size, degree, extent and type of lung emphysema and blood gas studies being our major concern.

MATERIAL AND METHODS

This contribution is based on 207 cases of postmortem studies with a retrospective review of their clinical records. The material was obtained from two health medical centres ; one centre was in a heavily industrialized area (St Louis, Mo.) and the other an area of light industry in a predominant agricultural community (Winnipeg, Canada). From St Louis there were 72 cases of pulmonary emphysema and 7 cases of cystic fibrosis, and from Winnipeg, Canada, 76 cases of clinically diagnosed cor pulmonale due to pulmonary emphysema and 42 cases of cystic fibrosis, and for comparison we reviewed 10 cases of congenital heart disease with pulmonary hypertension.

Out of these 207 cases, 58 had pulmonary function studies within a year before death performed while they were in clinically stable states. Of the 58 cases, 25 of the patients had complete arterial blood gas analyses obtained while they were free from multiple and acute clinical exacerbation of ventilatory failure. Few of the above cases of obstructive airway disease had been studied during life for pulmonary artery catheterization or angiography.

At postmortem the bronchi were insufflated with microcrystalline barium sulphate and the extent of chronic bronchitis was graded on the whole lung bronchogram. Lungs were inflated with formalin and multiple whole lung blocks were cut by the Gough method (1949). These multiple paper sections were classified and the anatomic extent of the disruptive emphysematous alteration was determined by our grid system and stereoscopic examination methods. In some cases, electronmicroscopic studies were performed. The heart was separated from the lungs and the infravalvular portions of the right ventricle, septum and left ventricle were separated from each other. The three components were weighed separately and the thickness of the walls measured after defatting the myocardium and cutting away the coronary arteries. Hearts showing the existence of valvular disease, a significant degree of coronary sclerosis or a protocol history of systemic hypertension were not considered in the final adjudication of our results. The evaluation of the problem of the cardiomegaly, in which left ventricular hypertrophy has been interpreted as a muscle response to chronic lung disease (Fluck *et al.*, 1966 ; Michelson, 1960) is the subject of another contribution. Right ventricular weights above a range of 65 grams, and a ratio of left ventricle plus septum to right ventricular weight below 2·5 or a right ventricular wall above 0·5 mm. in thickness were considered significant and a morphological expression of pulmonary hypertension.

RESULTS

In this survey cases originally considered as clinical examples of obstructive airway disease and at autopsy had enlarged right ventricles occasionally revealed on detailed morphologic analysis to be free of emphysema. In case #1 (Fig. 1) the lung macrosection is from a 55 year old man who had a marked kyphoscoliosis secondary to poliomyelitis. The vital capacity was found to be only 33 per cent. and maximum breathing capacity was 45 per cent. of

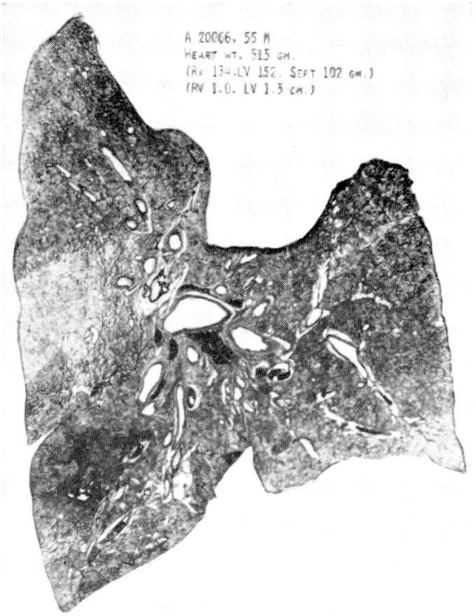

FIG. 1. *Case No.* 1—55 year old male, advanced cor pulmonale, kyphoscoliosis due to poliomyelitis, no emphysema of lung (original magnification 1/5). Heart weight: 515 gm., Right ventricle: 134 gm., Left ventricle plus septum to right ventricular weight ratio: 1·9.

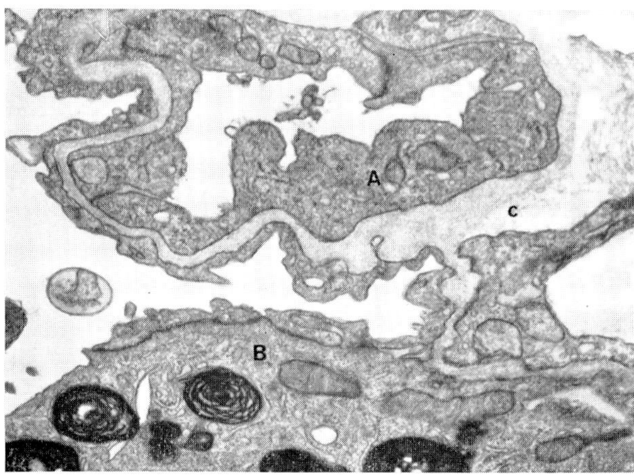

FIG. 2. *Case No.* 2—5 year old boy, congenital heart disease with right to left shunt. An electronmicrograph of the lung. The changes in the pulmonary microvascular channels are negligible. *A* (endothelial cell), *B* (epithelial cell with myelin inclusions), *C* (basement membrane). Magnification ×3,500.

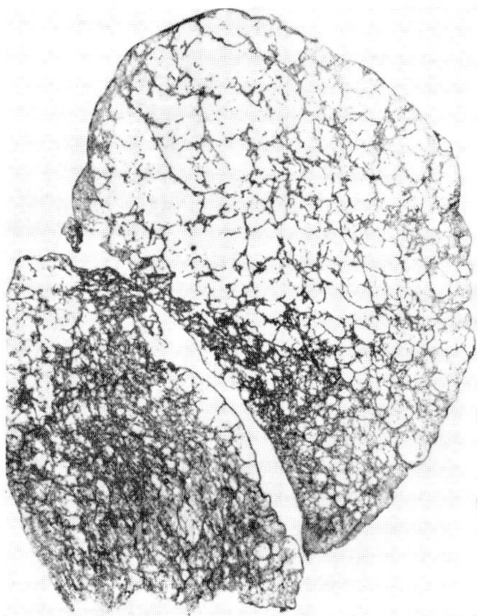

FIG. 3. *Case No.* 3—67 year old male, advanced emphysema (70%) (original reduction 1/5). No cor pulmonale. Right ventricular weight: 48 gm., Left ventricle plus septum to right ventricular weight ratio: 3·4.

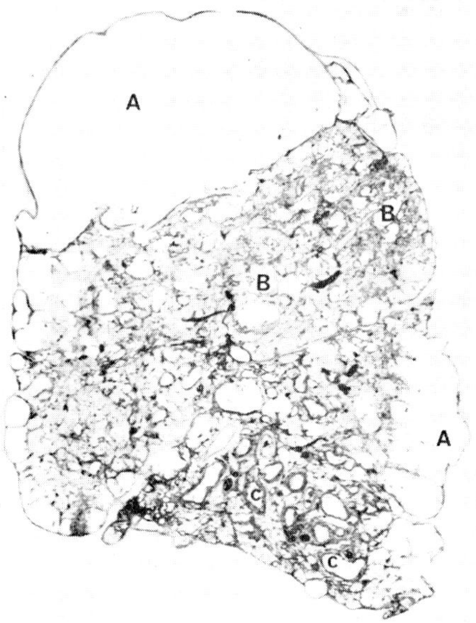

FIG. 4. *Case No.* 5—63 year old man, extensive bullous emphysema, cor pulmonale. Right ventricular weight: 67 gm., Left ventricle: 57 gm., Septum: 32 gm., Left ventricle plus septum to right ventricular weight ratio: 1·4. Paper macrosection showing advanced bullous formations (*A*), Centrilobular emphysema (*B*), and Bronchitis (*C*). Original reduction 1/5.

the predicted values and arterial Po_2 was 57 mm. Hg (oxyhemoglobin saturation was 85 per cent.). The heart weighed 515 G. and the split right ventricular weight was 134 G. with left ventricle weighing 152 G. The ventricular wall thickness was 1·0 cm. for right side and 1·3 for the left. Fishman has indicated that the distortion of the pulmonary arteries may be responsible for this type of cor pulmonale (Bergofsky *et al.*, 1959). The development of cor pulmonale is apparently not related to the aerating lung tissue which is intact but to distortion of the vessels at the lung root. Quasimodo, the hunchback of Notre Dame Cathedral may well be a literary example of such a cardio respiratory problem. The evaluation of the morphological complexities in encountering a ' Quasimodo heart ' demands a careful assessment of the lung relationships.

Figure 2 is an electronmicrograph of the lung biopsy from a child suffering from congenital heart disease associated with pulmonary hypertension demonstrated by pulmonary artery catheter studies (Case #2). Changes in the pulmonary microvascular channels from electron microscopic analysis are negligible suggesting that the pulmonary artery pressure elevations were not affected by significant organic lesions.

Figure 3 is a paper section of the lung (Case #3) obtained from a 67 year old man who had been diagnosed during life as having chronic bronchitis and emphysema and clinically supported by his pulmonary function tests. These physiological results showed total lung capacity of 120 per cent., vital capacity of 72 per cent., maximum breathing capacity of 30 per cent., of predicted values; the residual volume to total lung capacity ratio was 60 per cent. and the 7-minute washout of nitrogen was significantly elevated. The lung showed extensive disruption of the aerating lung structures. At least 70 per cent. of the entire lung field was destroyed. If the reduction of the air and blood interface is directly related to disturbance of gas exchange and diffusion, from this amount of lung destruction one might anticipate cor pulmonale but in fact the heart at autopsy showed right ventricular weight of only 48 g. and the ratio was normal at 3·4. Figure 5 shows the lack of association between right ventricular wall thickness and end tidal diffusing capacity or the dead space/tidal volume ratio in our series of emphysema cases. It is evident that there is no correlation between right ventricular wall thickness and dead space/tidal volume ratio or diffusing capacity.

In a 55 year old man (Case #4) with extensive panlobular emphysema of at least 60 per cent. of whole lung field, there was no morphological stigmata of cor pulmonale, (right ventricular weight

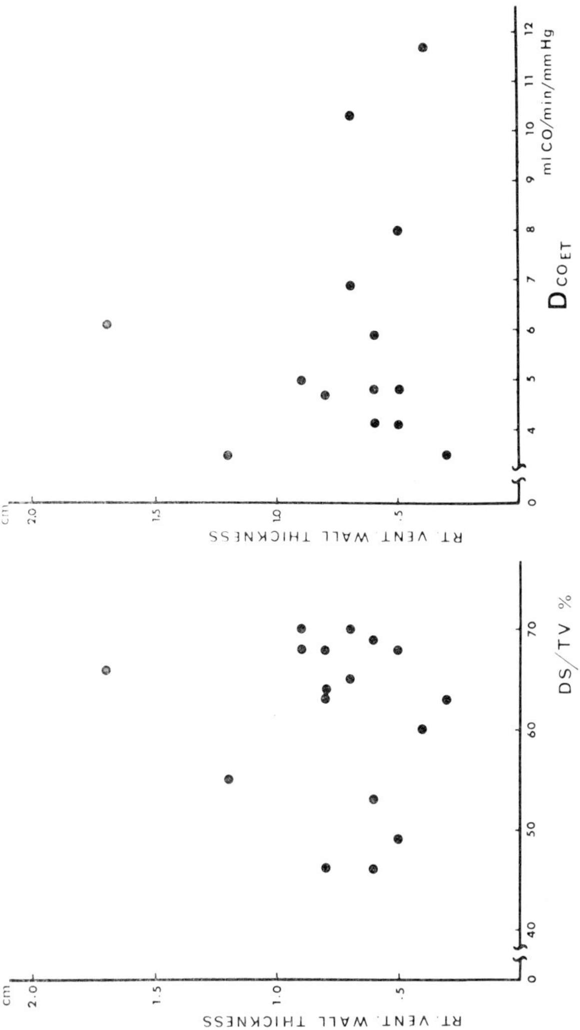

FIG. 5. Relationship between antemortem function and degree of cor pulmonale in cases of clinical emphysema. Left: Right ventricular wall thickness v.s. Dead space/Tidal volume ratio. Right: Right ventricular wall thickness v.s. Diffusing capacity. No correlation is apparent.

50 G. and the LV and S ratio of 2·6). Evidence of ' radiological bronchitis ' was ascertainable from the postmortem bronchogram. Probably because there was a limited degree of bronchitis and the lung capillary bed was adequate for the purpose of oxygenation of the haemoglobin, the resultant stimulus of hypoxia (desaturation) was not severe enough to produce pulmonary heart disease. A corollary of this human observation is the experimental studies of Harrison *et al.* (1957) on dogs ; these investigators demonstrated that some adaptive changes occur in the remaining lung after pneumonectomy. With a resection of as much as 75 per cent. of the total lung volume, there was initially an increase in pulmonary arterial pressure measured at rest but several years later this had fallen to normal levels.

Case #5 (Fig. 4) is that of a 65 year old man who had suffered from pulmonary heart disease for the last 10 years of his life. The lung showed advanced centrilobular emphysema with formation of giant bullae on both lungs. His heart was not markedly enlarged : total ventricular weight was only 151 G. but right ventricular weight was 67 G. and left was 57 G. This right ventricular weight appears to be at the upper limits of normal, but the ratio of left ventricle plus septum to right ventricular weight was 1·4. If one uses right ventricular weight only as a parameter of ventricular hypertrophy (Fulton, 1953) this case might have been labelled as free of hypertrophy. From our observations, a more accurate morphological reflection of cor pulmonale is the determination of ratio values.

An example of enormous right ventricular hypertrophy (161 G. with the ratio 1·4) is seen in case #6 (Fig. 6). This 49 year old man was diagnosed on the basis of clinical and pulmonary functional values as having ' clinical emphysema ' and cor plumonale. His vital capacity was 50 per cent., maximum breathing capacity 28 per cent and total lung capacity was 118 per cent. of predicted values. The residual volume to total lung capacity ratio was 58 per cent. and 7 minutes nitrogen washout was significantly elevated. There was no evidence of radiological bronchitis on postmortem study, but an extensive destruction of the lung tissue due to panlobular emphysema was observed. The left ventricular hypertrophy (142 G.) in this case is best explained on a multifactorial basis. The presence of hypoxia and influence of right side of the heart as well as an increase of the bronchopulmonary venous shunting which leads to an increase of left ventricular work or the hypertrophy of one ventricle might influence the muscular response of the other (Scott & Garvin, 1941).

Fletcher *et al.*, (1963) have found that patients with chronic bronchitis but without evidence of emphysema had more severe blood gas alteration changes and more right ventricular failure than did a group of patients with primary emphysema without chronic bronchitis. Ando (1965) has shown by animal experiments that chronic bronchitis plays an important role in the occurrence of cor pulmonale. Our case #7 (Fig. 7) is probably an example of this. The right ventricular hypertrophy (89 G. with the ratio 1·6) may be related to the extensive bronchitis with the lung showing only limited emphysematous disruption. The main problem was the airway blockage producing hypoventilation. The microvascular pattern was intact with the implication that perfusion was adequate apart from transient spastic influences on the vascular tree which would influence the ventilation-perfusion ratio.

The majority of the cases studied in this contribution had post-mortem evidence of chronic bronchitis. Although emphysema of any morphological type is not a common finding in females, there appears to be no sex difference in the development of cor pulmonale (Okinaka & Harasawa, 1964).

Case #8, a 47 year old white female (Fig. 8) had a right ventricular weight of 86 G. which was the same weight as the left ventricle (ratio 1·6). The precise placement of the emphysematous lesion in the centrilobular area is one of the distinctive features of this case. This lesion offers a lobular model for the consideration of difficulty in balancing ventilation and perfusion. Figure 9 shows a close-up view of one of the lesions from this example. At the centre of the lesion there is no perfusion but fresh air ; while at the margin of the lesion, one has a balance of ventilation and perfusion. At the periphery of the secondary lobule there is a good perfusion but no ventilation. It seems clear that a significant ventilation perfusion abnormality may occur in generalized centrilobular emphysema even though much of the total alveolar surface area is intact (Bates & Christie, 1964). It is also possible that lobular arteries compressed or distended by the pool lesion (Dunnill, 1961) may produce hypoxia but there is no way at this moment of quantitating this postulated functional derangement.

Figure 10 shows the presence of right ventricular hypertrophy in all forms of emphysema regardless of extent. There is a tendency to develop right ventricular hypertrophy in minor to moderate degrees of centrilobular emphysema at the early stage of the disease process. Our original commentary contended that generalized panlobular emphysema was more frequently associated with right ventricular hypertrophy. With the larger series now at hand and the obvious difficulties in morphological assessment of panlobular

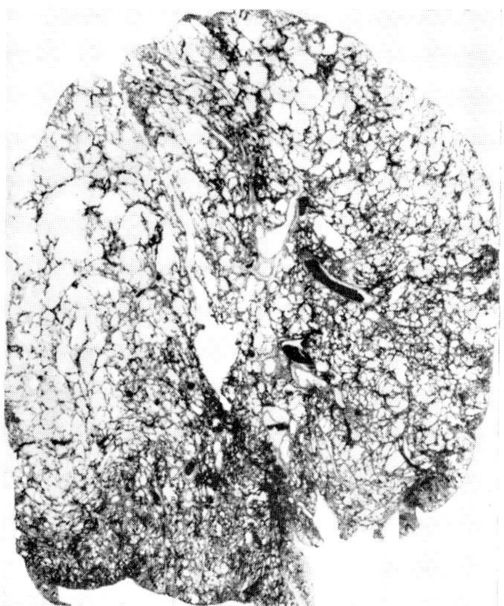

FIG. 6. *Case No.* 6—49 year old male, advanced panlobular emphysema (original reduction 1/5) and cor pulmonale. Right ventricular weight: 161 gm. Left ventricle plus septum to right ventricular weight ratio: 1·4.

[*To face page* 176

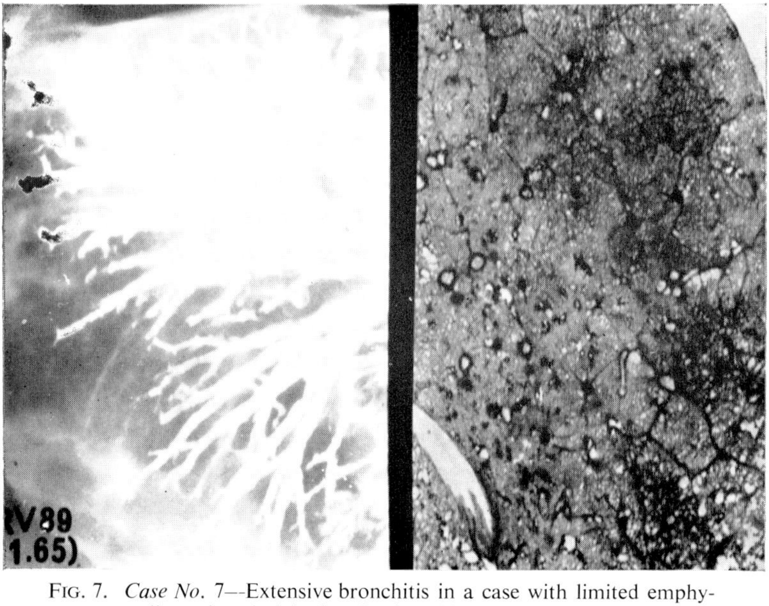

FIG. 7. *Case No.* 7—Extensive bronchitis in a case with limited emphysematous disruption (original reduction 1/5). Right ventricular hypertrophy (right ventricular weight of 89 gm. and ratio 1·6).

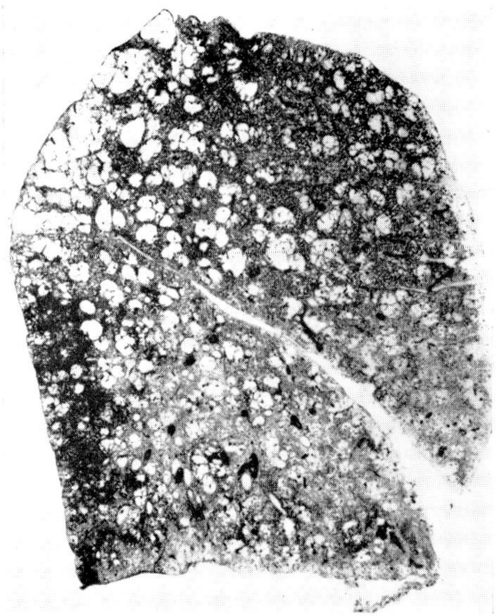

FIG. 8. *Case No.* 8—47 year old female, moderate degree of centrilobular emphysema (original reduction 1/5) and cor pulmonale. Right ventricular weight: 86 gm. Left ventricle plus septum to right ventricular weight ratio: 1·6.

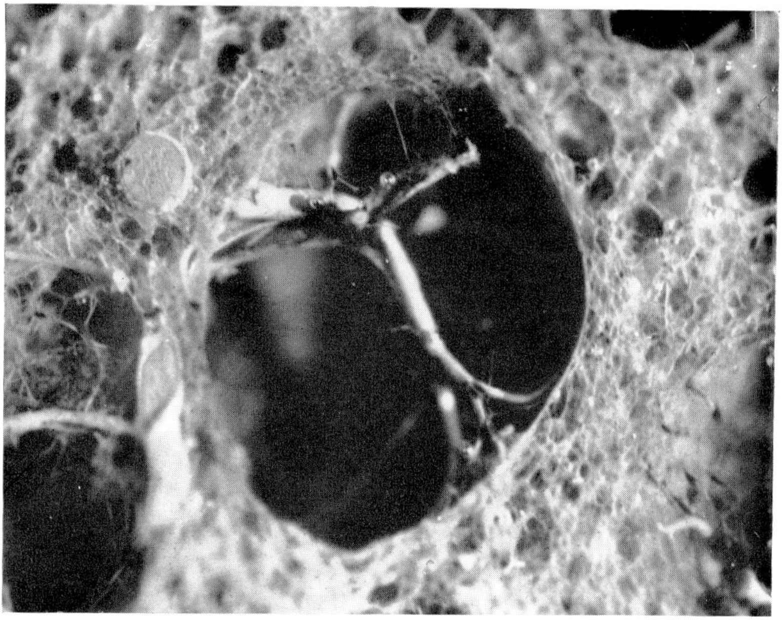

FIG. 9. Close up view of one of the centrilobular emphysematous foci from Case No. 8. Lobular arteriole traverses confluent air pool composed of fused respiratory bronchioles. Capillary network at periphery of secondary lobule intact. Magnification $\times 2\frac{2}{3}$.

emphysema in its early phases, our present attention is directed to the status of the bronchial conduits rather than the type of emphysema.

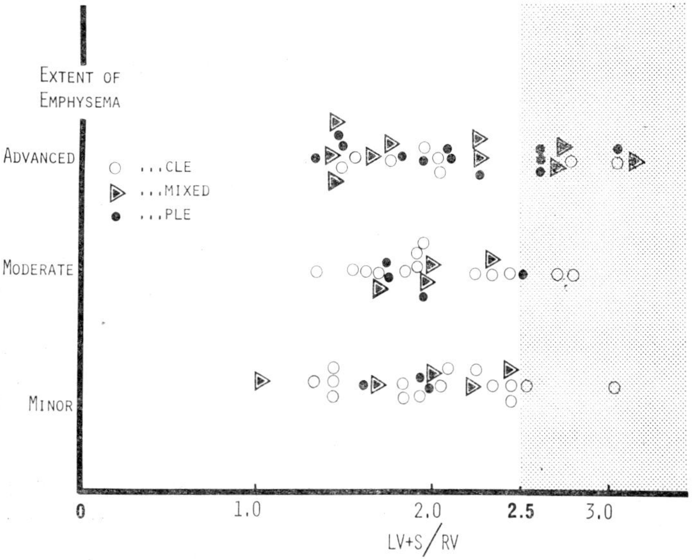

FIG. 10. The relationship between extent of emphysema and cor pulmonale. In the shaded area cases without evidence of right ventricular hypertrophy are shown.

CLE — centrilobular emphysema
PLE — panlobular emphysema
Mixed — mixed type of emphysema

Out of 76 cases of clinically diagnosed cor pulmonale secondary to emphysema, 25 cases had complete arterial blood gas analysis while they were at clinically stable state within a year prior to death. The relationship of the arterial oxyhemaglobin saturation and the right ventricular wall thickness of the case is shown in Figure 11.

There is a definite correlation between the right ventricular wall thickness and the degree of hypoxia. Exercise in some of the cases caused a further reduction of oxygen saturation. Although high correlation did not exist there were definite trends present between Po_2, Pco_2 and right ventricular wall thickness especially in centrilobular emphysema : the higher the Pco_2, the thicker the right ventricle and the lower the Po_2, the thicker the right ventricle. From randomly selected cases of centrilobular emphysema the oxyhemoglobin saturation index of 80 was usually associated with pulmonary arteriolar changes (Hicken *et al.*, 1965). The degree of disturbance of the blood gases could not be equated with the extent of the morphological emphysema or degree of bronchitis in our cases ; this conclusion agrees with the findings of Bates.

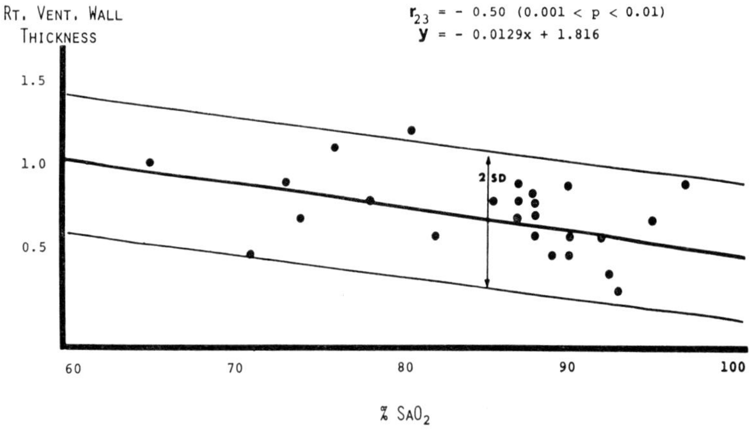

FIG. 11. The relationship of the arterial oxygen saturation and right ventricular wall thickness. The correlation is at a highly significant level.

For a pure model of bronchitis the best demonstration in the human lung is probably seen in cystic fibrosis. The majority of cases dying from cystic fibrosis have evidence of cor pulmonale. In all of these cases disruptive emphysema was eliminated and air blood interface was found to be intact. Marked dilatation of bronchioles and the stigmata of bronchiolitis and mucous plugs was consistently recorded. In the early cases of cystic fibrosis only the lesions of bronchitis-bronchiolitis were present. The complicating aspect of broncho-pulmonary artery communications were not demonstrated until the later phases of the disease.

Figure 12 is a paper section of lung from a case of a 12 year old child suffering from cystic fibrosis (Case #9). There is no evidence of disruptive emphysema but the end picture of multisegmental bronchiectasis is pronounced.

Measurements of airducts and airsac sizes in seven of our cystic fibrosis cases and six controls from a similar age group were compared. All of our cases studied showed evidence of airduct dilatation, but stereoscopic examination did not reveal airsac disruption. Measurements of the ventricles on these patients are shown in Table 1. Despite the small body surface area of the children, the

Table 1. *Measurement of cardiac weight and diameter of myocardial fibres for seven cases of cystic fibrosis. The diameter of right ventricular myocardial fibres are the same as those of the left.*

Age	Body surface area (M^2)	Cardiac weight (GM)		Diameter of myocardial fibres (μ)	
		Right ventricle	$\frac{LV+S^{**}}{RV}$	Right ventricle	Left ventricle
8·6±2·68*	·761±·230*	46·0±·230*	1·66±·125*	11·8±1·61*	11·5±1·30*

* Mean±1 standard error, ** Ratio of left ventricle+septum to right ventricle

right ventricular weight and wall thickness were in excess of the normal range. The diameters of the right ventricular myocardial fibers were the same as those of the left. The prominence of the right ventricular hypertrophy in this disturbance was probably initiated by chronic hypoxia (Goldring *et al.*, 1961) in the early phases of the disease. The *in utero* physiological hypertrophy of the right ventricle in the newborn disappears within a month or two and was not a complicating issue in these cases.

DISCUSSION

Although the exact mechanism of hypoxic pulmonary hypertension is not known, spasm of the precapillary vessels is the most likely explanation for this condition (Fishman, 1961). Clinical studies have shown reversibility of pulmonary hypertension in cystic fibrosis (Goldring, 1964) although other investigators have demonstrated that the mean pulmonary arterial pressure did not improve during 100 per cent. O_2 breathing (Moss *et al.*, 1965).

In emphysema catheterization has revealed evidence of the reversibility of pulmonary hypertension after treatment (Mise *et al.*, 1966). As shown in Figure 10 the development of cor pulmonale in emphysema was found to be independent of emphysematous lung destruction. Radiological studies have indicated that the largest hearts are often associated with lesser degrees of morphological emphysema. A few of the examples of far advanced emphysema on paper section appraisal had ratio values between 2 and 2·5 ; in lesser degrees of emphysema the heart often revealed a ratio of 1·5. These findings support the comments of Evans *et al.* (1963) that decreased pulmonary vascular bed might be of significance in other forms of lung disease but was less important in emphysema.

Of the types of anatomic emphysema examined, the centrilobular form of limited extent but with significant bronchitis-bronchiolitis often showed a remarkable degree of right ventricular hypertrophy.

Disturbances of function in the arterial tree are probably more important than structural changes in emphysema. Pulmonary hypertension caused by reactive arteriolar spasm due to anoxia (Liebow, 1959 ; Peñaloza *et al.*, 1963) with further aggravation by bronchial inflammation and perhaps increased packed cell volume all act in unison on the myocardium. The patency of the vascular bed in emphysema has been tested by timing the flow of fluid through it. It has been demonstrated that there was no consistent relationship between flow times and right ventricular weight suggesting that the aetiological factors in emphysema heart disease are functional rather than organic (James, 1966). A myocardial factor, possibly due to vascular narrowing, is an important cause of right heart failure (Hecht, 1956) and probably contributes to the overt manifestations of anatomical cor pulmonale.

Although Hicken *et al.* (1965) found abnormal pulmonary arterioles with distinct circular muscle media in all of their nine cases and James and Thomas (1963) found organic stenosis of small pulmonary arterioles in their series of cor pulmonale deaths, we did not observe distinctive inner muscle changes in pulmonary arteries and arterioles except in those cases which had significant degree of arterial oxygen desaturation (below 80 per cent.).

The difficulties which face the morphologist in arriving at a satisfactory explanation for the causes of vascular resistance in the complex problem of emphysema remind me of the Japanese proverb :

' A master who lived as a hermit on a mountain was asked by a monk,
" What is the Way ? "
" What a fine mountain this is ", the master said in reply.
" I am not asking you about the mountain but about the Way ".
" So long as you cannot go beyond the mountain, my son,
You cannot reach the Way " replied the master.'

CONCLUSION

1. The presence of right ventricular hypertrophy may be found in all forms of emphysema.

2. There is a tendency to develop right ventricular hypertrophy in minor to moderate degrees of centrilobular emphysema at apparently early stages of the disease.

3. There is a definite correlation between the right ventricular

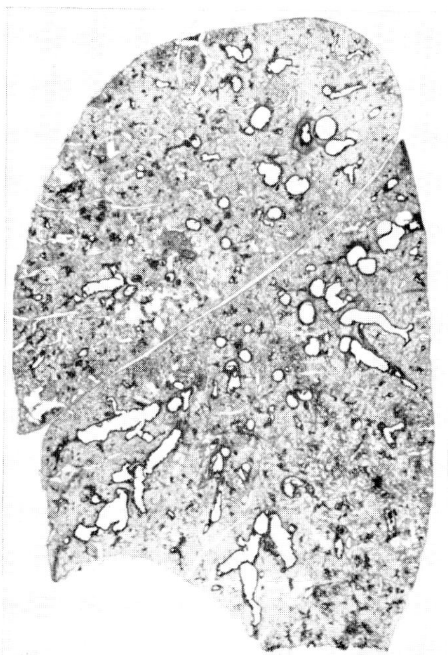

FIG. 12. *Case No.* 9—12 year old male, cystic fibrosis (paper section of the lung) (original reduction 1/5). There is no evidence of disruptive emphysema but there is marked multisegmental bronchiectasis.

[*To face page* 180

hypertrophy and the degree of arterial blood desaturation : the more severe the hypoxia, the thicker the right ventricle.

4. From randomly selected cases of centrilobular emphysema, the oxyhemoglobin saturation index of 80 or below was associated with pulmonary arteriolar changes.

5. The major factor for the development of cor pulmonale in emphysema is probably functional especially hypoxia due to air blockage. The complication of chronic bronchitis-bronchiolitis is probably of greater significance than the loss of aerating lung tissue.

DISCUSSION OF SESSION FOUR

Professor Arnott. Dr Heath, did you say there was a slight thickening of the intima in the small vessels amounting to only a tenth, which you thought was relatively unimportant ?

Dr Heath. Yes. In emphysema usually less than 10 per cent. of the internal diameter of the muscular pulmonary arteries is occupied by intimal fibrosis. This slight amount is comparable with the intimal fibrosis due to normal age changes described by Oscar Brenner (1935).

Professor Arnott. It is far less important than muscle, I am sure, but a reduction from 10 to 9 represents an increase in pressure, assuming flow to be the same, of 50 per cent., because it's a fourth-power relationship.

Dr Heath. I agree that from the Poisseuille formula one would expect small reductions in lumen to be important. Nevertheless we all have this mild degree of intimal fibrosis in our pulmonary arteries and yet we do not have pulmonary hypertension as a result.

Dr Bates. Did I understand that the histological changes you observed in Eisenmenger's Syndrome are similar to those found in emphysema or in patients with chronic lung disease ?

Dr Heath. No, they are not at all similar. Even at a very early stage in Eisenmenger's complex or in any large post-tricuspid congenital shunt, there is pronounced medial hypertrophy of the muscular pulmonary arteries. Secondly in these congenital cardiac shunts the type of intimal proliferation is different from that seen in emphysema in that it is in the form of coarse fibroelastosis. Finally later on in the course of these large shunts one can often find peculiar dilatation lesions such as angiomatoid or plexiform lesions which are never found in emphysema.

Dr Thurlbeck. Dr Heath, have you ever seen changes in the small veins and venules in patients with chronic bronchitis and emphysema, particularly those with a severe degree of right ventricular hypertrophy?

Dr Heath. No, I haven't. Generally speaking, I don't associate haemodynamic abnormalities with changes in the small veins but there are two outstanding exceptions to this. One of these is the acellular intimal fibrosis one finds in states associated with chronic high pulmonary blood flow like atrial septal defect. The other is the peculiar form of primary pulmonary hypertension called pulmonary veno-occlusive disease in which the brunt of the pathology falls upon the pulmonary veins.

Dr Whitaker. The problem that worries me in this form of hypertensive pulmonary vascular disease complicating emphysema is : where does the longitudinal muscle come from?

Dr Heath. This is indeed a problem. Presumably there must be some longitudinal muscle in the intima of the normal muscular pulmonary artery which becomes more prominent under the appropriate stimulus. However, I must say that we have searched for it in control material many times and never found it.

Dr Dunnill. One really can't say whether it's a metaplasia or a proliferation of muscle cells already there.

Chairman. Will someone else venture to say where it comes from?

Dr Filley. May I suggest the possibility that the muscularized arteriole may be a constricted muscular artery. We have to be careful in talking about constriction but I feel this possibility should be borne in mind when we are considering where the muscle comes from. I'm quite amazed at the reactivity in the postmortem vessels. When you take a lung and try to perfuse the arteries early after death and don't wait long enough, you have a lot of trouble forcing liquid into the vessels. If you wait a while they may relax. It usually takes about 30 hours. Perhaps we should review some of the questions about the size of these arteries, which ones we're looking at and so on, in the light of the possibility of postmortem contraction which has not been allowed to relax.

Dr Heath. Of course, all the lungs we observed were examined after they had been inflated and fixed by formalin steam, so the lung had assumed the size that it had in life, before the sections were taken. We generally assume that structures in lungs under these conditions have the same size as they had in life. A further point is that in the small arteries there is a formation of longitudinal muscle and I don't see how you can possibly explain that on the basis of constriction. It's a clear indication, I think, of muscular hyperplasia.

Dr Reid. I wonder if I might take up again a point mentioned relating to methods of fixation. The dry method for fixing lungs can let you down badly if you've got a bronchitic or a cystic fibrosis. It's for this reason that we have stopped using it. You get beautiful preparations of the normal and the more normal the lung the more beautiful the preparation but in disease it does not necessarily give you even or adequate fixation throughout the lung. For this reason we continue to fix the lungs inflated but wet.

A further technical point on which I would take issue with Dr Heath is that I feel that artery measurements done on undistended arteries have little meaning because we know that you get all degrees of crenation of the elastic laminae. For this reason all the work I mentioned this morning is done on vessels that are injected with micropaque barium down as far as vessels of about 15 μ. Although Brenner made a serious contribution his work was done more than 30 years ago and his measurements were done on uninjected arteries. We have been able to show that the extent of the muscular part of the blood vessel in the lung is much greater than was indicated by his studies. Even in a normal lung it's possible, in arteries below, say, 100 μ, to pick out the odd artery that is completely muscularized, the artery that is partially muscularized, and so on. So one can chart the population of arteries in the normal. In disease one gets a change in the population distribution of the arteries. A spread of muscle into arteries which normally do not have it changes the proportions of the different type of artery. The partially muscular vessels become fewer and the completely muscular become more numerous. It is important to inject the arteries if you want to measure them.

Dr Leopold. At what pressure ?

Dr Reid. I inject all of ours at 100 cm. of water because then we are injecting the normals at hypertensive pressures and will therefore minimise any difference between the normal and the hypertensive rather than the other way round. We put a lot of thought into this. It might be suggested that we do normals at normal pressures (do we choose systolic or diastolic ?) and the hypertensives at hypertensive pressures. But even if one had catheter studies on patients, which pressure would one choose ? So we stick to hypertensive pressures to inject both the normal and the diseased. Of course, we also measure medial area as well as percentage wall thickness so we've got some sort of double control on the degree of muscularity.

Dr Hasleton. Certainly the method of fixation we have used at Birmingham has some disadvantages but on the other hand it has more advantages. The first is a very important one and is that one can see the alveolar ducts in emphysema much better with formalin steam than with wet fixation. The second is that one gets much more accurate measurements of lung volumes. One advantage of fixation by formalin fluid is that one gets better cytological detail in the pulmonary blood vessels.

Dr Reid. It doesn't worry me that by my methods my lung volumes are smaller than by yours as long as when I compare my lungs prepared in formalin fluid I compare the normal volumes prepared by my method and not by yours.

Dr Dunnill. There is another objection against putting formalin fluid down the bronchial trees ; it tends to wash mucus down into the periphery. Standardization of preparation for examination of the arteries is very important and there's certainly no easy answer to it. I often wonder if you shouldn't tie the blood vessels off before you take the lung out.

Chairman. Although there may be differences of opinion about the best way to prepare lungs for study, it does seem that the affected vessels lie very close to the alveolar ducts and that there is nothing to distinguish these changes of ' emphysema ' from any other form of hypoxic pulmonary hypertension. Am I correct in this view ?

Dr Reid. Yes. But we found hypertrophy of vessels right up to the hilum just as in the smaller vessels.

Dr Heath. I agree with the Chairman. The form of hypertensive vascular disease one finds in states of chronic hypoxia is different from that which one sees in conditions like mitral stenosis or congenital cardiac shunts. In such diseases one finds hypertrophy throughout much of the pulmonary arterial tree but in emphysema and states of chronic hypoxia the muscularization occurs mainly in the distal portions of the pulmonary arterial tree.

Dr Reid. But once you get to the larger vessels, if you are to pick up these minor differences, you must have the arteries injected. If you do that you can find that right back to the hilar vessels you have got a significant degree of hypertrophy.

Dr Heath. I agree that to get absolute figures for these medial thicknesses is important, but I think it is more important to realise that there are different forms of hypertensive pulmonary vascular disease according to the mode of development of the underlying pulmonary hypertension. These various forms of hypertensive pulmonary vascular disease have striking individual qualitative differences allowing one to diagnose the particular type present. In this way there is a hypoxic form which is recognised by a group of qualitative changes.

Dr Strang. I am interested in the pulmonary hypertension of different cause at a different age. Everybody has a high pulmonary artery pressure in foetal life and this falls after birth. The greater part of this fall in the lamb is due to the changes in alveolar gas tensions which take place when breathing begins. This high vascular resistance in the foetal lung is associated with very muscular small vessels and there's very clear experimental evidence in the lamb that about 60 to 70 per cent. of the pulmonary vascular resistance is sensitive to the oxygen and carbon dioxide tension in the gas in the lung. This musculature of the pulmonary vascular bed gradually diminishes and disappears over the first few months of life. Can the anatomists tell us which vessels are involved in this process and whether the veins are involved as well?

Dr Heath. Presumably the intra-lobular arteries. The foetal lungs as you're well aware, are divided into well-demarcated lobules. Civin and Edwards (1951) showed that the inter-lobular arteries in the foetal lung develop into the elastic pulmonary arteries of the adult whilst the intra-lobular arteries develop into the muscular pulmonary arteries. They stated that the pulmonary arterioles are not visible at that stage, and in the same paper they also say that the pulmonary veins show no change.

Dr Strang. This must refer to a very early foetus. I'd like to know about the situation in the foetus at term when the lung is just ready to start exchanging gas. It's filled with fluid and has got a very low blood flow, but as soon as the fluid's got rid of and the blood flow increases, it's a perfectly good gas-exchanging organ.

Dr Mead. To what extent are the arterioles in the new-born muscularized?

Dr Reid. Surely an arteriole is not muscularized by definition or do the physiologists regard any small muscular artery as an arteriole?

Chairman. Pulmonary physiologists do not generally hold this view. The idea of an arteriole as a sphincteric vessels is a carry-over from the systemic circulation. I think that the word ' arteriole ' is more a function of size and location than of muscular endowment.

Dr Reid. And what sort of size do you want to give it?

Chairman. The size of those vessels which lead immediately to the capillary bed could qualify. Although these vessels arise from small muscular arteries, they are much smaller, *i.e.* of the order of 20 to 100 μ, and seem to contain very little muscle for vaso-constriction.

Dr Reid. We avoid the use of the word ' arteriole ' as it might connote a non-muscular small vessel or a highly muscular small vessel. To revert to the new-born then, here you've got very muscular small arteries. But because the lung grows at such a fierce rate—the growth of alveoli is particularly striking in the first four years of life—a complete remodelling of the pulmonary artery tree occurs producing a quite dramatic change in the distribution of muscle in the vessels in the first few years of life. Dr Davies in my department is establishing these patterns at various ages.

Dr Heath. To refer for one moment to the question of right ventricular hypertrophy. We believe that this can occur in either of the major forms of emphysema ; bronchiolar or alveolar, and follows the muscularization of the distal portion of the pulmonary arterial tree that we have just been discussing. It would appear that the cause of this muscularization is probably hypoxia, by analogy with the same thing that occurs at high altitudes.

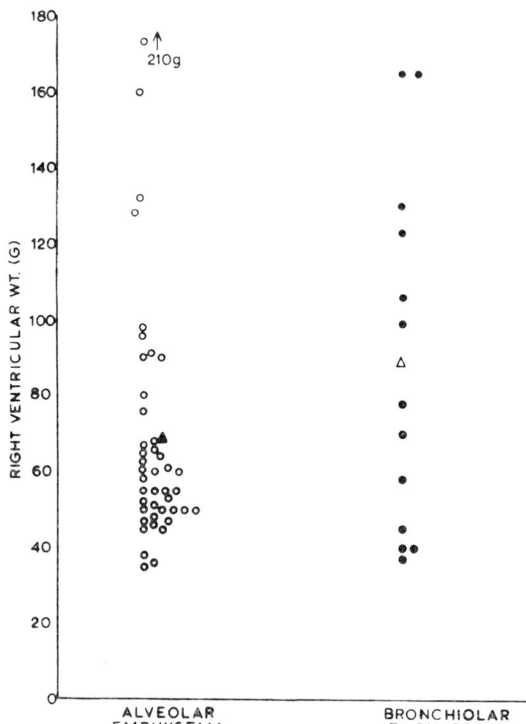

FIG. 1

Dr Fletcher. Could I suggest the words ‘ associated with ’ instead of ‘ cause ’ ? I see no evidence for the *causation* of the hypoxia by the emphysema. It’s not been presented anyway, at this meeting.

Dr Hasleton. May I take this opportunity to present some data on right ventricular hypertrophy in emphysema obtained from four years' combined work in the Departments of Pathology and Medicine at Birmingham University?

The lungs were fixed by the method of Weibel and Vidone (1961) and right and left ventricular weights were obtained by the method of Fulton *et al.* (1952). Figure 1 shows a graph of right ventricular weight in cases of alveolar and bronchiolar emphysema. The triangles represent mean right ventricular weight in both of these series. We see that 43 cases of alveolar emphysema had a mean right ventricular weight of 69 G. and 13 cases of bronchiolar emphysema had a mean right ventricular weight of 88·9 G. (Table 1). However,

Table 1

Type of emphysema	Number of cases	Mean right ventricular wt. (g.)	P
Alveolar . .	43	69·0	<0·1
Bronchiolar . .	13	88·9	

the problem arises that 14 of these 43 cases of alveolar emphysema had left ventricular hypertrophy and 6 of the 13 cases of bronchiolar emphysema were similarly affected. As soon as we pruned our series of these cases with left ventricular hypertrophy we found the mean right ventricular weight of the remaining 29 cases of alveolar emphysema was 67·5 G., just a trifle above the upper limit of normal (65 G.) as given by Fulton *et al.* and the mean right ventricular weight of the remaining 7 cases of bronchiolar emphysema was 58·4 G. (Table 2). In other words, the mean right ventricular weights in both forms of emphysema were roughly within normal limits.

Table 2

Type of emphysema	Number of cases	Mean right ventricular wt. (g.)
Alveolar . .	29	67·5
Bronchiolar . .	7	58·4

We then studied cases of alveolar and bronchiolar emphysema that had right ventricular hypertrophy and compared them with the amount of lung tissue affected by emphysema (Table 3). In 15 cases of alveolar emphysema with right ventricular hypertrophy the mean percentage of lung involved was 38·5 per cent. In the 8 cases of bronchiolar emphysema the mean percentage of emphysema found was 16·2 per cent. *p* was less than 0·01, so it seems that to produce right ventricular hypertrophy more lung tissue needs to be affected by the alveolar as contrasted to the bronchiolar form of emphysema.

Table 3

Type of emphysema	Number of cases	Mean % emphysema	P
Alveolar . .	15	38·5	0·01
Bronchiolar . .	8	16·2	

Dr Semple. I am a little sceptical of this magic figure of 65 G. as being the limit of right ventricular hypertrophy. Patients who have the centrilobular type of picture are probably heavier in weight than those who have the panacinar type. The latter seem to be lighter in weight and therefore would have the smaller heart size. It seems to me that without taking body weight into account, it's very risky to make comparisons of the presence or absence of right ventricular hypertrophy, using a single criterion of this sort.

Dr Heath. The way we get over this is to express right ventricular weight as the ratio : weight of left ventricle plus septum divided by the weight of the right ventricle. Right ventricular hypertrophy is present when the ratio is less than 2·0.

Dr Semple. And you've already excluded people with enlarged left ventricles. Is that right ?

Dr Heath. I have been looking forward to this discussion to seek advice on this point because this is a very practical problem with us. What do we do if we have an extremely good case of bronchiolar emphysema associated with slight left ventricular hypertrophy ? Do we study this case, or exclude it ?

Professor Stuart-Harris. About 20 per cent. of our cases of typical cor pulmonale have postmortem evidence of left ventricular hypertrophy but they may never have exhibited hypertension in life.

Dr Semple. Was it very significant as far as the morbid anatomists were concerned ?

Professor Stuart-Harris. Very gross. With a total heart weight of 600 G. in some cases.

Chairman. There seems to be no question that right ventricular hypertrophy and cor pulmonale do occur in some patients who have bronchitis and no emphysema and there seems little doubt that this must be related to changes in the small pulmonary vessels. Also, as Arias-Stella and Saldana (1963) have shown for native residents at high altitudes, the vascular changes are attributable as hypoxia. Clinically, patients who die during an attack of bronchitis are severely hypoxic. Why are we reluctant to pinpoint hypoxia in the pathogenesis of these smooth muscle changes when this is the one regular feature and common physiologic abnormality in the disease ?

Dr Reid. I can make two points which bear on your question and which also, I think, explain why we seem to be getting this relation between right ventricular hypertrophy and type of emphysema. In the first place, until you mentioned it in the present discussion, airways obstruction had not been referred to but this is probably what really matters in all of these cases. Secondly, let us consider the structure that is sensitive to hypoxia. It is out at the alveolar wall level, perhaps even at the capillary level. It is most likely to be found in blood vessels, shall we say, under 300 μ in diameter. In panacinar emphysema of the sort which is severe enough to disable and kill, it is this part of the vasculature that is gone. The actual detector and the responding region have both gone. In centriacinar emphysema (bronchiolar or centrilobular emphysema) on the other hand, the peripheral part of the pulmonary vascular bed is still intact ; the vessels which are going to detect and respond to hypoxia are still present.

Certainly cor pulmonale, right ventricular hypertrophy and hypoxia all occur in patients who have got bronchitis without any structural emphysema. If we group our fatal cases of chronic bronchitis according to the type and severity of emphysema we find that the ones with severe and widespread panacinar often do not have right ventricular hypertrophy and when they do it is usually mild or moderate. It is the other group who have bronchitis and airways obstruction without bad panacinar emphysema, who respond more often with both polycythaemia and, even in the absence of polycythaemia, with right ventricular hypertrophy.

Chairman. Would it be possible that those patients with panacinar emphysema who didn't have as much right ventricular hypertrophy just didn't have as much hypoxia ?

Dr Reid. This may be so ; we've got no conclusive evidence. But some of our cases have got hypoxia and they still don't seem to get pronounced right ventricular hypertrophy.

Professor Bishop. How many pathologists have encountered this situation of right ventricular hypertrophy without emphysema ?

Chairman. Dr Reid ? Dr Leopold ? Yes. Apparently everybody has seen it.

Dr Thurlbeck. No. One negative vote. Provided you exclude hypoventilators, bronchiectatics, fibrocystics and things like that, of course. Otherwise, no !

Dr Filley. I entirely agree with what Dr Lynne Reid has said about the tremendous importance of hypoxia as against structural emphysema in causing cor pulmonale. From our work in Denver, on the basis of 66 cases that we call pink, and 44 blue, it looks very much as if the presence of right ventricular hypertrophy and repeated episodes of cardiac failure, are closely related to the hypoxia of bronchitis and are almost independent of how much lung is destroyed by emphysema. Now to say that does not mean that loss of blood vessels to such an extent that there aren't enough for the right ventricle to pump blood without hypertension, is not important —it is. But what we find is that in pink patients in whom we think there is emphysema as a primary entity, such presumed vessel loss seems not to be important in producing right ventricular hypertrophy. There might be right ventricular hypertrophy in the last few months of life but this seems to be associated only with terminal heart failure. It is the blue cases who have right ventricular hypertrophy for years, and have much more mucous gland hyperplasia and less emphysema. In these cases pulmonary hypertension is significantly higher than in the cases with destroyed lung.

Dr Bates. It may be important that Dr Filley's data are taken from people living at 6,000 feet. Our findings at sea level are really quite different and it's possible that the hypoxia problem is made much worse by the mean reduction in oxygen tension of 20 mm.

Dr Heath. I think this diagnosis of chronic bronchitis has got to be made with extreme care because unless you are meticulous in your examination of the lungs at necropsy, you are very likely to miss minor degrees of bronchiolar emphysema which we are coming to think are extremely important. In Birmingham until we started using the method of formalin-steam inflation and fixation we used to have these cases of chronic bronchitis with right ventricular hypertrophy but since we've been looking at the lungs with extreme care, these cases of chronic bronchitis seem to be turning into examples of bronchiolar emphysema !

Dr Macklem. I wonder if you know of any measurements of airway resistance in cystic fibrosis and whether these patients do have obstructive airways disease which is severe ?

Chairman. Patients with cystic fibrosis of the pancreas have very severe obstructive airway disease.

Dr Bates. Although the surface area lost in centrilobular emphysema is not great, it has been a surprise to me to learn from Dr Thurlbeck's measurements that not uncommonly as much as 25 per cent. of the volume of lung is actually occupied by the holes of centri-lobular emphysema. That's a considerable volume and if the tidal volume goes into those holes, as I think Dr Leopold's studies amongst others suggest it must do, then an average tidal volume just about gets to them and goes nowhere else. This implies that the essence of the failure of ventilation in centri-lobular emphysema is the poor communication between the central hole, which has a low blood surface area in relation to its ventilation, and the relatively normal alveoli beyond it. We must regard the normal alveoli outside the holes as well-perfused and poorly ventilated and this must play a large part in the gas disturbance which this particular lesion causes.

As a second point, may I remind you of the study by Dr MacGregor in our department (Nakhjavan *et al.*, 1966), in which he demonstrated that it's possible to find patients with advanced pan-lobular emphysema affecting very considerable lung volumes, in whom the blood gases are still relatively normal but in whom, because of a complex defect at the level of the diaphragm, the heart is never capable of filling. These patients have not got pulmonary hypertension but they occasionally turn up with considerable oedema of the legs and hepatic enlargement. We have studied such a case : a man who was found to have a fixed, low cardiac output which he was not capable of increasing on exercise, normal pulmonary artery pressure, extensive emphysema and, using a complex dye cine-radiographic technique of looking at the inferior vena cava, it was clear that there was a mechanical problem of filling the heart through the diaphragm. Such a man has essentially got a heart with, as it were, constrictive pericarditis.

Dr Fletcher. I was very fascinated by Dr Wyatt showing us that there was no relationship between degree of emphysema and cor pulmonale. I wonder if Dr Heath and his group have made a similar quantitative study of emphysema and right heart weight. What is the correlation coefficient ?

Dr Brewer. The quantitative microanatomical methods are very time-consuming. It is important, therefore, to ask whether there are other less arduous methods of forming a quantitative assessment of the amount of emphysema present in the lungs. Figure 2 shows the relationship between the percentage of abnormal air space present as determined by the macroscopic point counting method and the internal surface area as determined by the mean linear intercept. The cases recorded are ones we have examined combined with those reported by Dunnill. There is a significant inverse correlation with a correlation coefficient of $-0{\cdot}52$.

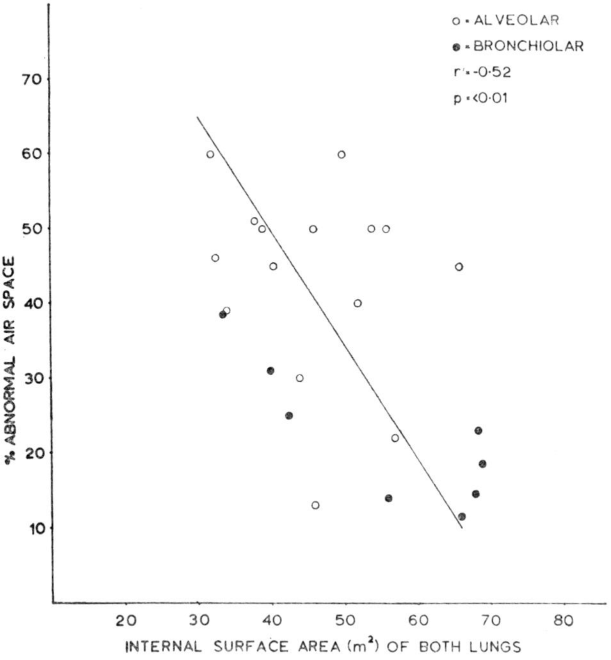

FIG. 2

It is not possible really to decide which parameter is the better measure of the disease until observations have been made on their correlation with some other, preferably clinical, manifestation of the disease.

Dr Fletcher. So you are showing us now that the lesion is *not* related to the right ventricular hypertrophy, yet earlier Dr Heath had suggested that centrilobular emphysema was in some way causally related.

Dr Dunnill. This shows that the *amount* of disease is not related. It does not refute the argument that a particular *type* of emphysema might be causally related to right ventricular hypertrophy. The number and distribution of the emphysematous spaces are also of the greatest importance.

Dr Thurlbeck. If we return to Dr Cumming's original statement: he made the calculation that if one had 25 per cent. centrilobular emphysema, it could involve every respiratory bronchiole although on a percentage point count only 25 per cent. of the lung volume would be involved. Mild panlobular emphysema, on the other hand, with 25 per cent. involvement, would involve a quarter of both lungs with three-quarters of the lung being entirely normal and this illustrates how misleading it can be to measure two different things using the same method.

Professor Harris. It seems to me quite clear that we're all wasting our time trying to relate the degree or nature of emphysema to the pulmonary hypertension we observe in this condition when it may be more strictly related to the degree of airways resistance. In fact, the work of Drs Segal, Green, Housley and myself has shown that there is a distinctive reciprocal relation between the pulmonary artery pressure and these patients' FEV1.

Dr Campbell. Whilst disagreeing fiercely about detail, many of the participants seem to be agreed that pulmonary hypertension and right ventricular hypertrophy matter. I am by no means convinced that they do. It seems possible to me that the abnormal blood gases are in some way due to a metabolic, not a purely mechanical defect. This metabolic process, whatever it is, causes fluid retention which goes to the lungs—there is some evidence for this—and causes changes in the lungs leading to pulmonary hypertension. Pulmonary hypertension should then be considered not a cause but a consequence of fluid retention.

Chairman. The possibility of water retention in the lungs in the cor pulmonale of obstructive lung disease has been under study in our laboratory by Edelman and Turino. During right ventricular failure, the injection of a potent diuretic may improve alveolar ventilation, decrease pulmonary artery pressure and leave the pulmonary water content unaffected.

Dr Campbell. What method did you use?

Chairman. We have used a double-dilution indicator technique, with T-1824 as the intravascular indicator and tritiated water as the extravascular one. This is a modification of the method originally developed by Chinard and Enns.

Dr Strang. Surely there's a lot of circumstantial evidence to suggest that the lungs are in general protected against oedematous states. When people get very oedematous with a nephrotic syndrome or any other cause of hypoproteinaemia, you don't see lung oedema.

Dr Campbell. I do not suggest that the cause of this oedema is the local effect of hypoxia or hypercapnia; I suggest there may be a metabolic factor which leads to general fluid retention and in the same way as you can get pulmonary oedema with over-transfusion or in acute nephritis, I think it possible that you can get fluid in the lungs in this condition.

Professor Bishop. I think there may be a lot in what Dr Campbell says and that the term cor pulmonale may have outlived its usefulness. We have been talking a great deal today about the mechanisms of pulmonary hypertension but we have to remember that it is not necessarily the cause of right ventricular failure. The patients we see with oedema are not necessarily in heart failure at all. Some of them are, certainly, but many are not.

Dr Whitaker. Surely we all recognise that if you give these patients a diuretic and they have a brisk diuresis, there is a tremendous improvement in their blood gases ?

Chairman. Could the improvement be related to Professor Bishop's demonstration earlier about the effect of blood volume as a contributing factor ? Or could it be due to improved alveolar ventilation with concomitant lowering of blood P_{CO_2} and increase in blood P_{O_2} ?

Dr Whitaker. I always thought it was because we removed oedema from the lungs and improved respiratory function.

Dr Permutt. There's been much written about this. Many of these patients are not very sensitive to diuretics but they have remarkable diuresis at some stage of their disease and they do get better. As to what causes the diuresis—it is generally associated with improvement in the state of hypoxia, administration of oxygen and many other factors. Our experience is that they don't respond very readily to diuretics until the hypoxia is corrected.

Dr Whitaker. You must be dealing with quite a different disease ! Dr Filley referred this morning to a paper which Charles Davies wrote from Sheffield many years ago, showing that if you gave these people mercurial diuretics they had a tremendous outpouring of urine and tremendous improvement in blood gases.

REFERENCES

ANDO, A. (1965). *Circul. J.* **29,** 755.

ARIAS-STELLA, J. & SALDANA, M. (1963). *Circulation* **28,** 915.

BATES, D. V. & CHRISTIE, R. V. (1964). *Respiratory Function in Disease.* Philadelphia : Saunders.

BERGOFSKY, E. H., TURINO, G. M. & FISHMAN, A. P. (1959). *Medicine, Baltimore* **38,** 263.

BOWDEN, D. H., FISHER, V. W. & WYATT, J. P. (1965). *Am. J. Med.* **38,** 2.

BRENNER, O. (1935). *Archs. intern. Med.* **56,** 211.

CIVIN, W. H. & EDWARDS, J. E. (1951). *Archs. Path.* **51.** 192.

DUKE, H. N. (1954). *J. Physiol., Lond.* **125,** 373.

DUNNILL, M. S. (1961). *J. clin. Path.* **14,** 246.

EULER, U. S. VON & LILJESTRAND, E. (1946). *Acta. physiol. scand.* **12,** 301.
EVANS, T. O., VAN DER REIS, L. & SELZER, A. (1963). *Am. Heart. J.* **66,** 741.
FISHMAN, A. P. (1961). *Physiol. Rev.* **41,** 214.
FISHMAN, A. P., FRITTS, H. W. & COURNAND, A. (1960). *Circulation,* **22,** 204.
FLETCHER, C. M., HUGH-JONES, P., MCNICHOL, M. W. & PRIDE, N. B. (1963). *Q. Jl Med.* **32,** 33.
FLUCK, D. C., CHANDRASIKAN, R. G. & GARDNER, F. V. (1966). *Br. Heart J.* **28,** 92.
FULTON, R. M. (1953). *Q. Jl Med.* **22,** 43.
FULTON, R. M., HUTCHINSON, E. C. & JONES, A. M. (1952). *Br. Heart J.* **14,** 413.
GOLDRING, R. M. (1964). *J. Pediat.* **65,** 4.
GOLDRING, R. M., TURINO, G. M., ANDERSEN, D. H. & FISHMAN, A. P. (1961). *Circulation,* **24,** 942.
GOUGH, J. (1949). *J. R. Microsc. Soc.* **69,** 231.
HANLEY, T., PLATTS, M. M., CLIFTON, M. & MORRIS, T. L. (1958). *Q. Jl Med.* **27,** 155.
HARRISON, R. W., ADAMS, W. E., BEUHLER, W. & LONG, E. T. (1957). Effects of acute and chronic reduction of lung volume on cardiopulmonary reserve, *A.M.A. Archs. Surg.* **75,** 546.
HARVEY, R. M. & FERRER, M. I. (1960). *Circulation,* **21,** 263.
HASLETON, P. S., HEATH, D. & BREWER, D. B. (1967). *J. Path. Bact.* In press.
HEATH, D. (1963). *J. Path. Bact.* **85,** 107.
HEATH, D. & BEST, P. V. (1958). *J. Path. Bact.* **76,** 165.
HEATH, D., HELMHOLZ, H. F., Jr., BURCHELL, H. B., DUSHANE, J. W., KIRKLIN, J. W. & EDWARDS, J. E. (1958). *Circulation* **18,** 1155.
HECHT, H. H. (1956). *Circulation* **14,** 265.
HICKEN, P., HEATH, D., BREWER, D. B. & WHITAKER, W. (1965). *J. Path. Bact.* **90,** 107.
JAMES, W. R. L. (1966). *Br. Heart J.* **28,** 512.
JAMES, W. R. L. & THOMAS, A. J. (1963). *Br. Heart J.* **25,** 583.
LAVENNE, R. (1951). *Revue belge Path. Med. exp.* **21,** Suppl. 6.
LEOPOLD, J. G. & GOUGH, J. (1957). *Thorax,* **12,** 219.
LIEBOW, A. A. (1959). *Am. Rev. resp. Dis.* **80,** 67.
LIEBOW, A. A. (1964). In *Aging of the Lung.* 10th Hahnemann Symposium. p. 99. Ed. Cander, L. & Moyer, J. H. New York : Grune and Stratton.
MCLEAN, K. H. (1958). *Australas. Ann. Med.* **7,** 69.
MICHELSON, N. (1960). *Dis. Chest,* **38,** 435.
MISE, J., MORIYAMA, K. & ITAGAKI, S. (1966). *Jap. Heart J.* **7,** 1.
MOSS, A. J., HARPER, W. H., DOOLEY, R. R., MURRAY, J. F. & MACK, J. F. (1965). Cor pulmonale in cystic fibrosis of the pancreas, *J. Pediat.* **67,** 5.
MOTLEY, H. L. & TOMASHEFSKI, J. F. (1950). *Am. J. Physiol* **150,** 315.
NAEYE, R. L. (1961 *a*) *Archs. Path.* **71,** 447.
NAEYE, R. L. (1961 *b*). *Am. J. Path.* **38,** 561.
NAEYE, R. L. (1967). *Am. J. Path.* **50,** 6.
NAEYE, R. L. & BICKERMAN, H. A. (1957). The effects of hypoxemia on the pulmonary arterial bed of humans and rats. Reported in *Fed. Proc.* **18,** 497. (1959).
NAKHJAVAN, F. K., PALMER, W. H. & MCGREGOR, M. (1966). *Circulation* **33,** 8.
OKINAKA, S. & HARASAWA, M. (1964). *Jap. Circul. J.* **28,** 3.
PEÑALOZA, D., SIME, F., BANCHERO, N. & GAMBOA, R. (1963). In *Normal and Abnormal Pulmonary Circulation.* p. 257. Fifth annual conference on research in emphysema. Aspen. Colorado. Karger. New York.
REEVE, R., SELZER, A., POPPER, R. W., LEEDS, R. F. & GERBODE, F. (1966). *Circulation* **33,** Suppl. 1, 4.
SCOTT, R. W. & GARVIN, C. F. (1941). *Am. Heart J.* **22,** 56.
VOGEL, J. H. K., CAMERON, D. & JAMIESON, G. (1966). *Am. Heart J.* **72,** 50.
WEIBEL, E. R. & VIDONE, R. A. (1961). *Am. Rev. resp. Dis.* **84,** 856.
WHITAKER, W. (1954). *Q. Jl Med.* **23,** 57.
WYATT, J. P., FISHER, V. W. & SWEET, H. C. (1964). *Am. Rev. resp. Dis.* **89,** 5.

SESSION FIVE

THE DIAGNOSIS OF EMPHYSEMA DURING LIFE

Chairman : D. V. BATES

A MATHEMATICAL MODEL OF PULMONARY GAS TRANSPORT[1]

GILES F. FILLEY, LUDOVIC M. LACQUET,[2] DAN E. OLSON,[3] RICHARD P. SPECK and INGVAR E. SODAL.

THE 'steady state' CO method for pulmonary diffusing capacity yields little or no difference between the values obtained in patients with probable reduction of diffusing surface because of emphysema and in patients without such reduction, their pulmonary disease being primarily chronic bronchitis (Bedell & Ostiguy, 1967 ; Filley *et al.*, 1967). The initial motivation for the present investigation was to determine the conditions under which CO transport, and hence perhaps O_2 transport, can be more impeded by failure to deliver the test gas to the alveolar surface than by interference with diffusion through the alveolar membrane.

Delivery of inspired gas to the alveolar surface takes place both by bulk flow and by diffusion in the gas phase. Since the former process is to some extent controllable (by varying the pattern of breathing) and the latter to some extent predictable (from equations based on knowledge of the geometry of the air spaces), it is possible to evaluate the importance of these processes by comparing the actual behaviour of inspired test gases under controlled conditions of breathing with the behaviour predicted from mathematical models of the lung.

The transport model formulated here includes many concepts from the past 75 years and is meant to be sufficiently general to form the basis for future modification. This paper will sketch how pulmonary gas transport has been conceived historically, develop a general mathematical lung model and show wherein it accounts and fails to account for the carbon monoxide uptake observed in two normal subjects.

[1] This investigation was supported in part by Research Grants : VRA Rehabilitation Research & Training RT–10, National Institutes of Health, HEO–3191 and HEO–5450, and U.S. Army DA 49–193 MD 2227.

[2] International Postdoctoral Fellow of the National Institutes of Health. Present address : University of Louvain, St. Barbara Hospital, Pellenberg, Belgium.

[3] Research Fellow of the National Institutes of Health.

HISTORY OF LUNG MODEL BUILDING

Since the actual transport paths from the trachea to the alveolar surface are too complex to be easily grasped, respiratory physiologists have formed simplified and usually non-quantitative concepts of the air passages of the lung (concepts which can be called non-mathematical models). The first quantitative formulation of gas phase transport was that of Bohr (1891) who visualized the lung as having only two compartments, (Fig. 1), a dead space and an alveolar space. The so-called Bohr equation or algebraic formulation of this concept is developed in the Appendix. Here we note the important

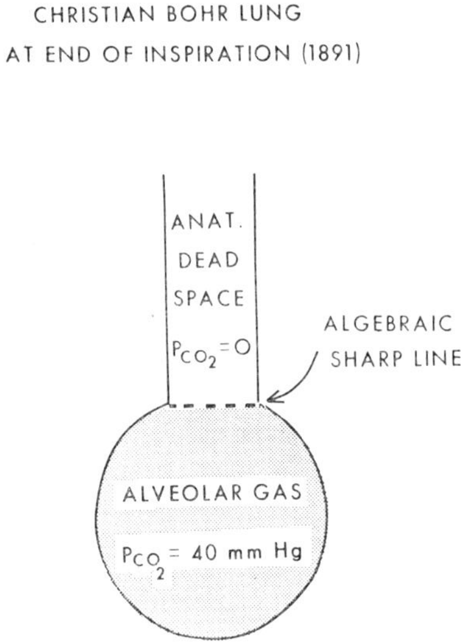

FIG. 1. The Bohr model.

fact that this first mathematical model of the lung implies (psychologically if not logically) that a sharp line or plane of demarcation exists between the dead space and an alveolar compartment of indefinite volume, that the gas leaving this compartment to become part of the expired tidal volume is representative of all alveolar gas and that alveolar gas is uniform in composition and does not vary during the respiratory cycle.

Clear evidence of non-uniformity of alveolar gas composition in normal lungs was obtained as early as 1916 by Sonne and has led to the most popular modification of the Bohr model—*i.e.* the model of ' parallel ' (somewhat less usefully called regional) non-uniformity shown in Figure 2. The concept that alveolar gas concentration differences (often called gradients), exist *between* lobes or segments and not within smaller lung units was supported by the calculations[1] of Rauwerda (1946) even though these were strictly applicable only to the breath-holding of gases not being transferred across alveolar walls.

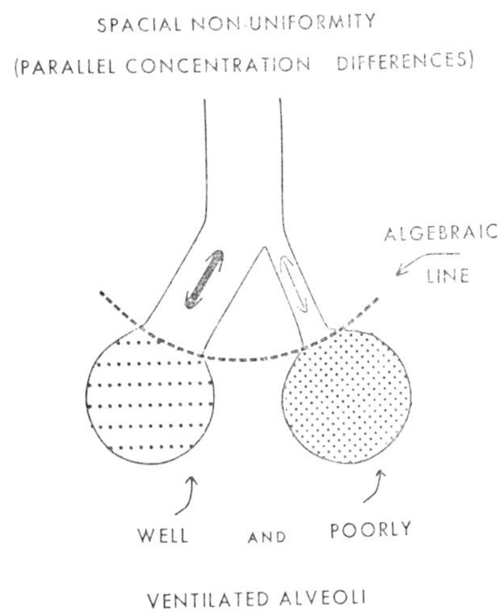

FIG. 2. The model of parallel non-uniformity. The dots can be thought of as CO_2 molecules being washed out of the lungs by fresh air.

Haldane (1922) considered that concentration gradients normally exist *along* the lengths of the small respiratory air passages and that the P_{O_2} in the distal ends of the alveolar ducts was lowered out of proportion to a P_{CO_2} rise. In modern terms, such a distribution of R suggests that inequalities of $\dot{V}/\dot{Q}$ may exist in the normal respiratory bronchiole-alveolar duct system and may be depicted by a model involving ' series ' (or stratified) non-uniformity (Fig. 3).

In contrast to these spatial models, a type of *temporal* non-uniformity has interested physiologists since Krogh and Lindhard's early efforts (1914) to quantitate the fluctuations of alveolar gas concentrations during the respiratory cycle. Du Bois' later work

[1] Rauwerda calculated that in a cylindrical respiratory tube 7 mm. long and 0·3 mm. in diameter a gas concentration difference would be reduced by diffusion in the gas phase to 16 per cent of its initial value in 0·38 sec. See Appendix.

(1952) stands almost alone among modern attempts to deal with these fluctuations and the temporal model (Fig. 4) has not achieved great popularity.[1]

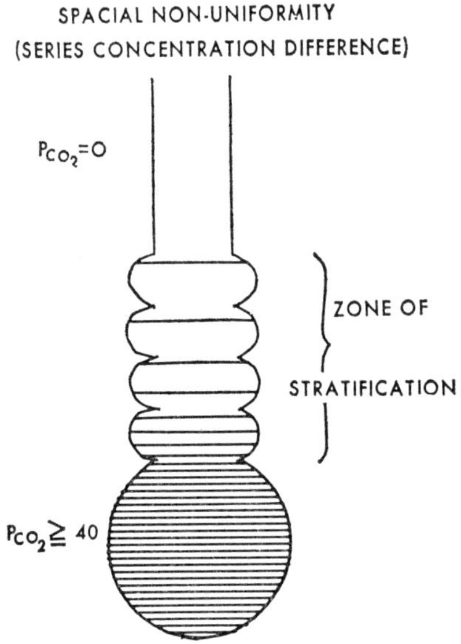

FIG. 3. Series or stratified non-uniformity illustrated with CO_2 pressures.

Two entirely different models which (probably to their advantage) bear little similarity to anatomical lungs were developed between 1945 and 1960. The first of these was devised by Riley and Cournand (1949) who simply assumed that ventilation was continuous because ' the cyclic nature of the ventilatory process tends to obscure certain fundamental relationships '. This model, until modified by later workers (Ross & Farhi, 1960) concerned with parallel non-uniformities of gas concentration, greatly clarified blood-gas exchange theory. By comparing our Figure 5 with Figure 1 in Riley & Cournand (1949), it can be seen how the elegant simplicity of the original model is lost by the introduction of a rebreathed dead space affected by such parallel non-uniformities. A contrasting model has been used by Altshuler *et al.* (1959) to account for the transport of aerosols into and out of the lung by bulk flow and by convective mixing. As

[1] In fact most gas exchange formulations assume that what is a periodic transient state can be considered a steady state. (See Appendix).

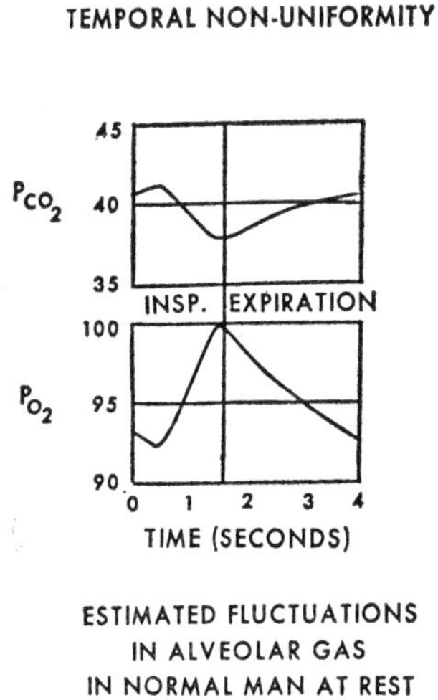

FIG. 4. The model of temporal non-uniformity. (After Krogh and DuBois.)

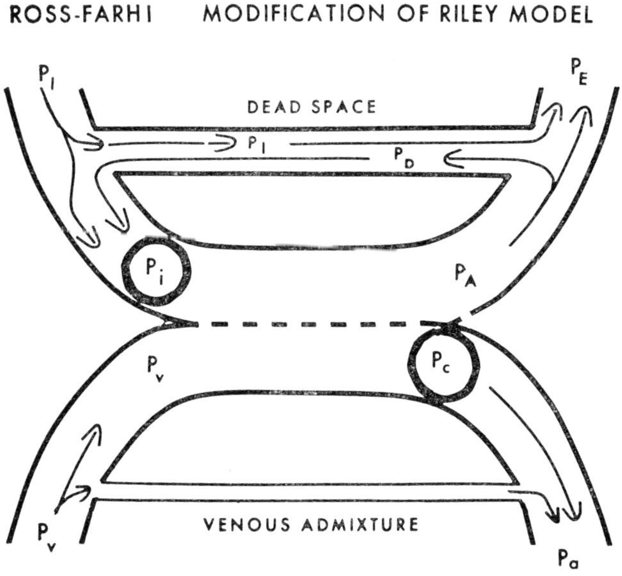

FIG. 5. The continuous ventilation model. Pi and Pc cannot be measured directly.

seen in Figure 6 this model illustrates the remarkably slight penetration of inspired aerosols into the alveolar gas and dramatizes the extent to which the transport of gases such as CO and O_2 must depend on diffusion in the gas phase.

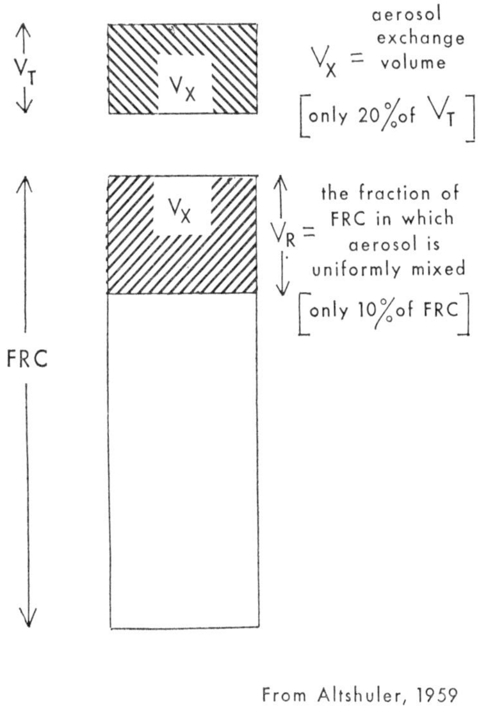

FIG. 6. The aerosol model

Current lung models are beginning to incorporate recent information on the contrasting ways in which gas molecules can be transported through the airways (Fig. 7) and to include concepts involving the mechanical properties of the lungs as affected by gravity and by the state of lung inflation (Fig. 8).

DEVELOPMENT OF THE PRESENT LUNG MODEL

It is first desired to predict the effects of simple changes in breathing pattern (Fig. 9) on the transport of a gas whose uptake

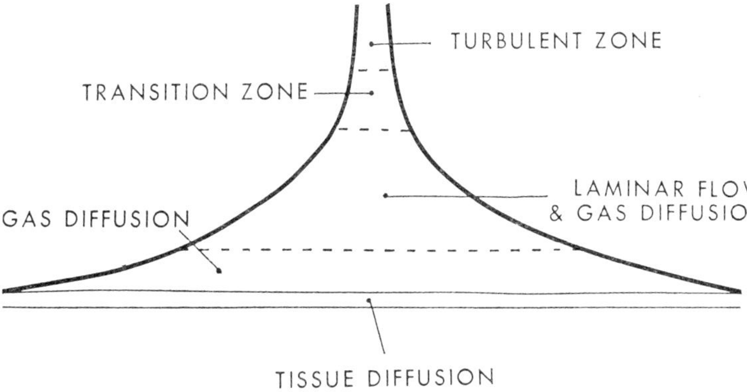

FIG. 7. The trumpet lung model. The shape suggests how the total cross section area of airways increases as the alveolar surface is approached slowing down flow but facilitating diffusion in the gas phase.

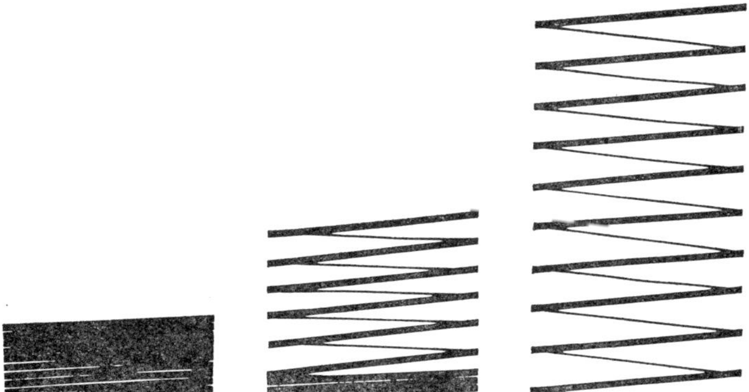

FIG. 8. The slinky lung model. The configurations suggest how, with partial lung expansion, the top of the lung inflates more than the bottom. It also suggests series non-uniformity.

is little affected by variations in pulmonary blood flow. We therefore consider how two contrasting types of controlled breathing affect the rate of CO absorption by a lung model based on four main assumptions listed below and indicated in Figure 10.

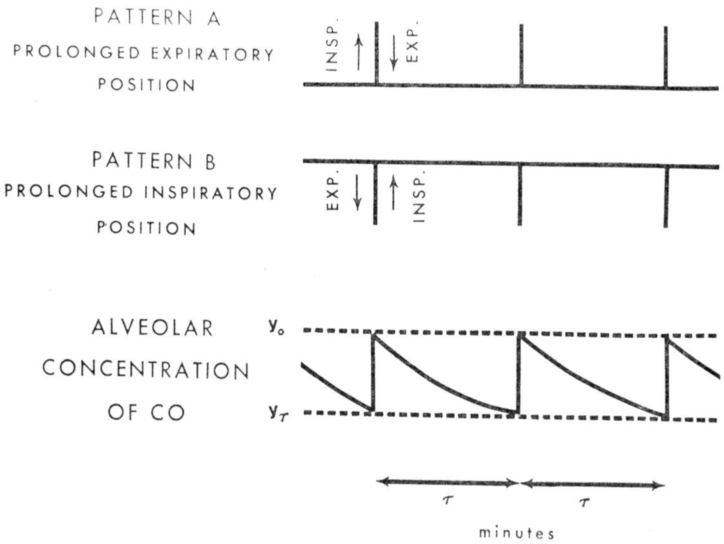

FIG. 9. Two breathing patterns A and B. In A, inspiration is instantaneously followed by expiration and the breath is held in expiration for the period, τ, of the respiratory cycle. In B, breath-holding is in the inspiratory position. In both patterns, the alveolar CO concentration falls exponentially at different rates during the period, τ.

1. The tissue conductance *D*, including both membrane and chemical kinetic factors, is independent of the alveolar gas volume.
2. The tissue conductance *D* is independent of tidal volume, *V*.
3. Once an initial CO concentration, y_o, has been established in alveolar gas after an inspiration, the concentration y (t) remains spatially uniform regardless of changes in lung volume but varies with time. This admission of temporal non-uniformity is the main feature distinguishing the present model from that of Bohr (1891).
4. The dead space, δ, is constant both during a respiratory cycle and for different cycles. This implies (4.1) that δ has the same volume whether inspiration is an instantaneous process or whether it is a slow enough process to allow complete mixing to occur between inspired gas and the gas already present in the initial alveolar volume

A, and (4·2) that once a plane has been established between dead space and alveolar gas, the position of this plane does not change during breath-holding. Implications (4·1) and (4·2) are equivalent to assuming instantaneous mixing in the alveolar compartment and no exchange between δ and alveolar gas.

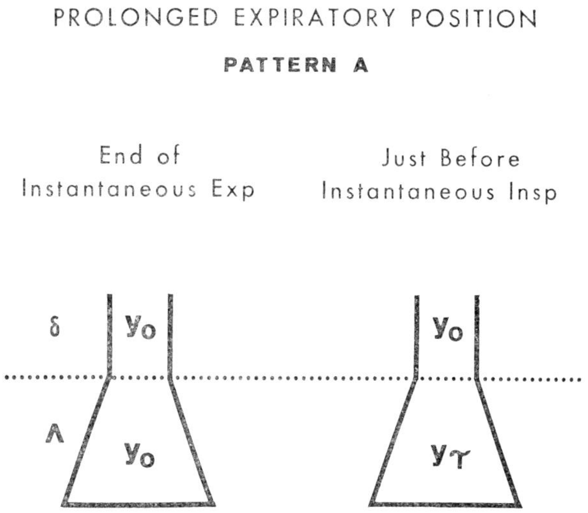

$$y_{\Upsilon} = y_0 e^{-\frac{D}{A}\Upsilon}$$

FIG. 10. The lung model for A breathing. The inflated state of the lung at end inspiration is not shown. The concentration y_0 exists at the beginning of every respiratory cycle.

If a lung with these assumptions breathes CO in a low[1] concentration long enough to establish a state such that the mixed expired gas concentration is constant, the rate of CO uptake measured at the mouth will depend on the alveolar concentration y and on the tissue conductance, D. This statement and the deductions from it which the assumptions permit are expressed in prediction equations in the Appendix. The significance of these deductions (*i.e.* the meaning

[1] Low enough so that CO uptake does not appreciably affect the gas volume of the lung or the CO tension in the blood.

of the prediction equations) can, perhaps must, be grasped with the help of words and diagrams.

Consider two contrasting breathing patterns : A, in which the lung at end-expiration is held throughout the respiratory cycle in the expiratory position so that CO is removed from the volume Λ ; and B, in which the lung at end-inspiration is held throughout the respiratory cycle in the inspiratory position so that CO is removed from the volume $\Lambda + V$.

Prolonged expiratory position (Pattern A)

The rate at which CO is absorbed from the alveolar gas, given the above features of the lung, can be mathematically predicted for this pattern of breathing and the total impediment to CO uptake expressed as a dimensionless ratio equal to the sum of two impediments : a tissue term involving the tissue conductance (D) and a gas phase term dependent on the ratio of the dead space (δ) to the tidal volume V. The prediction equation describing these impediments is shown in Figure 11. This Figure also shows graphically how the

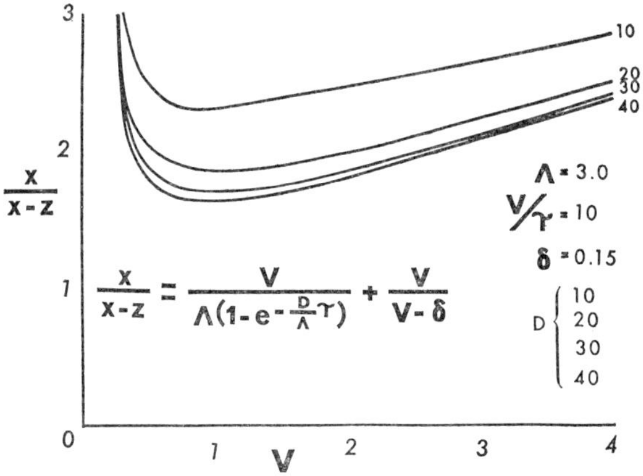

FIG. 11. Prediction equation and prediction curves for Pattern A breathing when total ventilation is held constant at 10 L/min, Λ at 3 L and δ at 0·15 L; D is allowed to vary from 10 to 40 L/min.

total impediment, $x/(x-z)$, varies with V and D when the total ventilation V/τ is held constant along with the two parameters Λ and δ.

A most important prediction of this model is that with deep breathing, when the ratio δ/V decreases, the total impediment is almost entirely dependent on the tissue term and the effect of δ

becomes negligible. On the other hand, with shallow breathing almost all the impediment to CO uptake depends on the gas phase term. How these two impediments add up to the total is shown in Figure 12.

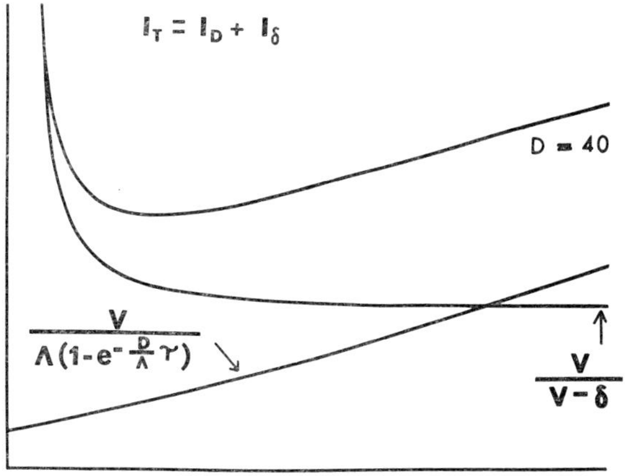

FIG. 12. Total impediment, I_T, plotted for D = 40, along with plots of the tissue impediment I_D containing the parameter D and the gas phase impediment I_δ containing the parameter δ to show how these two impediments add up to the total with Pattern A breathing.

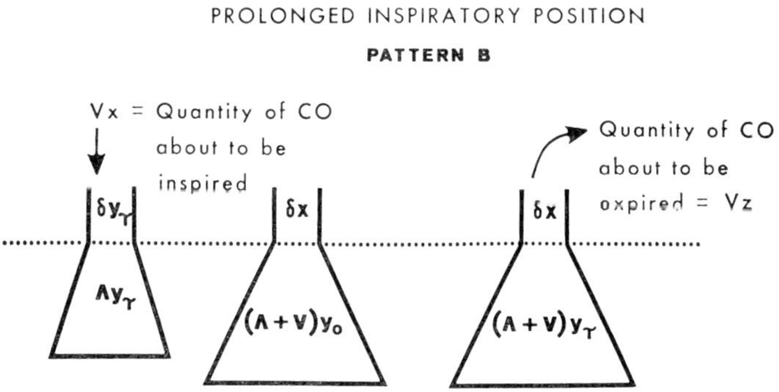

FIG. 13. In Pattern B breathing the lung inspires immediately after an instantaneous expiration and the breath is held throughout the period, τ, of the respiratory cycle. All the symbols used for volumes and concentrations are illustrated.

Prolonged inspiratory position (Pattern B)

With this pattern of breathing, CO is taken up from a larger volume than with Pattern A because the breath is held during inspiration. As shown in Figure 13, expiration is delayed until the alveolar concentration of CO has reached its lowest point, namely y_T Stated otherwise, the ' time of exposure ' of an inspired breath is as long as possible with this pattern of breathing while with Pattern A this exposure time was made as short as possible. As seen in Figure 14, the total impediment consistently (monotonically)

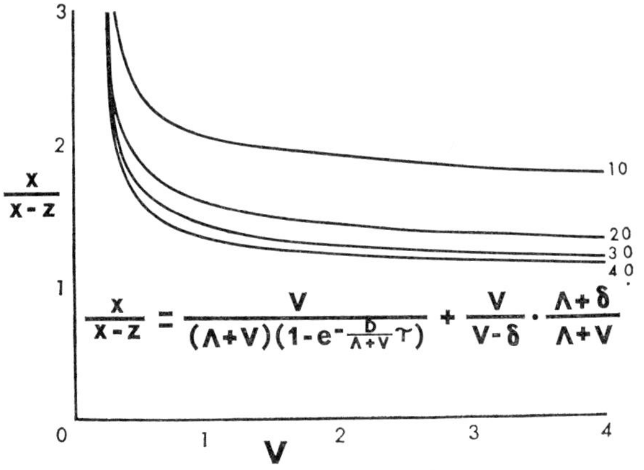

FIG. 14. The prediction equation for Pattern B differs both in the tissue and the gas phase term from that for Pattern A.

decreases with deep breaths and does not go through a minimum as in Pattern A. In other words prolonged breath-holding in inspiration, at a given ventilation, allows for a greater extraction of CO, than if the expiration follows immediately after inspiration.

EXPERIMENTAL

Two healthy men, *DH* (age 22, 91 Kg., 184 cm.) and *LH* (age 22, 75 Kg., 175 cm.), breathed 0·1 vol per cent. CO in air through a Rudolph directional valve for 6-minute periods either sitting or standing. The gas to be inspired flowed at a rate of 6·5 *L*/min. (STPD) from a cylinder through an anesthesia bag. The subjects emptied this bag at the end of each inspiration. Because the subjects breathed in time to a metronome, the requirement that the anesthesia bag be emptied with each breath insured a reasonably constant inspired tidal volume. The expired tidal volume was not controlled nor was the FRC measured during the test but the subjects attempted to maintain their lung volume constant at FRC at the end of each expiration.

No more than four 6-minute periods of CO breathing were allowed in one day to avoid significant increases in (COHb) in the blood. Expired gas was collected in a Douglas bag for the last three minutes of each experimental period. The volume of the bag was measured with a precision of $\pm 1{\cdot}0$ per cent. in a large Tissot spirometer. The CO concentration was measured by a Liston-Becker infra red meter with a precision of 2×10^{-3} as volume per cent. of CO. (This involves a 2 per cent. error in the analysis of 0·1 vol per cent. inspired gas and a 4 per cent. error for an expired sample containing 0·05 vol per cent.). Oxygen and CO_2 concentrations were measured by the Scholander $\frac{1}{2}$ cc. analyzer.

The attempt was made to vary the tidal volume and the frequency over as wide a range as possible from one 6-minute run to another while still maintaining the total ventilation constant at 10 L/min.

CALCULATIONS

The inspired tidal volume, V, was calculated from the 3-minute expired volume of the Douglas bags as follows :

$$V = \frac{\text{Bag vol. in liters (BTPS)}}{\text{Resp. freq. per min.} \times 3} \times F_{E_{N_2}} / F_{I_{N_2}}$$

The mean period, τ, of the respiratory cycle, was expressed as the reciprocal of the frequency per minute.

The impediment to CO uptake, $x/(x-z)$, is derived as shown in the Appendix. It is simply the reciprocal of the fraction of CO removed from inspired gas

$$\frac{x}{x-z} = \frac{F_{I_{CO}} F_{E_{N_2}} / F_{I_{N_2}}}{F_{I_{CO}} F_{E_{N_2}} / F_{I_{N_2}} - F_{E_{CO}}}$$

where the symbols in the right hand term are those customarily used in respiratory physiology (Pappenheimer, 1950). The fit between measurements and predictions was determined by the least squares procedure.

RESULTS

The data are collected in Table 1. Measurements for Pattern A breathing in the two subjects are plotted as single points in Figures 15 and 16. The curve which best fits the data for subject *DH*

Table 1. *Data in two normal subjects. The tidal volume* V, *is in liters* (*BTPS*), *the period,* τ, *of the respiratory cycle is in minutes, and the impediment to CO uptake is the dimensionless ratio* $x/(x-z)$.

	Pattern A			Pattern B		
	V	τ	$x/(x-z)$	V	τ	$x/(x-z)$
	1·028	0·098	1·91	1·019	0·098	1·40
	0·861	0·093	1·71	1·000	0·098	1·46
	0·944	0·094	1·73	0·979	0·101	1·38
	0·438	0·049	1·68	0·996	0·101	1·39
	0·475	0·049	2·25	1·985	0·203	1·27
	0·447	0·046	1·89	1·955	0·203	1·30
	0·527	0·049	1·68	1·825	0·203	1·27
	0·483	0·049	1·83	1·868	0·202	1·26
	0·519	0·048	2·05	1·879	0·203	1·28
	0·615	0·053	1·89	1·867	0·203	1·24
	0·552	0·051	1·84	0·489	0·051	1·64
	0·552	0·047	1·92	0·513	0·051	1·64
	0·571	0·047	2·00	0·540	0·051	1·59
	2·102	0·195	1·79	0·540	0·051	1·58
	1·912	0·195	1·84	0·511	0·051	1·71
DH	2·114	0·196	1·94	0·480	0·151	1·90
	2·131	0·196	1·91	2·422	0·253	1·21
	2·122	0·195	1·87	2·338	0·253	1·23
	2·117	0·195	1·85	2·418	0·253	1·21
	2·189	0·196	1·86	2·356	0·253	1·22
	2·207	0·196	1·86	2·338	0·253	1·22
	1·517	0·152	1·73	2·337	0·253	1·22
	1·488	0·152	1·74	2·341	0·254	1·22
	1·506	0·151	1·69	2·407	0·253	1·23
	1·460	0·151	1·89	2·367	0·253	1·23
	1·052	0·097	1·98	1·076	0·098	1·51
	0·940	0·109	2·09	1·092	0·098	1·55
	1·067	0·098	1·45	1·450	0·152	1·35
				1·491	0·152	1·36
				1·023	0·098	1·43
	2·080	0·195	1·76	0·984	0·098	1·43
	2·087	0·195	2·15	1·456	0·152	1·35
				1·484	0·152	1·37

	Pattern A			Pattern B		
	V	τ	$x/(x-z)$	V	τ	$x/(x-z)$
	0·694	0·093	1·83	1·081	0·101	1·59
	0·745	0·093	2·03	1·028	0·101	1·68
	0·720	0·089	1·84	1·059	1·101	1·52
	0·678	0·093	1·85	1·012	0·101	1·59
	0·843	0·098	2·00	1·018	0·101	1·58
	0·421	0·049	2·02	1·000	0·101	1·64
	0·516	0·049	2·05	1·094	0·101	1·57
	0·490	0·049	2·47	1·094	0·101	1·58
	0·508	0·047	2·38	0·586	0·051	1·90
	0·536	0·050	2·18	0·612	0·051	1·78
	0·492	0·051	2·24	0·613	0·050	1·78
	0·468	0·047	2·21	0·596	0·051	1·81
	0·492	0·047	2·35	0·772	0·051	1·70
LH	0·512	0·047	2·39	0·750	0·050	1·90
	0·495	0·047	2·54	2·157	0·202	1·49
	2·131	0·197	2·39	1·972	0·202	1·39
	2·130	0·196	2·05	2·016	0·202	1·38
	2·102	0·197	2·05	2·011	0·202	1·46
	2·048	0·196	1·99	2·199	0·202	1·33
	2·266	0·196	2·07	2·165	0·202	1·39
	2·119	0·196	2·03	2·102	0·202	1·40
	1·475	0·151	1·94	2·154	0·202	1·35
	1·378	0·151	1·98			
	1·440	0·152	1·92			
	1·423	0·152	1·93			
	1·489	0·152	1·93			
	1·415	0·152	1·92			
	1·044	0·147	1·68			

indicates that D is approximately 28·5 L/min. and δ 0·162 L. When these numbers are converted to the usual expressions, DH has a

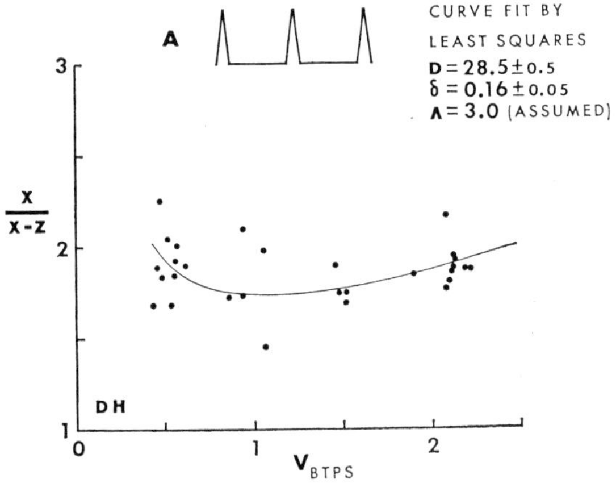

FIG. 15. The data obtained for Pattern A breathing by DH are plotted as solid circles. The prediction equation for Pattern A was fitted to the data by computer analysis according to the theory of least squares, (courtesy of Mr. Dan Olson), and yielded the D and σ values shown.

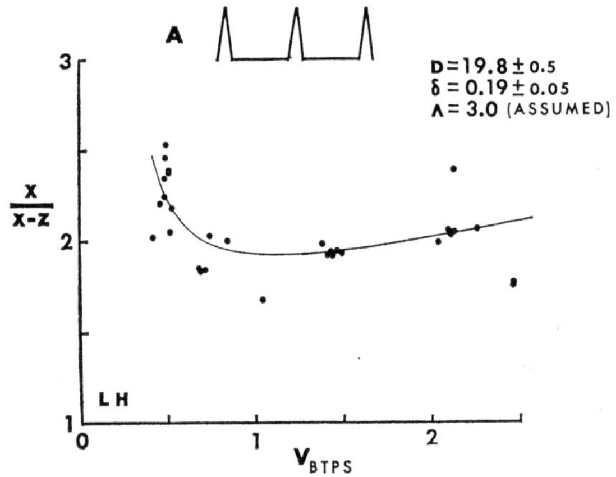

FIG. 16. The data and prediction equation fit for LH yielded a lower D and a higher δ for this subject.

$D_{L_{CO}} = D/0{\cdot}863 = 33$ cc. CO/min./mm. Hg. and a personal dead space for CO of 160−85 = 75 ml. Subject LH had a smaller D and a larger δ.

In Pattern B breathing, the data cluster much more closely about the lines of best fits as shown in Figure 17 and 18. In both subjects the *D* which resulted from the least squares curve fitting

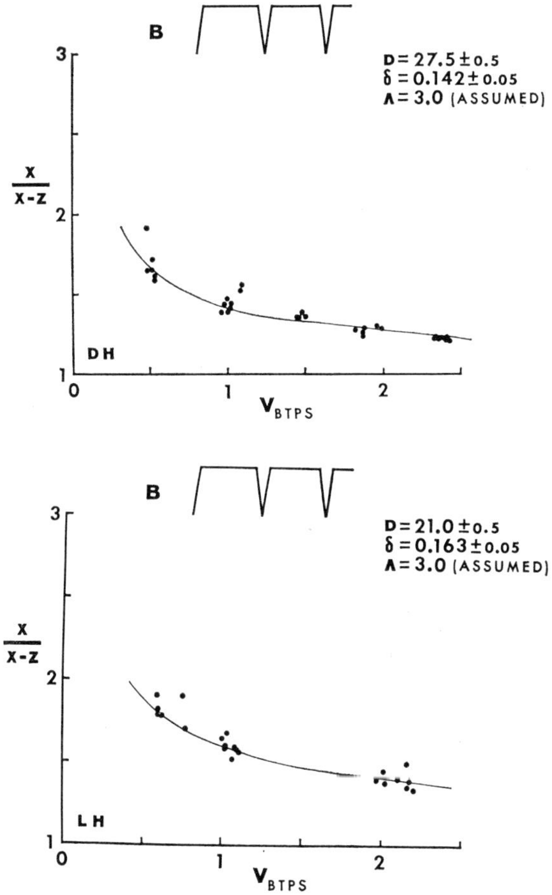

FIGS 17 and 18. The scatter of the data is less in Pattern B than in Pattern A breathing because the analytical error in determining z is less noticeable when the difference x—z is relatively large. In a given subject virtually the same D accounts for the data of both breathing patterns but B required a smaller δ than A.

procedure was approximately the same as calculated from Pattern A measurements. However, the δ needed to account for the data was lower in both subjects in Pattern B breathing.

DISCUSSION

The findings will first be discussed in relation to normal values found by other methods.

1. The average tissue conductances found in the two subjects were 28 and 20·4 *L*/min. When these are converted to the usual units (see Appendix), these subjects had $D_{L_{CO}}$ values of 32·5 and 23·7 ml./min./mm. Hg—values higher than usual for normal resting subjects. The reason for the discrepancy is not known. Possibly the effort to breathe in time to a metronome, and to empty an anesthesia bag in accordance with the experimental procedure may have increased pulmonary blood flow thereby filling the capillary bed more than under more restful conditions. Possibly the usual relaxed state of resting subjects causes portions of the lung to be underventilated so that the present values may more truly represent the tissue conductance for CO than the $D_{L_{CO}}$ measured by the usual steady state method.

2. How tidal volume *per se* affects diffusing capacity has not been adequately studied. In most papers on pulmonary physiology, the tidal volume is not even reported,—a rather remarkable omission since the depth of a breath must have a bearing on the distribution of inspired gas. The present findings indicate that the tissue conductance is normally independent of tidal volumes between 500 and 2,500 ml.

3. How alveolar volume affects $D_{L_{CO}}$ when measured by usual methods has been studied but the matter is not settled (Cadigan *et al.*, 1961 ; Marshall, 1958 ; Ross *et al.*, 1959 ; Forster, 1965). Most evidence indicates that when the breath is held for 10 seconds for the single breath test, the value of $D_{L_{CO}}$ increases with alveolar volume, but no clear explanation for this has been offered. The present finding that *D* is not affected by the alveolar volume suggests that the shorter breath-holding times of the present technique or the fact that the lung is cyclically inflated and deflated may be important in eliminating the volume-dependency of *D*.

4. The dead spaces for the two subjects were smaller than when determined by inert gas or CO_2 methods. No obvious explanation is at hand. The particularly low dead space found in Pattern B is explainable by diffusion in the gas phase since breath-holding in the inspiratory position favours such diffusion. It is possible that such diffusion also occurred, though to a lesser extent, with Pattern A since the subjects probably could not always keep the total duration of inspiration and expiration as short as desired to hold diffusion from dead space to alveolar gas to a minimum.

The experimental data will next be considered as a test of the validity of the four main assumptions of the model developed above and in the Appendix.

1. Is the tissue conductance, D, actually independent of lung volume ?

The data obtained in a given subject could be explained by a constant D for that subject whether CO was being transferred through the alveolar membrane whose configuration (area ?, thickness ?) was maintained for most of the respiratory cycle at FRC or at FRC plus tidal volume.

2. Is the tissue conductance, D, actually independent of tidal volume ?

For Pattern A breathing, this feature could not be examined both because the alveolar membrane was only maintained at peak tidal volume very briefly and because of the large data scatter (Figs. 15 and 16). For Pattern B breathing, D was probably not influenced by the depth of breathing.

3. What is the effect of volume of alveolar compartment on CO transport ?

The exponential decay of CO concentration proceeded as predicted whether the gas was absorbed from A (FRC-dead space) or from $A+V$ (FRC+tidal volume−dead space). This is evidence that CO concentration non-uniformity was more temporal than spatial under the conditions of these experiments—at least in ' distal ' alveolar gas not exchanging with dead space gas.

4. Is the dead space actually constant ?

Only in this feature were the data incompatible with the model. In Pattern A breathing the dead space was larger than in Pattern B breathing in both subjects. One reason for this may be that the very brief inspirations followed immediately by rapid expirations in Pattern A allowed only very incomplete mixing of inspired with alveolar gas. In this case Assumption 4·1 given earlier would be invalidated. Another explanation for the lower δ in B is that since the breath is held in inspiration with this Pattern, the dead space contains a higher CO concentration than in Pattern A during most of the respiratory cycle ; because of this, a larger concentration gradient exists from δ to $A+V$ than from δ to A in Pattern A so that more CO leaves δ by diffusion in the gas phase in Pattern B. In this case Assumption 4·2 given earlier would be invalidated.

Finally the present model will be discussed as a basis for future investigations of pulmonary disease.

Since the process of oxygen extraction is the lung's main function and since respiratory failure can result from disturbances in any of several components of this process, both physiologist and clinician should be able to assess the adequacy of these several transport components. Certain ' overall ' indices, for example the oxygen ventilation equivalent ($\dot{V}_E / \dot{V}_{O2}$/, O_2v, essentially the reciprocal of the fraction of O_2 removed from inspired gas), have proved useful but more as a measure of over breathing than as an index of pulmonary efficiency (Filley, 1967). This is mainly because such an overall index is affected by stimulus-response complexities involving the central nervous system.

To measure separately the several components of the oxygen extraction process is extremely difficult since they are so closely integrated. Ventilatory and circulatory function, for example, are normally constantly being adjusted so that normal oxygenation of arterial blood is maintained ; how such adjustment fails in disease is not understood because methods involving only oxygen measurements do not permit separate assessment of these functions.

The present model not only separates the transport components mathematically but permits their individual assessment. The components of the model are arranged as the sum of dimensionless impediments to gas transport ; hence a series rather than parallel distribution of gas concentration differences is assumed. This is extremely convenient mathematically and is simple conceptually ; the experimental data of this report tends, furthermore, to support the validity of the series type of lung model.

With the present model, each transport component can be individually assessed by studies of the behaviour of other gases whose transport properties depend predictably on changes in airway function, gas phase diffusion, membrane permeability and pulmonary blood flow. Carbon monoxide is the first such gas studied. It is believed that the mathematical structure of the present model will allow useful predictions to be made for other gases and eventually for the understanding of pulmonary oxygen transport in health and disease.

SUMMARY

A modified Bohr model is adequate to account for CO transport in normal men breathing under the conditions of these experiments if temporal non-uniformity is assumed for distal alveolar gas (adjacent to alveolar walls) and if both spatial and temporal non-uniformity are permitted in proximal alveolar gas (in contact with dead space gas). The present investigations indicate that series non-uniformity of CO concentration in the gas phase can be detected even in the normal human lung and that methods for quantitating this non-uniformity will be useful in accounting for gas transfer abnormalities in pulmonary disease.

APPENDIX

Symbols and definitions

Gas Volumes (liters, BTPS)

- V The volume of a single inspiration or expiration ; a tidal volume.
- Λ A volume of intrapulmonary gas from which CO is absorbed ; sometimes called ‘ alveolar volume ’.
- δ The volume of dead space ; $\Lambda+\delta =$ FRC or functional residual capacity.

Carbon Monoxide Concentrations (volume fractions, dimensionless)

- x inspired concentration
- y alveolar concentration
- z expired concentration

Tissue Conductance (liters (BTPS)/min.)

- D The rate of uptake of CO per unit alveolar CO concentration in alveolar gas. The units may be written (cc CO$-$min.$^{-1}$)/(cc CO$-$L alv gas^{-1}). This is dimensionally equivalent to L alv gas/min.

Periodically repeated transient state (PRTS).

A state in which the CO concentration in a given region of the lung is the same at equivalent times in every respiratory cycle. For example, the alveolar CO concentration has, for a given PRTS, the same value at the end of each inspiration. It is convenient to consider the end of every inspiration to be the beginning of a respiratory cycle and to designate the alveolar CO concentration at any such point in time as y_o.

Mathematical derivation of lung model

Pattern A breathing. The rate at which CO is absorbed from Λ in the periodically repeated transient state defined above depends on the CO concentration $y(t)$ in Λ and on the tissue conductance D.

$$\Lambda \frac{dy}{dt} = -Dy \tag{1}$$

If y_o denotes the CO concentration at the beginning of each respiratory cycle and y_τ the concentration after τ minutes, the integrated form of (1) may be written

$$y_\tau = y_0 e^{-\frac{D}{\Lambda}\tau}. \qquad (2)$$

To specify y_0 we consider that at the beginning of each respiratory cycle an inspiration of volume V washes into Λ the quantity δy_0 of CO in the dead space[1] followed by the quantity $(V-\delta)x$. These quantities are added to and instantaneously mixed with the quantity $\Lambda y/$ remaining in Λ at the end of the previous cycle. Thus in the total volume $\Lambda + V$ the initial concentration at the start of each respiratory cycle is

$$y_0 = \frac{\Lambda y_\tau + \delta y_0 + (V-\delta)x}{\Lambda + V}; \qquad (3)$$

By combining (2) and (3) we can obtain

$$\frac{1}{y_0 - y_\tau} = \frac{\Lambda}{(V-\delta)x} + \frac{1}{x\left(1 - e^{-\frac{D}{\Lambda}\tau}\right)}. \qquad (4)$$

Since the uptake of CO per breath is

$$\Lambda(y_0 - y_\tau) = V(x - z), \qquad (5)$$

we combine (4) and (5) to get

$$\frac{x}{x-z} = \frac{1}{\Lambda\left(1 - e^{-\frac{D}{\Lambda}\tau}\right)} V + \frac{V}{V-\delta}. \qquad (6)$$

Pattern B breathing. With this pattern of breathing, CO is taken up from the volume $\Lambda + V$. The alveolar CO concentration at the end of the breath hold is

$$y_\tau = y_0 e^{-\frac{D}{\Lambda + V}\tau}. \qquad (7)$$

In this case, the gas rebreathed from the dead space has the concentration y_τ rather than y_0. Hence, instead of (3) we write

$$y_0 = \frac{\Lambda y_\tau + \delta y_\tau + (V-\delta)x}{\Lambda + V} \qquad (8)$$

Combining the uptake equation for the inspiratory position

$$(\Lambda + V)(y_0 - y_\tau) = V(x - z)$$

[1] Since expiration is assumed to occur immediately ' after ' (strictly speaking ' concurrently with ') inspiration as shown in Figure 9, the concentration y_0 will be in δ as well as in Λ at the end of expiration. This is illustrated in the left drawing of Figure 10 ; this figure also shows how the concentration y_0 remains unchanged in δ during the period of breath holding.

with (7) and (8) we obtain

$$\frac{x}{x-z}=\frac{1}{(\Lambda+V)\left(1-e-\frac{D}{\Lambda+V}\tau\right)}V+\frac{V}{V-\delta}\cdot\frac{V+\delta}{\Lambda+V}. \tag{9}$$

The Bohr Model. Equations (6) and (9) will now be shown to be very closely related to the original Bohr model in which alveolar gas was assumed not to vary during the respiratory cycle. Bohr (1891) showed that in such a state of uptake of a gas, its alveolar concentration, y, could be calculated from the amount of the gas, Vz, in an expiration, the amount, δx, in the dead space and the difference $V-\delta$ according to the formula

$$y=\frac{Vz-\delta x.}{V-\delta} \tag{10}$$

Define the tissue conductance

$$D=\frac{V}{\tau}(x-z)/y. \tag{11}$$

From (10) and (11) we find

$$\frac{x}{x-z}=\frac{1}{D}\frac{V}{\tau}+\frac{V}{V-\delta} \tag{12}$$

This equation is what (6) reduces to as τ approaches zero, since $1-e^{-\xi}\rightarrow\xi$ as $\xi\rightarrow 0$. In other words, with rapid shallow breathing, ($\tau < 0{\cdot}025$ min., $D/\Lambda < 10$ min.$^{-1}$), alveolar gas composition changes so little during a respiratory cycle that the original Bohr model adequately describes CO transport.

Special features of the present model

Equations (6), (9) and (12) are all dimensionless expressions. Since $x/(x-z)$ is the reciprocal of the fraction of CO removed, it might be called an over-all resistance equal to the sum of two separable resistances arranged in series. However, it seems wise to reserve the term resistance for a dimensional concept whose reciprocal is a conductance, and to use the new term, impediment, for the dimensionless ratios of the present development.

Dividing (12) by V/τ results in the equation developed by Hatch (1952),

$$\frac{1}{U}=\frac{1}{D}+\frac{1}{L},$$

where $U=V(x-z)/x\tau$ is the overall conductance, D is the tissue conductance and $L=(V-\delta)/\tau$ the ‘ effective rate of lung ventilation ’ or what we prefer to call the gas phase conductance. All these conductances are in liters (BTPS) per minute. While it is easy to see how these dimensions apply to L, it is less obvious for U and D.

The overall conductance U can be thought of as the uptake of a tracer gas per minute per unit concentration of the gas in the inspired mixture ; it can also be thought of as a clearance, *i.e.* the number of liters per minute of respired gas cleared of the tracer. Similarly D is the uptake per minute per unit concentration in ' alveolar ' gas and can be thought of as the liters of alveolar gas cleared per minute of tracer. Thus D is in L(BTPS)/min.

Since Krogh's time it has been customary to express the diffusing capacity for carbon monoxide in ml. CO per min. per mm. Hg. partial pressure of CO in alveolar gas ; these units are

$$\frac{\text{ml. (STPD, CO)/min.}}{(P_B\text{-}47)\ \text{ml. (STPD, CO)/ml. (STPD, alv gas)}} = \frac{\text{ml. (STPD, alv gas)}}{(P_B\text{-}47)\times \text{min.}}.$$

To convert this to L (BTPS, alv gas)/min, we multiply the above expression by

$$\frac{P_B\text{-}47}{1000}\times\frac{310}{273}\times\frac{760}{P_B}\times\frac{P_B}{P_B\text{-}47} = 0{\cdot}863\ ;$$

hence

$$D = 0{\cdot}863\ D_{L_{CO}}.$$

The relevance of Rauwerda's calculations to CO uptake

Rauwerda (1946) calculated the time required for a gas confined to one portion of a *single cylinder closed at both ends* to diffuse into the entire cylinder. These calculations are not entirely applicable to the lung for several reasons : (1) the actual arrangement of the alveolar ducts is more suggestive of a rapidly flaring cone than a cylinder, (2) the walls are permeable to gases like CO, (3) the gas in the upper airways affects the diffusion of gases in the distal portions of the bronchial tree, (Cumming *et al.*, 1966), and (4) no consideration was made for a temporal variance of concentration imposed at the upper end of his cylinder (the terminal bronchiole). Recent calculations in this laboratory indicate that the time required for 90 per cent. of the CO gradient between the average terminal bronchiole and the average alveolar sac to disappear is in the order of ·75 and 1·5 seconds (depending on the pattern of the breath).

ACKNOWLEDGMENTS :

The authors wish to thank Dr D. Boyd Bigelow for his assistance and Dr David Hutchison and Dr Louis Hagler for being the subjects of these experiments and for their help in the gas analyses.

DISCUSSION

Dr Fishman. If I understand your model, Dr Filley, it consists of three different compartments with different characteristics : in one compartment diffusion would be limited *to* the membrane as opposed to *through* the membrane. May I ask, what are the distinguishing characteristics for the three compartments ?

Dr Filley. I think the first compartment is variable and under experimental control because it is mainly concerned with bulk flow. How *fast* you breathe in as well as how *deeply* you breathe will determine how far the gas goes into the airway. The bulk flow is the upper compartment. In the last compartment, of course, is the alveolar membrane which may or may not change its surface area ; it may be like an accordian opening without an actual change in surface. The middle compartment has never been under control before. But with carefully controlled breathing patterns we have found that between the membrane and the bulk flow compartment there is an area, even in normals, where diffusion in the gas phase can be measurably modified experimentally. This area urgently needs exploration in patients with disturbances in oxygen transfer.

The whole issue of diffusion in the gas phase is a paradoxical situation, because in one sense, diffusion in the gas phase is all important, while in another sense, it can be neglected. Why is it all-important ? It is all-important because if we did not have diffusion in the gas phase we would not live, because we would never get the oxygen to the alveolar membrane fast enough. On the other hand, this process has been neglected by physiologists as not important, apparently largely because of Rauwerda's calculations (1946). These calculations are now being examined here in Birmingham as not being necessarily correct and certainly not directly applicable to patients with disturbed air space function.

Dr Fishman. Recognising the three compartments, where does maldistribution fit into the model of either the normal or the diseased lung ?

Dr Filley. The maldistribution will be both in parallel and in series, and it will be a maldistribution of concentration gradients in the gas phase. In other words, oxygen will be higher towards the mouth and lower towards the membrane in the series model and it will be hyper-ventilated and hypo-ventilated in the parallel model and both will be important. As Dr Cumming has said, the question is what proportion of the non-uniformity is series and what proportion is parallel in what disease ?

Dr Cumming. If I can summarise what we currently feel about this situation as applied to disease : I think it is important to separate distribution of ventilation into two types. One is that type which depends on transit time and the second is that which depends on gaseous mixing by diffusion. And in the transit time there are all the questions of lung elasticity, lung anatomy, altered resistance and compliance in disease, which Dr Mead has said is not particularly relevant in health, but I am sure is in disease ; the blocked small bronchioles have been referred to—all these affect the transit time and produce regional differences in ventilation. So we end up, if we could get the distribution of gaseous interfaces at zero time, with a potential wide distribution of concentrations through the lungs, not yet established because diffusion has not yet taken place. Then diffusion occurs, with the establishment in time of a uniform concentration. If, however, there is a defect in gas mixing, a concentration gradient will remain. Now, the important thing is what in disease particularly, will cause this second type of stratified inhomogeneity ? It is a simple, single fact. It is the distance that the gas interface has to diffuse from where it is established in the airway by bulk flow to the end of the alveolar sac where exchange across the membrane occurs. Any situation in disease or in health which increases diffusion distance, will increase stratified inhomogeneity and will make gas mixing efficiency worse or, as Dr Filley has said, its delta will increase. Now we can perhaps subject this to an analysis on the basis of prediction. If it is true that the distance of diffusion is important, let us in a normal establish a long distance of diffusion. Gareth Jones (1966) has recently carried out an experiment to do just this. He has measured gas mixing efficiency, using the decay curve technique, in normal subjects. Tidal volume was similar in all studies, and washout was effected from residual volume, from functional residual capacity and at total lung capacity. The greatest gas mixing efficiency was found at FRC. At the greater lung volume, the interface distance from the end of the alveoli would be expected to be greater, so that in a given time mixing would be less complete. This would explain the observation made that a significant diminution in mixing efficiency was found at TLC.

At RV the opposite would be the case, so that efficiency should be greater at RV than at FRC. In fact it was slightly worse, and we attribute this to the important effect of regional inhomogeneity when breathing from residual volume.

The main problem in disease is which of these two types of ventilatory disturbance plays the dominant role. In the majority of patients having cough, sputum and shortness of breath whom we have studied, the decay curve is practically rectilinear, indicating a dominance of stratified factors. In some however, the curvature of the decay curve is greater than in normals, indicating a greater than normal amount of regional inhomogeneity.

How to put figures on these two factors is at the moment, beyond us.

MORPHOLOGIC AND FUNCTIONAL STUDIES IN EMPHYSEMA

W. M. THURLBECK, D. V. BATES, R. G. FRASER, and J. HENDERSON

THE data I would like to present have been obtained from patients who had routine tests of pulmonary function and subsequently died, and whose lungs were studied in detail at necropsy. Patients with heart disease and lung disease, other than emphysema and bronchitis, likely to affect tests of pulmonary function have been excluded. The common reasons for exclusion were mitral stenosis, fibrosing alveolitis, lung cancer involving major airways, asthma and bronchiectasis.

The material is presented as group data. The primary division is made by a simple subjective grading system (Thurlbeck, 1963) derived from a Ciba symposium (1959). The patients with emphysema are divided into five groups which reflect increasing extent and severity of emphysema. The results are shown in Tables 1—4 which tabulate pathological data, clinical data, pulmonary function test data and data referring to pulmonary vascular disease respectively.

Table 1. *Pathological data*

Group	N	Units	Lm. mm.	ISA_5 m^2	% E
0	5	0	·294	61	0
I	10	1–5	·304	62	14
II	7	6–10	·337	53	21
III	12	11–15	·386	47	54
IV	9	16–23	·458	43	53
V	11	24+	·568	35	70

Group O : Patients without emphysema.
Units : Subjective assessment[1].
Lm : Average interalveolar distance[3].
ISA_5 : Internal surface area at arbitrary lung volume of 5 liters.
% E : Percentage of lung parenchyma involved by emphysema.

Table 2. *Clinical data*

Group	N	Bron- chitis	Smok- ing	Dys.	Hb. gm.	Radiology Over inf.	Emph.	PA	Obstr. lung dis. c.o.d.
O	5	1/5	3/5	0/3	13·4	·4	0/5	0/5	0/5
I	10	6/10	8/9	2/8	14·7	·8	4/10	2/10	0/10
II	7	6/7	7/7	3/4	14·9	1·6	4/7	3/6	2/7
III	12	11/12	11/12	9/11	14·4	2·1	10/11	4/12	7/12
IV	9	9/9	9/9	7/7	14·6	2·3	9/9	5/9	7/9
V	11	10/11	9/9	11/11	15·5	3·0	11/11	9/11	11/11

Dys. : Dyspnea considered due to bronchitis and/or emphysema.
Hb. : Haemoglobin.
Over inf. : Over inflation assessed on a 0–4+ scale.
Emph. : Diagnosis of emphysema.
PA : Enlargement of major pulmonary arteries.
Obstr. lung dis. c.o.d. : Emphysema and/or bronchitis considered the cause of death.

The *pathological data* indicate that other measurements of emphysema alter appropriately with the subjective assessment of emphysema. The objective measurements of emphysema (Thurlbeck, 1967)—mean cord (Lm) and alveolar surface area measurements (ISA_5)—of the patients with grade I emphysema fall within the normal range. There is considerable overlap in these values between individual groups.

The *clinical data* (Table 2) show that patients without emphysema or patients with grade I emphysema did not die of obstructive lung disease. The great proportion of patients with emphysema had bronchitis, rather higher than would be anticipated from a random necropsy population. *Radiologically*, there is a progressive increment of over-inflation of the lungs as assessed on a subjective 0–4+ scale. Emphysema—either of arterial deficiency pattern or increased marking pattern (Thirlbeck *et al.*, 1965)—was not diagnosed in patients without emphysema and was progressively more commonly diagnosed in patients with increasing amounts of emphysema. Enlargement of pulmonary arteries (PA) was absent in patients without emphysema, uncommon in grade I emphysema, and commonly found in patients with severe (grade V) emphysema. The intervening grades showed no striking difference in enlargement of pulmonary arteries.

Standard *tests of pulmonary function* (Table 3) were close to predicted normal in patients without emphysema. Severe emphysema (grade V) revealed the pattern well known to be typical of

Table 3. *Tests of pulmonary function*

Group	N	Int. mo	VC	FRC	RV	TLC	RV/TLC	ME	MMFR	FEV	DCO	CO%
O	5	2	101	94	105	102	0	106	99	110	121	99
I	10	5	80	108	133	100	13	102	45	72	122	89
II	7	7	65	123	177	103	24	75	33	42	86	86
III	12	8	60	126	168	101	25	68	18	31	76	72
IV	9	14	54	133	178	102	28	72	16	27	64	64
V	11	20	47	162	241	116	36	54	9	16	46	57

Int. : Interval between tests and death.
Tests are expressed as % of predicted except for RV/TLC which is expressed as % over predicted.
DCO : Steady state diffusion of carbon monoxide.
CO% : Fractional uptake of carbon monoxide.

severe clinical emphysema. The one patient with bronchitis but no emphysema had normal tests of pulmonary function. The striking findings were abnormalities of flow rates and subdivisions lung volumes in patients with grade I emphysema. These were present in patients with this degree of emphysema whether they had bronchitis or not. Gas mixing efficiency and steady state diffusion of carbon monoxide were normal in grade I emphysema. In fact, the latter test was uniformly higher than the normal in the individual cases in the group although fractional uptake of carbon monoxide was not. We believe that these results indicate that there is a general correlation between increasing amounts of emphysema and disturbances of pulmonary function tests but that no one single test will predict precisely the amount of emphysema. There was considerable overlap between the groups and, in general terms, the patients that died of obstructive lung disease in grade II and III emphysema had disproportionate alterations of tests of pulmonary function, particularly of flow rates.

Table 4. *Effect on pulmonary circulation*

Group	N	C.P.	Radiol.	ECG			Path	RV weight gms.
				Inc. P.	RVH	RVH>1		
O	5	0/5	0/5	0/5	0/5	0/5	0/3	...
I	10	0/10	1/10	0/10	0/10	0/10	0/9	48
II*	7	1/6	2/5	1/6	1/6	1/6	2/6	54
III	12	3/12	2/11	5/12	1/12	0/12	7/10	77
IV	9	2/8	4/9	5/9	4/9	2/9	6/9	86
V	11	7/11	9/11	11/11	8/11	5/11	10/10	104
B'esis	5	3/5	3/4	3/5	3/5	3/5	4/4	116

* Excludes one case with bronchitis, emphysema and multiple pulmonary emboli.
B'esis : Patients with widespread bronchiectasis.
C.P. : Heart failure thought due clinically to bronchitis and/or emphysema.
Inc. P. : All ECG abnormalities, including P pulmonale, suggesting right heart disease.
RVH : Any ECG evidence of right ventricular hypertrophy.
RVH>1 : Right ventricular hypertrophy greater than grade 1.
Path. : Right ventricular hypertrophy at necropsy. Doubtful cases excluded.
RV weight : Weight of right ventricle at necropsy.
Radiol. : Radiologic enlargement of right ventricle.

Analysis of our data related to the *pulmonary circulation* (Table 4) came as somewhat of a surprise. Heart failure, considered clinically due to obstructive lung disease (CP), was absent in our patients without emphysema and was common in patients with severe emphysema. Radiological evidence of right ventricular hypertrophy was absent in patients without emphysema, uncommon in patients with grade I emphysema and common in patients with grade V emphysema. Similar trends were apparent in electrocardiograms whether these referred to any abnormalities involving the right heart (inc. P), any right ventricular hypertrophy using the classification devised by Goodwin and Asdin (1959) (RVH) or right ventricular hypertrophy more than grade I (RVH $>$ 1). Similar trends were noted in the postmortem examination of the heart.

This striking departure from conventional wisdom is accounted for by the fact that our series includes a large number of patients in groups O, I, II and III who did not die of obstructive lung disease. Right ventricular hypertrophy and pulmonary hypertension was strikingly present in a group of five patients with widespread bronchiectasis which have been included by others as ‘ bronchitics ’ (Burrows *et al.*, 1966). However, our data do not support the concept that chronic bronchitis, without underlying structural disease such as emphysema or bronchiectasis, commonly produces severe pulmonary circulatory disease. Nor does it support the concept that patients with severe pulmonary emphysema are free from right ventricular disease. The tables do not include an analysis of blood gas disturbances but these in general closely parallel pulmonary circulatory disease.

In summary then, we believe that the extent of emphysema in the lungs can be predicted adequately by the use of radiology and pulmonary function tests. However, occasional cases were encountered in which emphysema was either considerably worse or considerably less than anticipated. For example, we have one patient who was predicted to have grade V emphysema but found to have grade II emphysema and a patient with grade IV emphysema who was predicted to have grade I or grade II emphysema. But these were exceptions. Our study also underlines the critical importance of the nature of selection of cases. If only patients with fatal obstructive lung disease were included and if patients with bronchiectasis, mitral stenosis and multiple pulmonary emboli were included, then one might come to a very different conclusion. The belief that pulmonary hypertension is unrelated to, or unassociated with, emphysema has been derived from studies on patients with symptomatic obstructive lung disease ; these conclusions cannot be extrapolated to the population as a whole.

SOME OBSERVATIONS ON THE BRONCHIAL AND EMPHYSEMATOUS TYPES OF PATIENT WITH SEVERE GENERALISED AIRWAYS OBSTRUCTION

C. M. FLETCHER

MY concern in this paper is with the clinician's diagnostic problem, which is to determine as accurately as possible the morbid anatomical basis of the disability of patients with airways obstruction. What is the lesion which disables our patients ? We must have some idea in order to guide treatment and prognosis. Furthermore, as an epidemiologist, I appreciate the need to improve diagnostic techniques so that we may recognise the various forms of disease that cause airways obstruction at an early stage so that we can study means of prevention.

We have now learnt to recognise two main types of abnormality in our patients. The first is emphysema for which I accept the definition put forward by the World Health Organisation (1961). 'Enlargement beyond the normal in the size of air spaces distal to the terminal bronchiole, with destruction of their walls.' I do not regard as emphysema the simple reversible enlargement of respiratory air spaces which Woolcott and Read (1965) have shown can occur in an acute asthmatic attack when the lung volume goes up right above normal limits. Now the fascinating thing about emphysema, of course, is the hypnotic effect the word had and still has on most morbid anatomists and many clinicians. Perhaps this is because it is often easy to see, even though, as we have heard during this symposium, it can be very difficult to quantitate in type, distribution or amount. Whatever the reason, there has certainly been an overwhelming concentration on emphysema in our thinking and writing on chronic airways obstruction.

The second lesion with which we are concerned is something hitherto unidentified : something which must presumably lie in the bronchioles and which, even in the absence of emphysema, can cause expiratory slowing to a degree which may be fatal and which is also, presumably because it is unevenly distributed, associated with grossly abnormal ventilation-perfusion ratios.

On the basis of clinical and physiological tests, we are now able to make a rough estimate of how much emphysema our pathological colleagues will find at autopsy in our disabled patients. We can at least distinguish those cases in which emphysema is the predominant and overwhelming lesion from those cases in which it is largely, if not wholly, unimportant. The important point which must be stressed is that there are cases with severe bronchiolar disease which may have a fatal outcome in which destructive emphysema appears to play no significant part.

We took our first steps towards this conclusion some years ago now when we began to recognise cases dying of respiratory failure in whom, at autopsy, emphysema appeared to be very slight. We next looked at the characteristics of patients with airways obstruction who had obvious radiological emphysema but no bronchitis, and compared them with patients who had chronic bronchitis (by which we implied simply productive cough) some of whom had and some had not got radiological emphysema (Fletcher *et al.*, 1963). And we found, briefly, that the cases with severe emphysema as shown on the radiograph had relatively normal blood gases, were relatively free from cor pulmonale, had a low transfer factor and had an increased total lung capacity, whereas in cases with what we thought was ‘ pure ’ bronchitis we found gross hypoxia and hypocarbia, frequent cor pulmonale, a fairly normal transfer factor and a normal or low total lung capacity.

There was, of course, considerable resistance to the idea that the cases we called ‘ pure ’ bronchitis could have no emphysema and in our Chairman’s book on Respiratory Function in Disease, written jointly with Professor Christie, we read (p. 217) : ‘ it seems likely that in many of these (patients) some degree of morphologic emphysema was present and in our view, it is less confusing at the present time to classify them as patients with a disproportion between $\dot{V}/\dot{Q}$ disturbance and the degree of morphological emphysema, rather than to describe them as having only “ chronic bronchitis ”.’

There are two interesting points in that quotation : the first is the ‘ disproportion between $\dot{V}/\dot{Q}$ disturbance and morphologic emphysema.’ This implies that there was something causing the $\dot{V}/\dot{Q}$ disturbance other than emphysema, so that agreement is at least implied that there is some other lesion which can cause this most important disproportion. The second point is some confusion about ‘ only ’ chronic bronchitis. We did not intend to suggest that these patients had only simple chronic bronchitis (defined as chronic productive cough.) What they had was severe airways obstruction of the kind which we believed was due to chronic bronchial inflammation, or bronchitis, and it was this which was causing gross disproportion between emphysema, which was absent or insignificant, and severe airways obstruction causing the $\dot{V}/\dot{Q}$ disturbance. Five of the 17 cases of bronchitis have come to autopsy since that paper was written and in none of them was more than 5 per cent. of the area of a whole lung section affected by emphysema.

Since then we have extended our understanding of the morphological basis of the abnormality in our patients by comparing clinical and physiological studies made during life on 32 male patients in London and Chicago on whom autopsy studies have been made by Dr Brian Heard and Dr John Wootcliffe in the Department of Pathology at Hammersmith. The results have been published (Burrows *et al.*, 1966) but I propose to demonstrate them here with the addition of some findings on patients studied since these were published.

To assess severity of emphysema Dr Heard divides a sagital lung slice into six areas of equal size and in each area he rates the severity of the emphysema on a scale 0 to 3, taking into account both the amount of lung involved and the severity. Since there are six areas and a possible three marks for each area the maximum score is 18. (Heard & Izukawa, 1964.)

Since all our cases had severe obstruction the FEV is low in all of them and there is no relationship between FEV and severity of emphysema. In Figure 1 the cases are divided into those with

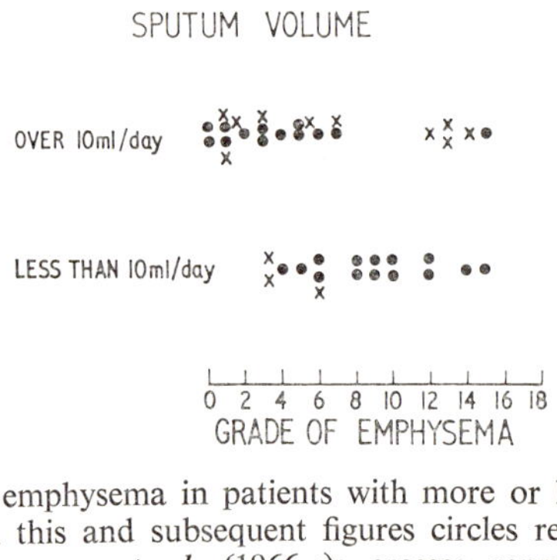

FIG. 1. Grade of emphysema in patients with more or less than 10 ml. sputum daily. In this and subsequent figures circles represent patients published by Burrows *et al.* (1966 *a*); crosses represent additional patients.

more and those with less than 10 ml. of sputum per day. On the whole the cases with less sputum have more severe emphysema but we have recently added four cases with severe emphysema and bronchial hypersecretion. Sputum volume is a weak indicator of the presence or absence of emphysema.

The X-ray is fairly helpful in diagnosing severe emphysema. When you have got more than two-thirds of the lung destroyed

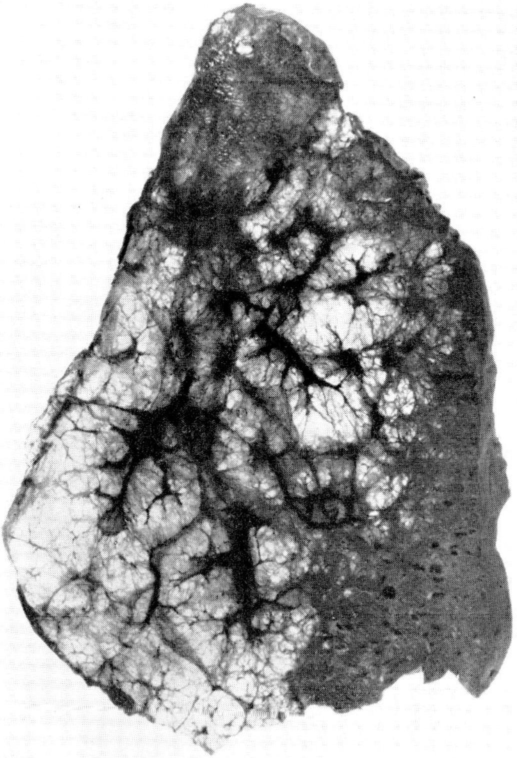

FIG. 2. Lung of man aged 34 who died of respiratory failure with cor pulmonale (for details see text).

[*To face page* 232

nearly all the cases have radiological evidence of it. The open circles in Figure 3 are patients suspected of having a minor degree of emphysema on the X-ray and this has not been very helpful. We are using here the criteria of Laws and Heard (1962) and are looking only for impairment of the vascular pattern.

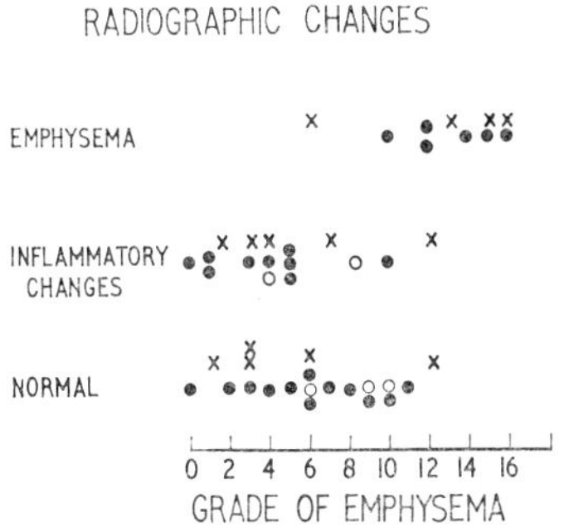

FIG. 3. Grade of emphysema in patients with evidence of emphysema, with inflammatory change or neither in chest X-ray. Open circles indicate patients with 'suspected emphysema'.

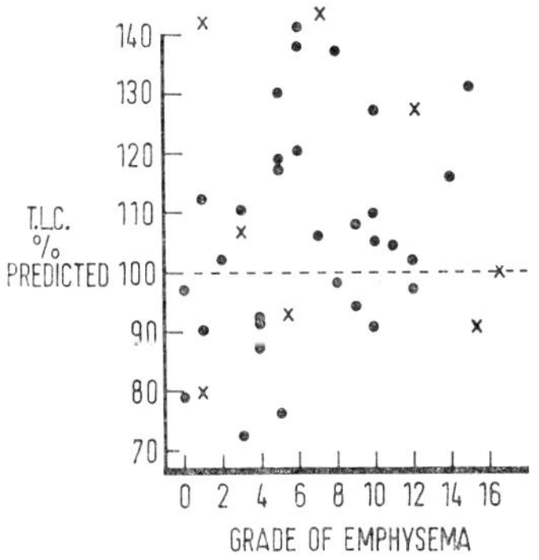

FIG. 4 Relationship of total lung capacity 1 per cent. (predicted) to grade of emphysema.

Total lung capacity, which in our first study seemed to be useful, now appears to be much less useful (Figure 4). Although it is true that most of the severe emphysema cases have a total lung capacity above the expected level we have recently acquired two very severe ones with reduced TLC and we have some cases with very little emphysema who, nonetheless, have high TLC. Although there is some relationship it is not close.

In Figure 5 we have expressed the gas transfer factor as DL/VA. Again, the relationship with emphysema is evident but

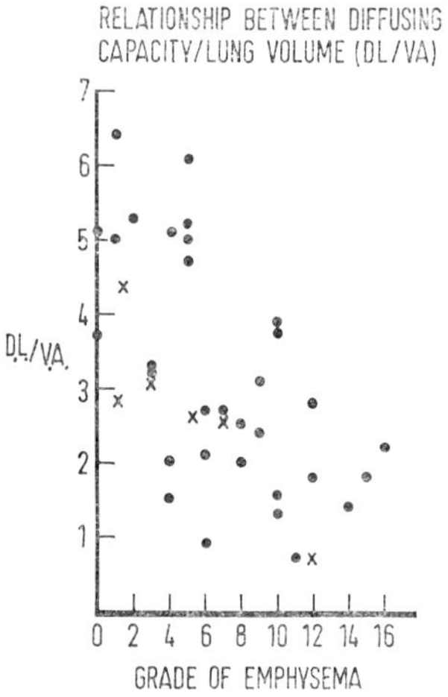

FIG. 5. Relationship of transfer factor (DL/VA) to grade of emphysema.

pretty poor. We can say, however, that if the value is high there is very little emphysema ; if it is low, there may be any amount. Some of the cases with little emphysema have a lesion which may greatly reduce gas transfer.

Burrows *et al.* (1965) have shown a relationship between mixed venous Pco_2 and FEV in cases with airways obstruction expressed by the formula $P/co_2 = 11{\cdot}5/FEV + 30{\cdot}7$. We have calculated the expected Pco_2 in our cases from this formula and Figure 6 shows the values of the deviation of the observed from the predicted Pco_2 Since we originally published this figure, you will notice, we have had two patients with severe emphysema who had relative under-ventilation. These patients also had profuse sputum. But there is a strong tendency for patients with severe emphysema and little bronchitis to have relative over-ventilation, and those with little emphysema and marked bronchitis to have relative under-ventilation. One of these patients with severe emphysema and bronchitis was a man who developed a productive cough at the age of 24 and first became breathless two years later. He came up to out-patients at the age of 31 with cyanosis and oedema and was already in cor pulmonale. He had hypercarbia and hypoxaemia which became more marked on exercise. His X-ray showed gross emphysema. He came into hospital several times in cor pulmonale, with increasing blood-gas disturbance. He died at the age of 34 and his lungs were almost totally destroyed by emphysema (Fig. 2). It is of interest that this man had a complete absence of alpha 2 antitrypsin in his plasma.

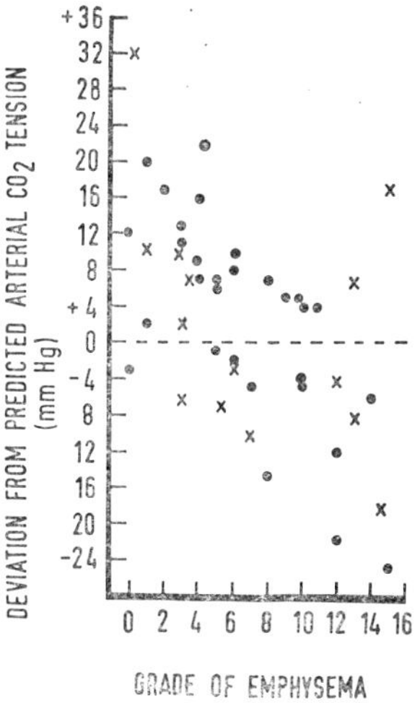

FIG. 6. Relationship of relative hypercarbia (difference between observed and expected Pa_{CO_2}) to grade of emphysema.

It is thus possible to have very severe emphysema and have recurrent cor pulmonale, but this is unusual ; cor pulmonale, in our experience, occurs almost solely in those with gross abnormality of PCO_2 and PO_2

When we classify all our patients into Types A, B and X, as we have defined them (Burrows *et al.*, 1966), the amount of emphysema in each group is shown in Figure 7. Type A patients all have moderate or severe emphysema (6 per cent. or more). All but one of the type B patients have less emphysema than this and the type X patients have intermediate amounts. The case of severe emphysema I have just described is classed as type X in Figure 7. He is really type A since there was obvious radiological emphysema but clinically he was type B and so I have called him type X. By using fairly simple criteria we appear to be able to make a reasonable estimate of the amount of emphysema that is present.

Dr Norman Jones (1966) has shown that the effect of exercise on arterial oxygen provides additional diagnostic evidence. In Figure 8 it is interesting to note that in type B patients on exercise there

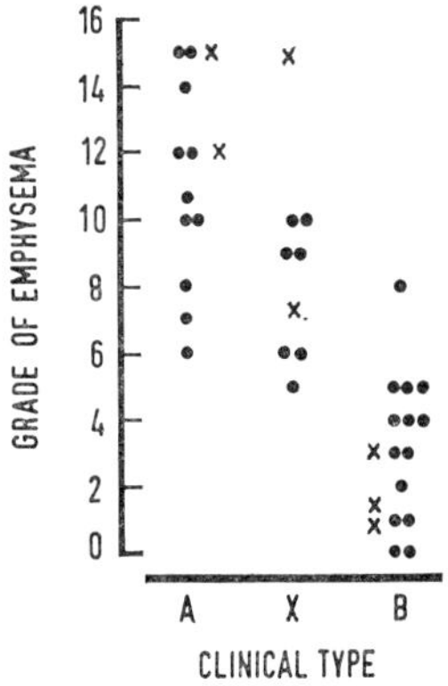

FIG. 7. Grade of emphysema in patients divided into Types A, B and X.

is a tendency for the PaO_2 to improve. And seeing that this is taking place in the presence of a widening A-V difference and an increase in arterial CO_2 it represents a very considerable improvement in $\dot{V}/\dot{Q}$ balance. Type A patients, on the other hand, show a fall in arterial oxygen on exercise. One man of type A showed an improvement in PaO_2 and is of special interest. He was a man who first presented with wheeziness at the age of fifty-one. He had recurrent episodes of bronchial infection characteristic of type B, but his total lung capacity was increased at 140 per cent. of expected, his mixed venous P_{CO_2} and arterial P_{CO_2} were within normal limits, and his diffusing capacity was considerably impaired and so we rated him, at that time, as type A. When he died he had relatively little emphysema—6 units, (about 30 per cent.) on Dr Heard's scale.

At autopsy, his bronchi were plugged with mucus which was full of eosinophils and there was tremendous hypertrophy of the bronchial muscles. He was in fact an infected asthmatic, and he died of this widespread plugging of his bronchi which, together with the moderate emphysema may also perhaps account for his low diffusing capacity. But the emphysema was not enough to prevent his improving his $\dot{V}/\dot{Q}$ balance on exercise.

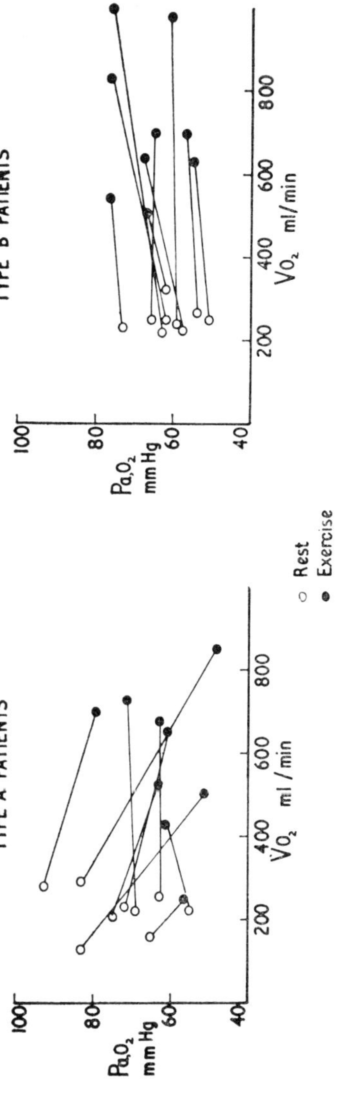

FIG. 8. Change of arterial oxygen tension on exercise in patients diagnosed as Type A and Type B by criteria of Burrows *et al.* (1964).

Table 1. *Main differential characteristics of patients with severe irreversible airways obstruction with and without severe emphysema.*

Characteristic	With Severe Emphysema (Type A)	With Little Emphysema (Type B)
Body Build	Asthenic	Stocky
Sputum	Slight, mucoid	Profuse, often purulent
Dyspnoea	Late onset, severe	Early onset, often mild
X-ray Vasculature . .	Attenuated	Normal or congested
Heart	Long, narrow	RV & PA +
CID	Infrequent	Frequent
$PaCO_2$	Low for FEV level	High for FEV level
SaO_2	Normal at rest	Low at rest
	Falls on exercise	Rises on exercise
Oedamatous Cor Pulmonale	Infrequent. Terminal	Frequent. Remittent
Compliance	High	Low
Inspiratory AWR . .	Normal	Increased

To summarise (Table 1) we can say that emphysema is likely to be severe in a patient of asthenic build, with slight sputum, with a late onset of ultimately severe dyspnoea with attenuated vasculature and a long narrow heart in the X-ray, with Pco_2 low in relation to the FEV level, with normal oxygen saturation at rest which falls on exercise and without cor pulmonale. In addition there is evidence that compliance is relatively high and inspiratory airways relatively normal (B. Burrows, F. B. Sakensa & C. F. Diener, (1966) unpublished). On the other hand there is likely to be little emphysema in a broad, stocky type of man with profuse sputum, with an onset of disease early in life, with a normal X-ray or one with evidence of chronic infection or vascular distension, with an enlarged heart, with retention of CO_2 and a low oxygen saturation which improves on exercise, with remittent cor pulmonale, a low compliance and increased inspiratory airways resistance.

I want now to raise the question of the significance of the small degree of emphysema which we see in some of these type B cases. We have been told that it is most important. Dr Heath scrutinizes the last bronchiole to find a little bit of dilatation to which he attributes the cor pulmonale in his cases. Dr Cumming shows us beautiful casts of dilated respiratory bronchioles and bronchi in centrilobular emphysema and maintains that this is the thing that really matters. Dr Jack Howell, in his Goulstonian Lecture, recently said that in type B patients it was the centrilobular emphysema that interfered with gas exchange and produced the hypercarbia and hypoxia. On the other hand, we have heard Lynne Reid telling us

Table 2. *Men with severe airways obstruction without emphysema and with moderate centrilobular emphysema*

	Case	Age	Hb%	FEV	TLC %	RV/TLC	DL/VA	$PaCO_2$	$PaCO_2$ Dev^n	RV mm	Emphy. %
No Significant Emphysema	F1	43	17·0	·65	79	58	5·1	62	+12	9	0
	H29	51	16·7	·74	97	51	3·7	43	−3	6	0
	H40	47	20·0	·70	112	58	5·0	67	+20	9	6
	Mean	47	17·9	·70	93	56	4·6	57	10	8	2
Moderate Centrilobular Emphysema	H23	60	17·0	·65	30	60	5·2	47	−1	8	28
	H16	68	13·0	·60	117	65	5·0	57	+7	9	28
	H44	61	10·7	1·20	138	66	2·1	48	+8	5	33
	Mean	63	13·6	·82	128	64	4·1	51	+5	7	30

that she thinks this can occur in perfectly normal, undisabled people. Heard and Isukawa (1964) have shown a lot of centrilobular emphysema occurring in routine postmortems in men without any clinical evidence of respiratory disease and Pratt (1963) has found that in lungs with up to 25 per cent. destroyed by centrilobular emphysema there may be no delay in expiratory airflow measured after death.

I thought it would be interesting to look at this point by comparing three men in our series, whom we rate as having no emphysema, with three men who have moderate centrilobular emphysema (Table 2). There are only three cases in our series whom Dr Heard rated as having pure centrilobular emphysema. Once it gets more severe than this, it inevitably begins to be rated as panacinar.

Figure 9 shows the appearance of the lung in case H 40 which Dr Heard rated as having one unit of panacinar emphysema. This area is characteristic of the whole of both lungs and the alveolar structure really does look pretty normal almost everywhere although there is some dilatation. Figure 10 shows the lungs of H 44. There is obvious centrilobular emphysema. This was rather less marked in the lower lobe but the total amount was rated as 6 units or 33 per cent. on Dr Heard's scale.

Table 2 shows that the patients with no significant emphysema are younger than those with centrilobular emphysema. They are more polycythaemic. The FEV levels are similar, their total lung capacity is lower and the RV as a percentage of TLC is less increased. The diffusing capacity is very similar, the arterial P_{CO_2} is higher, the right ventricular thickness (the only measure we have of heart involvement) is similar. If anything, those with centrilobular emphysema have *less* disturbance of blood gases but there is nothing very much to choose between them. I can see no reason for attributing the respiratory failure in any of these men to centrilobular emphysema since those with none of it are worse than those who have it. Our main task is to identify in these cases the lesion which causes the severe airways obstruction which disables them. It produces a clinical and physiological syndrome quite different from that which we see in the cases with severe emphysema.

I conclude, then, that we can roughly estimate the severity of emphysema ; we can distinguish patients with severe from those with little or no emphysema. We have no evidence, only presumption, that centrilobular emphysema is an important lesion. Cor pulmonale appears to occur in those cases with severe abnormality of blood gases so that it is uncommon in patients with severe emphysema. I am sure our severe emphysema cases have a greatly increased alveolar pressure during expiration but they do not get cor

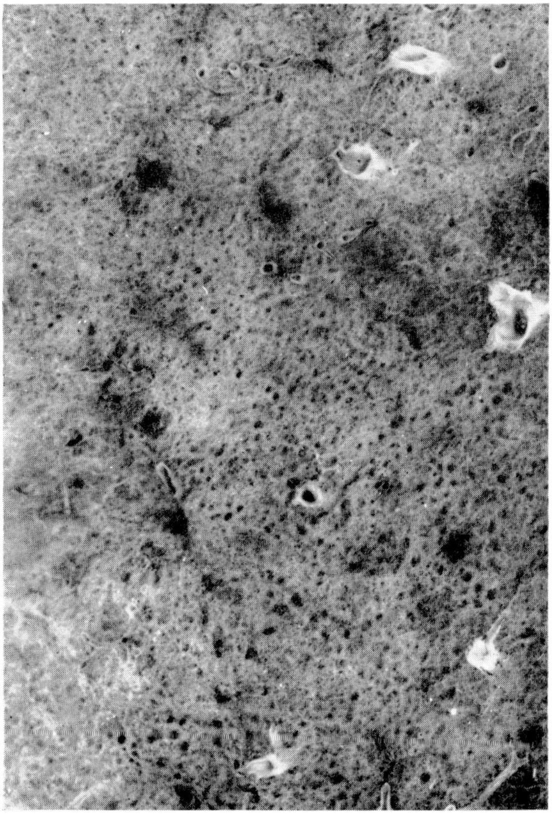

FIG. 9. Section of lung of Case H 40 (Table 2) showing only minor evidence of emphysema.

[*To face page* 240

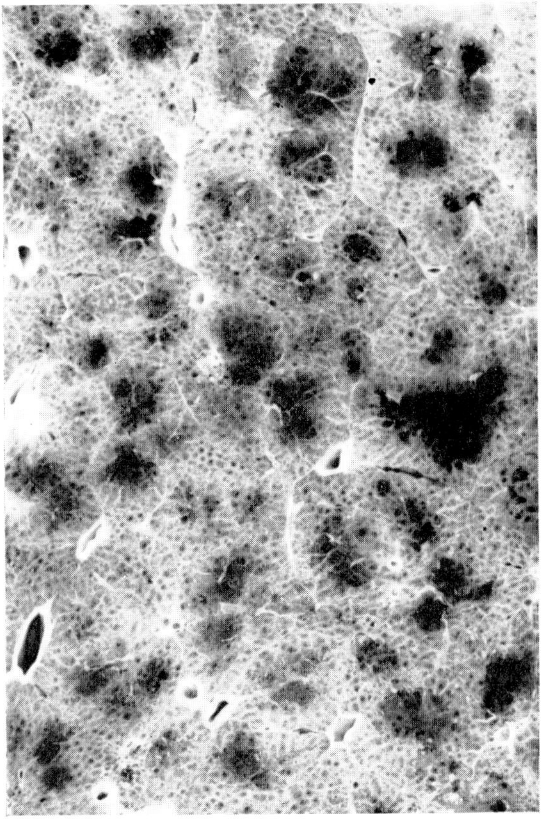

FIG. 10. Section of lung of Case H 44 (Table 2) showing centrilobular emphysema with well preserved intervening respiratory tissue.

pulmonale ; they only get it if their blood gases are disturbed. I am mystified by the effect a minor degree of emphysema has on so many people's minds. There is now so much evidence that it can be unimportant when present in small amounts. I suppose it is the stranglehold of tradition. Our real challenge is to find the nature and pathogenesis of the lesion which causes the airways obstruction which, in the absence of emphysema, may be fatal and to develop our diagnostic techniques so that we may study the development of these two different types of disease at an earlier stage, when it may be possible to delay progression in some cases.

DISCUSSION

Dr Dunnill. Dr Fletcher says that centrilobular emphysema is of no significance, but the reasons he gives for this are not entirely adequate. Centrilobular emphysema is a condition where there is dilatation of the respiratory bronchioles in the lung, accompanied by some destruction. Each centrilobular space is served by a terminal bronchiole ; the respiratory bronchiole in the normal lung is approximately 500 μ in diameter ; if that bronchiole dilates, say to four times its diameter, to form a centrilobular space, its volume will increase 64 times. Now, if each of the 64,000 terminal bronchioles in the lung leads into such a centrilobular space, the actual volume of emphysema in the lung will only be of the order of 15–20 per cent. of the total lung volume, but every single gas molecule going to or coming from the alveolar membrane will have to pass through one of these spaces. I do not think that we can say categorically that such a state of affairs will occur without very profound patho-physiological consequences.

Dr Fletcher. There are ample theoretical grounds for supposing that centrilobular emphysema must disturb function. I only say that the disturbance may be unimportant since the lesion can be present in subjects with no obvious respiratory disease and absent in those with severe degrees of the abnormality attributed to it in theory. There is a lesion in these people which kills them and which we haven't yet identified. They have severe mucous gland hypertrophy but I do not think this causes the obstruction, for its severity has not been shown to be correlated with airways obstruction. This should be looked into.

Dr Heath. May I comment on the method of examination of the lungs reported on by Dr Fletcher ? They were graded from 0 to 3 on six areas of lung and I presume that one slice of lung only was examined. Such a method, in my opinion, does not bear comparison with examination of the whole of the lung.

Dr Fletcher. In the case I showed you with no emphysema (F1 and H29) emphysema was absent from all the lung slices. I am not a morbid anatomist but Dr Heard reported that the alveoli in these lungs were uniformly normal throughout.

Dr Horsfield. If we represent a normal bronchial tree as in Figure 1 *A* with cones distally for the acini, then the dilatations

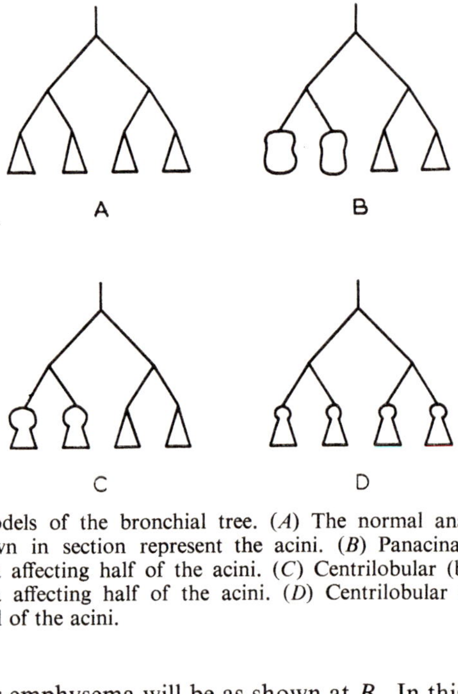

FIG. 1. Models of the bronchial tree. (*A*) The normal anatomy. The cones shown in section represent the acini. (*B*) Panacinar (alveolar) emphysema affecting half of the acini. (*C*) Centrilobular (bronchiolar) emphysema affecting half of the acini. (*D*) Centrilobular emphysema affecting all of the acini.

of panacinar emphysema will be as shown at *B*. In this case, 50 per cent. of the lung volume is involved in the dilatations. These patients can live perfectly well—it's just the same as if they had had a pneumonectomy—but on point counting of the lung surface 50 per cent. of the lung is involved. *C* represents a case of centrilobular emphysema in which 20 per cent. of the lung is affected with big dilatations but the rest is normal. Such a patient will not be very severely breathless.

What I believe to be of particular importance is the significance of widely distributed centrilobular emphysema of apparently minor degree. In this case, *D*, *all* the respiratory bronchioles have a dilatation on them but the total amount involved may only be 10 per cent. of the lung volume. If the lung volume were 5,000 ml. the dilations would add up to 500 ml. When the patient took a breath in, the inspired gas would not reach the alveolar ducts and there would be a severe degree of blood gas disturbance. Thus in the examples shown here, those lungs which have the smallest amount of emphysema are those with the greatest degree of functional disturbance and those with the greatest degree of emphysema have the smallest degree of functional disturbance. This may explain some of the difficulties we have had in trying to correlate the structural and functional abnormalities.

Dr Fishman. Could the type of ventilation play any part in helping to overcome the functional handicap imposed by the localised dilatations ?

Dr Horsfield. I don't think patients with panacinar emphysema can do very much to improve their ventilation. Those with centrilobular emphysema on the other hand may hyperventilate and thus move the inspired gas front further down the dilatation. This will decrease the diffusion distance and thereby improve their alveolar ventilation.

Dr Reid. I have been very concerned to note the complete contradiction over some of the results that have been presented and in this connection there is a question relating to the use of terms by pathologists which should be cleared up. It doesn't matter whether we use the terms centriacinar, centrilobular or bronchiolar emphysema. These are all being applied to the same condition and, as we were shown yesterday, its essential feature is that there are normal alveoli round the ' hole '. I will only use the term centriacinar when in fact we do observe the conditions demanded by the definition, *i.e.* that there is a centriacinar accentuation of emphysema and that there is lung recognisable at the periphery. Then we come to the panacinar group where there is virtually even change throughout the acinus which may go on to complete loss of any tissue represented either in an acinus or in a lobule.

Some of the slides that were put up yesterday afternoon and were called centrilobular or centriacinar, in fact showed virtually a complete ' candy cotton ' change right through the whole of the lung. Now I would call this panacinar. What happens is that when pathologists talk to each other they will admit that there are a large number of cases in which, perhaps because there is so much destruction, it is not possible to decide how a lesion started. What happens, you see, is that into the terms centrilobular (or centriacinar) and panacinar (or panlobular), as they are often used, an element of interpretation tends to come in. That's where the confusion very largely arises. Cases showing complete destruction of a large part of lung, anatomically panacinar, are classified as centrilobular lesions because the pathologist is interpreting them as having started as centrilobular. We must use the anatomical terms to describe the anatomical lesions we see and then discuss as a separate problem whether or not centriacinar ever goes on to panacinar change or not.

If we want to find out what recognisable centriacinar emphysema can do, it is necessary to pick out a group of these cases in a pure form and study them. My own view, as you know, is that centriacinar emphysema of itself is not important, and in support of this view I would cite the group of patients who die from obstructed airways disease ; who die without any cough and sputum, without any evidence of gland hypertrophy and, what is more important, without any evidence of bronchiolitis. I have never seen one of these patients with a lesion which is recognisably centriacinar. All of them have got a panacinar lesion. I have never seen an abnormal X-ray, or a patient die from airways obstruction but without bronchitis, in whom the predominant lesion in their lung is recognisable centriacinar emphysema.

Chairman. These divisions, as far as we can see them, are not in any sense absolute. Pure one or the other is not, in our experience, very common. Commonly we find both panlobular change in some parts and centrilobular in others. In this extremely muddled and complex situation the dominant fact is the tremendous overlap between what you choose to study.

Dr Filley. I disagree vigorously. The pure case is an extremely important subject for study. The method of science is to set up an hypothesis and test it and pure cases make this possible. Dr Reid says that she has never seen a patient die from lung disease without bronchitis and only centrilobular emphysema. Now, it's up to others to test the hypothesis suggested by this important observation on pure cases.

Chairman. Dr Reid, do you mean simple bronchitis ? What criteria would you like us to use ?

Dr Reid. I demand three things : clinical evidence that there was no cough and sputum in life, the fact that the glands are not hypertrophied and the fact that there are no goblet cells or fibrosis or any peripheral bronchiolar lesions.

Chairman. No cough or sputum ?

Dr Reid. No sputum. I don't mind a dry cough.

Dr Cumming. Mr Chairman, I feel the story of F. E. Smith, who later became the Lord Chancellor of England would fit in appropriately at this point. When he was an undergraduate at Oxford, he became engaged in a fracas with the police—not an altogether uncommon event for him ! When he came to court and was prosecuted for making an affray, he was cross-examined by a barrister and the question at issue was : was what the police sergeant who observed the episode said, true or not ? So they said to F. E. Smith : ' Do you agree with what the sergeant said ? '

He said : ' No, I don't.'

Barrister : ' You mean you're calling the sergeant a liar.'

F. E. Smith : ' No, I'm not.'

Barrister : ' That is the only interpretation.'

Upon which F. E. Smith spread out five fingers and pushed them under the barrister's nose, and shouted : ' No ! Not one ; five ! Firstly, he was lying ; secondly, I was lying ; thirdly, he was mistaken in his observation ; fourthly, I was mistaken in my observation, although we honestly believe them to be true, and, fifthly, although we cannot yet see it, there is an adequate compromise which fits all the facts ! '

I want to make an attempt to get some kind of a compromise solution. There seems to be, in the model we are all building up about emphysema, the concept that the thing which is really wrong is the structural deformity. These cases either accept the consequences of their structural deformity, *i.e.* do not adapt to it, in which case they will have disturbed blood gases or they can adapt to their structural deformity by some physiological means in which case their blood gases will not be disturbed. You would predict also, on the basis of what Dr Dunnill and Dr Horsfield have said, that there'd be no real correlation between the quantity of the lesion and their morphological nature.

There are many things we don't know. If we take centrilobular emphysema, when you breathe in, does the centrilobular space dilate or is it fixed ? This is a fabulously important fact which we cannot at the moment know. And all models are based upon apportioning compliance equally between the two. If it's a fixed space it's almost insignficant. If it's a dilated space, with a compliance greater than the distal one, it's tremendously important. This we do not know. We are short of facts, but the model is not denied by any of this data. But we must certainly take into account both morphological deformity, and the presence or absence of functional adaptation.

Professor Wade. I've been listening very carefully to what people have said about human bronchitis and this assessment of emphysema because, as some of you may know, Dr Elmes in my department has in the last three of four years had two colonies of rats : one of specific-pathogen-free rats and one of the same strain of rats kept in ordinary conventional situations (Wheeler, S. M., 1963). Now there's no doubt whatsoever that in the life span of these animals, the ordinary rats develop many of the things which Dr Lynne Reid has described and when you kill them you see an enormous development of goblet cells, a great increase in mucous secretion, and also a lot of lymphocytic cuffing of bronchi. Now the specific-pathogen-free rat is completely free of this lesion but nevertheless it is our impression that as far as the parenchyma of the lung is concerned, holes in the lung occur in both these colonies of animals and as far as we can see they occur in about the same proportion of animals.

Dr Macklem. Dr Fletcher talked about patients dying with chronic obstructive airways disease without morphologic emphysema. Yet most other people have been describing dilatation of the bronchioles and it hardly needs to be said that dilatation does not lead to destruction. Now the question comes up, have we seen patients with obstructed airways disease who have normal parenchyma and I think that I can say that we have. I have personally studied two such lungs. One was a patient with bronchiectasis ; a lady who died with chronic respiratory failure and cor pulmonale but had a very high peripheral resistance with small airways disease in addition to bronchiectasis. Similarly, another lady who died from a cerebral haemorrhage we thought had a normal lung, but when we removed it and partitioned her resistance, we found she had an increase in peripheral resistance and histology showed that she also had small airways disease. So I think there is no question that you can get chronic airways obstruction in the presence of normal parenchyma.

The question then arises whether you can get blood gas disturbances as a result of this. I personally think you can but have no idea how common it is. There are two additional cases that I'd like to describe : one is a man who had bronchogenic carcinoma. He had a pneumonectomy on this account, and following this he was more dyspnoeic than he should have been but the reason for this was not apparent. He went home where he developed a cold and over a three-day period became acutely dyspnoeic. He was unable to walk across the room and was readmitted to hospital with P_{O_2} in the 40's and P_{CO_2} in the high 50's and low 60's. At that time we measured his airway resistance which was about 3·5 cm. H_2O/LPS and for a man with one lung, this is virtually what you would predict, as a normal value. His chest X-rays showed that he had a diffuse pulmonary infiltration in his remaining lung and we thought at that time that we would then go and review the pathology of the lung that was removed. He had a minor degree of emphysema in that lung but he had a lot of small airways disease. We thought that he had an acute exacerbation of the bronchiolitis so we treated him with corticosteroids and over a two-week period his dyspnoea disappeared and his blood gases returned to normal, his diffuse infiltration disappeared radiologically, and his airways resistance fell from 2·5 to 3·3. An insignificant change. Obviously his respiratory failure was not due in any way to destruction of lung tissue because it was reversible and so was the diffuse pulmonary infiltration. Similarly, there is another young man in his twenties who has chronic respiratory failure and cor pulmonale, in whom a lung biopsy did not reveal any evidence of parenchymal destruction but he also had a diffuse bronchiolitis. It could be that the common lesion in all these cases is in fact disease in small airways. Until we know more about what causes this we can only speculate but is it possible that we may be seeing bronchiolitis in association with emphysema in Montreal but bronchiolitis occurring without parenchymal destruction in London ? I simply proffer this as a suggestion to reconcile the opposing points of view.

REFERENCES

ALTSHULER, B., PALMES, E. D., YARMUS, L., & NELSON, N. (1959). *J. appl. Physiol.* **14,** 321.

BEDELL, G. N. & OSTIGUY, G. L. (1967). *Clin. Sci.* **32,** 239.

BOHR, C. (1891). *Skand. Arch. Physiol.* **2,** 236.

BURROWS, BENJAMIN, STRAUSS, RICHARD H., and NIDEN, ALBERT H. (1965). Chronic Obstructive Lung Disease. III. Interrelationships of pulmonary function data. *Amer. Rev. resp. Dis.* **91,** 6.

BURROWS, B., FLETCHER, C. M., HEARD, B. E., JONES, N. L. & WOOTLIFF, J. S. (1966). *Lancet* **1,** 830.

BURROWS, B., NIDEN, A. H., FLETCHER, C. M. & JONES, N. L. (1964). *Amer. Rev. resp. Dis.* **90,** 1.

CADIGAN, J. B., MARKS, A., ELLICOTT, M. F., JONES, R. H. & GAENSLER, E. A. (1961). *J. clin. Invest.* **40,** 1495.

CIBA SYMPOSIUM. REPORT (1959). *Thorax,* **14,** 286.

CUMMING, G., CRANK, J., HORSFIELD, K. & PARKER, I. (1966). *Resp. Physiol., Neth.* **1,** 58.

DU BOIS, A. B., BRITT, A. G. & FENN, W. O. (1952). *J. appl. Physiol.* **4,** 535.

FILLEY, G. F. (1967). *Pulmonary Insufficiency and Respiratory Failure,* Philadelphia : Lea & Febiger.

FILLEY, G. F., BECKWITT, H. J., REEVES, J. T. & MITCHELL, R. S. (1967). *Am. J. Med.* In press.

FLETCHER, C. M., HUGH-JONES, P., MCNICOL, M. W. & PRIDE, N. B. (1963). *Q. Jl Med.* **32,** 125.

FORSTER, R. E. (1965). In *Handbook of Physiology,* Sec. 3, Vol. II, p. 1455. ed. FENN, W. O. & RAHN, H. Washington D.C. : American Physiological Society.

GOODWIN, J. F. & ASDIN, J. F. (1959). *Br. Heart J.* **21**, 523.
HALDANE, J. S. (1922). *Respiration*, p. 41. New Haven : Yale University Press.
HATCH, T. F. (1952). *A.M.A. Archs. ind. Hyg.* **6**, 1.
HEARD, BRIAN E. & IZUKAWA, B. (1964). *J. Path. Bact.* **88**, 423.
JONES, N. L. (1966). *Clin. Sci.* **31**, 39.
KROGH, A. & J. LINDHARD. (1914). *J. Physiol.* **47**, 431.
LAWS, J. W. & HEARD, B. E. (1962). *Br. J. Radiol.* **35**, 750.
MARSHALL, R. A. (1958). *J. clin. Invest.* **37**, 384.
PAPPENHEIMER, J. R. (1950). *Fedn. Proc. Fedn. Am. Socs. exp. Biol.* **9**, 602.
PRATT, P. C. (1963). *Acad. Med. New Jersey Bull.* **9**, 204.
RAUWERDA, P. E. (1946). Thesis Groningen University.
RILEY, R. L. & COURNAND, A. (1949). *J. appl. Physiol.* **1**, 825.
ROSS, J. C., FRAYSER, R. & HICKAM, J. B. (1959). *J. clin. Invest.* **38**, 916.
ROSS, B. B., FARHI, L. E. (1960). *J. appl. Physiol.* **15**, 363.
SONNE, C. (1916). "Ueber die Homogenität der Lungen luftmischungen". *Pflügers Arch. ges. Physiol.* **163**, 75.
THURLBECK, W. M. (1963). *Am. Rev. resp. Dis.* **87**, 206.
THURLBECK, W. M. (1967). *Thorax*. In press.
THURLBECK, W. M., FRASER, R. G. & BATES, D. V. (1965). *Med. Thorac.* **22**, 295.
WHEELER, S. M. (1963). *J. Anim. Techns. Ass.* **14**, 1.
WOOLCOCK, ANN J. & READ, J. (1965). *Lancet* **2**, 1323.
WORLD HEALTH ORGANIZATION (1961). *Tech. Rep. Ser. Wld Hlth Org.* No. 213.

SUMMING UP AND CONCLUSION

ALFRED P. FISHMAN

THIS conference was designed to explore our present levels of understanding of the relationships between Form and Function in the Human Lung. To fulfill this purpose our hosts provided a delightful setting, not only for the meetings but also for dining and relaxation between scientific sessions. Before beginning my interpretation of the scientific proceedings of the last few days, I should like to take the liberty of speaking directly to our hosts on your behalf: Professor Arnott, Dr Cumming and Dr Hunt, we are all grateful to you for the considerable thought and effort which you have expended in arranging this meeting and for your generosity and hospitality.

For the sake of convenience, I have sorted the various papers which comprised the programme under several distinct headings. By this type of grouping, it became possible for me to express personal points of view about general topics rather than about particular papers. Since the original papers and the discussions that followed are also contained in this volume, the reader will be in a position to compare his own conclusions, drawn from the preceding printed accounts, with the interpretation that I gained not only as a participant but as a member of the audience who had been charged to listen attentively and critically.

Form

The first three papers dealt with the anatomy of the normal (Brewer) and abnormal lung (Heppleston ; Dunnill). In clear and succinct ways, they depicted the anatomical lessons to be learned from classical approaches. There can be no doubt that the anatomy of the airways is better understood now than ever before and that ' quantitative morphology ' has provided a new approach to the anatomy of the lungs. But I must confess that these detailed morphological descriptions of the airways and air spaces seem to have become more of an end in themselves than a device for promoting the understanding of the relationships between pulmonary structure and function. It is true that some of the inadequacies of anatomical observations with respect to function are inherent in the available anatomical methods. For example, sampling is always a problem in non-homogeneous disease of the lungs and airways ; bronchial obstruction may be obscured in the process of preparing the lungs for anatomical study ; the pathogenesis of bronchitis and emphysema is difficult to infer from sections obtained at autopsy. However, there are other more tractable problems, of major interest to physiologists, which have not yet been seriously examined by anatomists. One such problem is the relation of blood vessels to airways and air spaces. This is a pressing problem since the natural history of bronchitis and/or emphysema is strongly influenced by the interplay of alveolar ventilation and perfusion. In effect, anatomists seem to be concentrating on either the air phase or the blood phase but not on both simultaneously.

This conference has also reaffirmed that the anatomical changes which are found in the lungs at autopsy often fail to explain either the clinical or physiological derangements of bronchitis and emphysema, or their pathophysiological consequences. For example, right ventricular hypertrophy does not correlate well with either the degree of bronchitis or the degree of emphysema (Heath ; Dunnill ; Wyatt) ; mixed forms of bronchitis and emphysema are common and their respective contributions to the clinical or physiological picture are generally difficult to quantify ; neither localized ballooning nor disruption of the airways nor holes in the lungs at autopsy correlate well with specific functional abnormalities during life. Indeed, the increasing awareness that morphological observations have not provided a full explanation has served to emphasize that derangements in the blood gases from subtle anatomical changes, are more apt to shape the untoward clinical consequence of emphysema than are the conventional anatomical evidence of pulmonary disease.

The poor correlation between anatomical findings at autopsy and pulmonary or cardiac performance has also tended to undermine confidence in the anatomical classification of bronchitis and emphysema as the reliable basis for physiological or clinical classification. For example, although the present conference repeatedly returned to the question of the functional significance of centrilobular emphysema, the opinions remained as strong and divergent at the end of the meeting as at its start.

To obtain answers to particular questions concerning structure and function, physiologists are taking anatomy into their own hands. Thus, to explore some anatomical determinants of the mechanical performance of the lungs, Macklem has put lungs obtained at autopsy through their mechanical paces. It is true that such lungs are somewhat abnormal simply as a consequence of being removed from the chest (West ; Milic-Emili). Nonetheless, they do provide a realistic model to answer particular questions, such as the ones that he posed concerning the partition of airway resistances in the normal lung and in the lung which is the seat of obstructive disease of the airways.

The need for pure forms of disease

It has been mentioned above that bronchitis and emphysema usually coexist so inextricably that the effect of each one separately on pulmonary performance may be exceedingly difficult to assess. In some respects, the importance of distinguishing between these two entities has been somewhat obscured by the popular designation ‘ chronic, non-specific respiratory disease.’ Consequently I welcomed the remarks of several speakers, particularly Wyatt and Heath, who pointed out the need for examining pure forms of pulmonary disease both in anatomical and in physiological terms.

Several years ago our laboratory addressed itself to this problem by picturing a spectrum of broncho-pulmonary disease with pure bronchial obstruction at one end and with pure emphysema at the other (Fig. 1). Although these ‘ pure forms ’ are relatively uncommon, they do make it possible to analyze the more common types as mixtures of the pure forms. Also, they do provide a basis for rational forms of therapy based on the reversibility of bronchitis and the irreversibility of emphysema. But only few such observations have been made and there is still a critical need for seeking out and studying pure forms of disease as a next step in the understanding of bronchitis and emphysema.

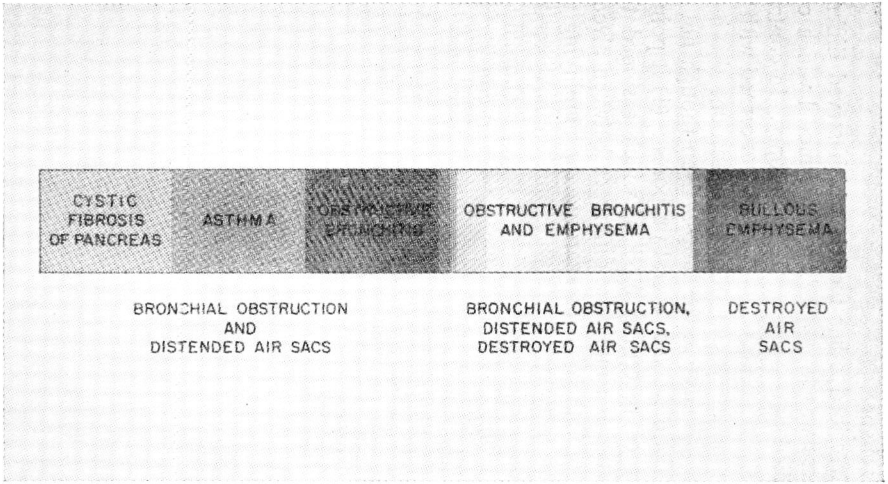

FIG. 1. The spectrum of bronchopulmonary disease ranging from bronchial obstruction (cystic fibrosis of the pancreas; asthma; obstructive bronchitis) to emphysema. The spectrum illustrates the therapeutic importance of distinguishing between bronchial obstruction (potentially reversible) and emphysema (irreversible). Also, although the entities are sharply defined at either end, they become blurred as the centre of the spectrum is approached; this central band is broad and consists largely of obstructive bronchitis and emphysema, the most common clinical group. [Reprinted, with permission, from the *Ann. N.Y. Acad. Sci.* (1965) 121, 657].

Models

In a delightful preamble to a consideration of his own model, Filley dealt with the history of pulmonary models, expounded the reasons why modelling was necessary, and then presented his own mathematical model as a natural outgrowth of those which had previously been developed by others. His model was primarily concerned with gas exchange.

Other speakers described other models which served different purposes. One of these was Macklem's realistic model which consisted of a lung, studied out of the chest, at autopsy. In contrast, Dr Mead's model was a conceptual one. It was concerned with the elastic behaviour of the lungs and took into account the interdependent behaviour of spaces in the lungs. Even though not yet in final form, the model did serve several purposes : (1) it pointed out the inadequacies of preceding models, which assumed that transpulmonary pressure is simply the difference between alveolar and pulmonary pressure, thereby disregarding the amplifying and the distorting effects of the intervening architecture on the distending pressures of blood vessels, airways and airspaces, (2) it showed that if this model applies to the lung, static properties exert considerable effects on the distribution of air and (3) it demonstrated how this interdependence makes lungs more rigid, how the amplification of distending pressures opposes alveolar collapse and how local distortions of distending pressures operate to reverse the distortion and, thereby, to relieve atelectasis.

Reverting to realistic models, Heath has taken advantage of the fact that disorders other than intrinsic pulmonary disease may serve as models to promote understanding of diffuse pulmonary disease. For example, the alveolar hypoventilation of obesity and kyphoscoliosis has been shown to be associated with pulmonary vascular changes comparable to those which exist not only in bronchitis and emphysema but also in native residents at altitude with Monge's disease. The observations on alveolar hypoventilation (in patients with normal lungs) emphasize that the pulmonary vascular changes associated with bronchitis may be more characteristic of hypoxic pulmonary hypertension that of the broncho-pulmonary disease, *i.e.* that they are mainly functional rather than anatomical in origin.

Distribution of inspired gas

The several different experimental approaches which were described in the present meeting seemed to converge and provide a unified concept concerning the mechanisms by which inspired gas is non-uniformly distributed throughout the normal and abnormal lungs. The cumulative evidence seemed to settle that regional inhomogeneity (Milic-Emili), a consequence of unequal rates of gas flow down the bronchi, as well as stratified inhomogeneity (Cumming), from inadequate mixing of gas in the airways, contribute importantly to variations in gas concentrations throughout the lungs. It also seems clear from combined morphological and physiological observations (Cumming), that the role of stratified inhomogeneity is exaggerated by disease of the airways or of the air-spaces which enlarges distances for molecular diffusion of gases. Supporting these physiological and anatomical observations was the spectacular demonstration of the ‘ slinky ’, a toy well-known to children and now destined to serve adult physiologists as a model of the mechanical behaviour of the lungs (Milic-Emili ; Filley). However, despite this remarkable accord, not all is settled. For example, the quantitative partition of inhomogeneity into its regional and stratified components has yet to be accomplished.

Gravity

Never since Newton has gravity been of such grave concern. Pulmonary physiologists share in this concern and the present conference reflected their interest. Under the influence of gravity, pleural pressures vary from top to bottom of the lung (Milic-Emili) ; alveoli vary accordingly in size (West) ; ventilation-perfusion relationships become non-uniform ; and even interstitial pressures involved in fluid exchange must vary and may become more negative around vessels than in the pleura (West). The preoccupation with the effects of gravity promises to continue unabated as it extends from man on earth to gravity-free subjects in space, to aquatic mammals and to man spinning on the centrifuge.

Form and function

Physiologists are well aware that meaningful estimates of the balance between alveolar ventilation and perfusion require that these two functions be measured simultaneously. In a serious attempt to detect early functional abnormalities of ventilation and perfusion in early bronchitis, Bates and his co-workers used $Xenon^{133}$ by injection and by inhalation. In providing this fresh approach to the problem of bronchitis, these studies also pointed up two fundamental problems : (1) the difficulties in obtaining reliable morphological information in live patients in whom anatomical changes are more easily inferred than proved and (2) the limitations imposed by a non-homogeneous pulmonary disorder on the interpretation of surface counting of radioactivity, which can only provide *mean* values for relatively large parts of the lung. In consideration of the first problem, the discussants seemed inclined to believe that refinements in roentgenographic techniques may soon make possible quantitative estimates during life of anatomical abnormalities in the air-spaces and the air sacs. But they were much less sanguine about coping with the distorting effects of non-homogeneous disease on the radioactivity viewed by the scanner.

It has been noted above that considerable evidence was presented to indicate that the effect on the blood gases predominates over the anatomical lesions in the airways and lungs in determining the outcome of bronchitis and/or emphysema. The effect of the blood gases is mediated largely by way of the vascular changes of hypoxia, resulting in hypoxic pulmonary hypertension (Bishop). Whether acidosis aggravates these anatomical changes is unclear but, on experimental grounds, it certainly seems capable of intensifying hypoxic pulmonary vasoconstriction. From such observations, it seems clear that the bronchitic, who develops hypoxemia and respiratory acidosis, is a likely candidate for pulmonary hypertension, cor pulmonale and heart failure. On the other hand, the emphysematous patient, with normal blood gases may continue in a breathless state for many years but will remain free of right heart enlargement and failure unless alveolar hypoventilation from a bronchitis supervenes (Fletcher). From the point of view of therapy, this distinction is of major importance since clinical experience dictates that the patient with hypoxemia and hypercapnia from imbalance of alveolar ventilation and perfusion is usually suffering from a bronchitis, which may respond to antibiotic and bronchodilator therapy (Fig. 1). On the other hand, the emphysematous patient, with near-normal blood gases, is usually suffering from irreversible disease, in which perfusion as well as ventilation is curtailed, so that the lung operates as through parts of it had been amputated thereby exerting a greater effect on its reserve than on its performance in arterializing the blood.

Conclusion

This conference fulfilled its mission of considering form and function in the human lung. How the interplay of form and function can be fruitfully examined was clearly demonstrated with respect to the distribution of inspired gas and with respect to the role of hypoxic pulmonary vascular disease in the genesis of cor pulmonale. However, the conference also indicated that the next step, *i.e.*, relating abnormalities in ventilation and perfusion to structural abnormalities, will be more difficult. But, in helping to define the problem, the conference has also perhaps helped to point the way to its solution.

GLOSSARY OF SYMBOLS AND ABBREVIATIONS

Subdivisions of lung volume

I.R.V. = inspiratory reserve volume

V_T = tidal volume

E.R.V. = expiratory reserve volume

R.V. = residual volume

The sum of these is the total lung volume.

T.L.C. = total lung capacity

Inspiratory capacity = I.R.V.+tidal volume (at rest)

Vital capacity (V.C.) = I.R.V.+tidal volume+E.R.V.

Functional residual capacity (F.R.C.) = R.V.+E.R.V. (at rest)

Symbols

(*a*) General variables

V = Gas volume (state conditions of pressure, temperature and saturation with water vapour)

$\dot{V}$ = Gas volume per unit time

P = Gas pressure in general

F = Fractional concentration in dry gas phase

$\dot{Q}$ = Volume flow of blood in unit time

S = saturation of haemoglobin

f = Respiratory frequency

R = Respiratory quotient $\dfrac{CO_2 \text{ output}}{O_2 \text{ consumption}}$

D = Diffusing capacity in general (volume per unit time per unit pressure difference)

$\dot{V}/\dot{Q}$ = Ventilation/perfusion ratio

(*b*) Symbols for the gas phase (small capitals)

I = inspired gas
E = expired gas
A = alveolar gas
T = tidal gas
D = dead space gas
B = barometric

(*c*) Symbols for the blood phase (lower case letters)

b = blood in general
a = arterial (specify location)
v = venous (specify location)
c = capillary (specify location)

(*d*) Special symbols

$\bar{X}$ = dash above symbol indicates a mean value
$\dot{X}$ = dot above symbol indicates a time derivative

Thus, for example:

$P\text{A}_{O_2}$ = partial pressure of oxygen in the alveolar gas
Pa_{O_2} = partial pressure of oxygen in the arterial blood
$S\bar{v}_{O_2}$ = mixed venous saturation
$\dot{V}_{O_2}$ = uptake of oxygen in unit time

SUBJECT INDEX

PRINTED BY NEILL & CO. LTD., EDINBURGH